FIGHTING FIT

FIGHTING FIT

David Mitchell

Published in association with
The Martial Arts Commission of
Great Britain

London
UNWIN PAPERBACKS
Boston   Sydney

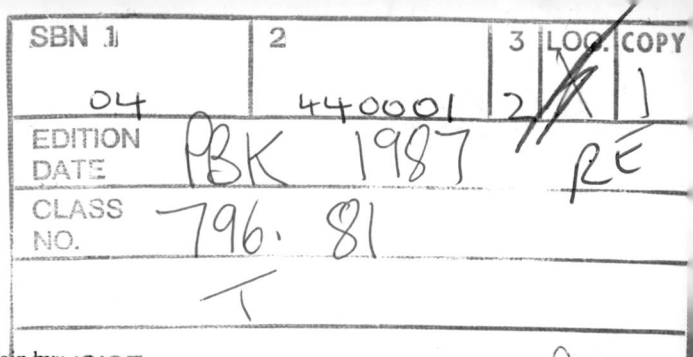

First published in Great Britain by
Unwin Paperbacks 1987
Designed by Bob Vickers
Produced by the Bowerdean Press
London SW11
© Copyright The Bowerdean Press

The photograph on p12 is from Sport
and General. All other photographs are
by Sylvio Dokov. Drawings and diagrams
by Amanda Barrett

UNWIN PAPERBACKS
Denmark House, 37–39 Queen Elizabeth Street
London SE1 2QB
and
40 Museum Street, London WC1A 1LU

Allen & Unwin Australia Pty Ltd
8 Napier Street, North Sydney, NSW 2060,
Australia

Unwin Paperbacks with Port Nicholson Press
P O Box 11–838 Wellington, New Zealand

British Library Cataloguing in Publication Data
Mitchell, David
   Fighting fit.
   1. Martial arts 2. Physical fitness
   I. Title, *1944*
   613.7'1   GV1111
ISBN 0 04 440001 2

Typeset by TJB Photosetting Ltd.,
South Witham, Lincolnshire.

Printed and bound in England by
RJ Acford
Chichester, Sussex.

Contents

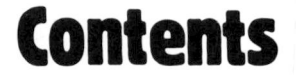

Acknowledgements

I would like to thank the following who helped me with this book:

Doctor James Canney for his advice on the Injury Management and Drugs chapters.
Brian Robinson of Bulmershe College, Reading for extensive help with several chapters. His contribution to the book has been indispensable.
Tony Gummerson of the College of Ripon and York St John for reading and commenting on the manuscript.
St Mary's College, Twickenham, for the use of their sophisticated facilities.
The United Kingdom Seiki Jukyu Karate Organisation for supplying the models for our photographs.
The National Coaching Foundation for the impact they have had upon martial arts practice.
The Martial Arts Commission for their progressive approach to coaching, an unusual and praiseworthy attitude in an activity so dependent upon traditions.

David Mitchell
London 1987

What is Fitness?

Even when you are lying quietly in bed, your heart beats, the muscles of your respiratory system pump air in and out and your stomach and intestines are busy processing food. Your blood transports oxygen and food and your brain monitors the whole system. Although things may look fairly inactive from the outside, they are not. Even when you are just lying around in bed, the complex systems of your body require energy and a certain level of fitness

Energy consumption increases when you decide to get out of bed to visit the bathroom. Your breathing deepens and your heart pumps more frequently and with greater force as it responds to the working muscles' need for additional oxygen. To achieve all this, the body must have a degree of fitness greater than that required for lying in bed. You need a still higher degree of fitness to carry weights, climb stairs or run around.

The tissues of your body respond to the physical stresses of life. To realise the importance of these daily stresses, consider what happens to a fractured limb in plaster. The unused muscles quickly lose their protein content and become smaller and weaker in a process known as 'muscle atrophy'. In a similar way, if you are confined to bed for a long period, your bones weaken as minerals are removed and not replaced. Regular physical stress is therefore important in securing a level of fitness.

Observations of children show that without any external motivation, they enjoy running, jumping, skipping etc and by this means develop their fitness.

As a martial artist, you will know that the stresses of training exceed those required for everyday life. You probably suffered after your first few training sessions, feeling stiff and achey the next day or so. This happened because the tissues of your body were not fit enough to withstand the physical requirements of training. Had you trained a little more sedately, you might not have suffered but think yourself lucky that you weren't actually injured by the training.

Do develop your level of fitness before you train in the martial arts and *do not* use a martial art as a means of developing your fitness.

What actually is fitness? If we consider three top athletes – a shot putter, a marathon runner and a gymnast – each will produce a good performance in their own sport yet be unable to give an equivalent performance in another. Although they all have high levels of fitness, they are all different. Let's look at how they compare (see Table 1)

As you can see, each performer has developed certain aspects to a high degree but because of the nature and requirements of their sport, it has not been necessary to develop all the aspects to the same high level. However, the athletes would still outperform untrained persons even in those low rated aspects.

Table 1

	Gymnast	Marathon Runner	Shot Putter
Aerobic Endurance	Low	Very High	Low
Anaerobic Endurance	Medium	Low	Low
Local Muscular Endurance	High	High in legs	Medium
Strength	High	Low	Very High
Power	High	Low	Very High
Flexibility	Very High	Low	Medium
Agility	Very High	Low	Medium
% Body Fat	Low	Low	High
% Lean Tissue	Very High	Very High	Medium

Fitness is different things to different athletes

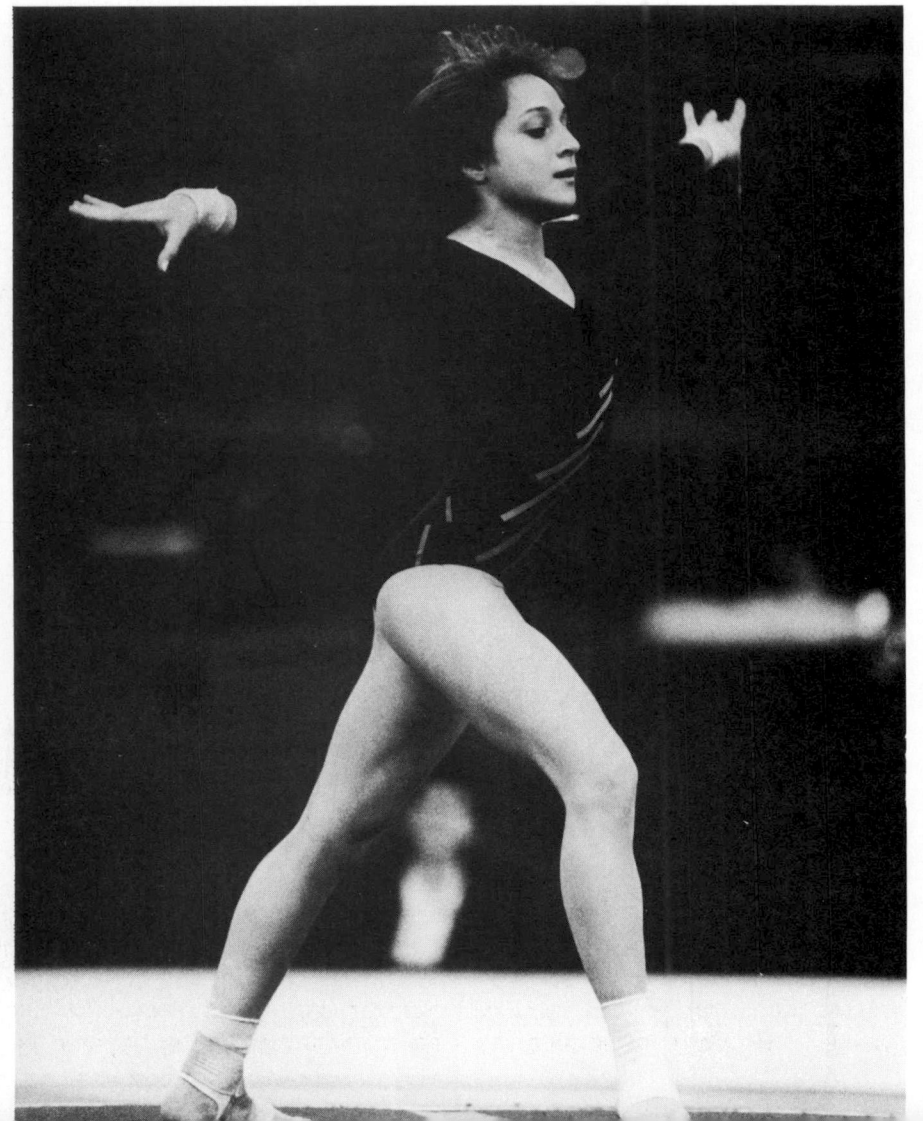

Three minutes can be a long time at maximum speed even for a world champion

Though body tissues respond to stress, the limit of this response is determined by such factors as age, sex and heredity. The top marathon runner or gymnast could never develop the required physique to attain excellence in putting the shot.

Let's consider the various components of physical fitness.

Endurance

Some people say they are unfit because they soon tire when running, cycling, climbing, swimming or merely walking fast. The ability to keep going in any of the above activities for an extended period of time is known as 'endurance'. There are basically two types of whole-body endurance, aerobic and anaerobic.

Aerobic endurance is also known as 'cardiovascular endurance', 'cardio-respiratory endurance' or 'stamina'. It relies upon the ability of the heart, blood, bloodvessels and lungs to transport oxygen and food to the tissues of the body and in particular the working muscles. The muscles use these to form *adenosine triphosphate* which provides the energy to contract and relax.

Improving aerobic endurance requires a training programme which improves the condition and efficiency of the lungs, heart, blood, blood-vessels and the ability of muscles to use the oxygen provided. A good level of aerobic endurance is important because it underpins extended activity and ensures fast recovery from exercise.

If insufficient oxygen is available to meet demand, the working muscles can still make adenosine triphosphate by using a process which works in the absence of oxygen, ie, an *anaerobic* process. However, this results in a build-up of *lactic acid* which produces symptoms of fatigue. Most people stop exercising before discomfort becomes too great but anyone who has completed a 400 metre race flat out all the way will have sampled the limits of anaerobic endurance in the final straight.

Improving anaerobic endurance is the painful part of training and is best entered into only after a period of aerobic training. It is accomplished by the various forms of interval training which repeatedly engage the lactic acid-producing process during a training session.

As the name implies, 'local muscle endurance' is not a whole-body aspect. It is the ability of a muscle, or group of muscles to contract and relax repeatedly over a period of time in an ever-increasing climate of fatigue at local level. Press-ups for example, test the local muscular endurance of the upper arms, shoulders and chest.

Strength

Strength is linked to local muscular endurance in that strong muscles generally have good local endurance. Strength is measured during one maximum contraction of the muscle(s). It helps to support and protect some of the more delicate skeletal structures such as the knee and elbow joints and the spine.

Both strength and local muscular endurance are important to the successful martial artist and are developed by working the muscles against body weight, by weight training, or other activities which increase the resistance against which muscles work.

Power

Strong muscles need not be powerful. Power is a combination of strength and the speed at which a muscle can contract. Muscles basically contain two types of fibre. These are the 'white' and 'red' fibres, the proportions of which in a muscle vary from individual to individual. It appears that the ratio of one type to another cannot be altered.

White fibres contract more quickly ('fast twitch') than red fibres ('slow twitch'), though the latter are better at aerobic endurance activities.

Even if you are low in white fibres, you can still improve your power by selecting an appropriate training method.

Flexibility

Flexibility is also called 'suppleness' and refers to the range of skeletal movement at a joint, or series of joints. This movement must be full, without being excessive since excessive flexibility can lead to joint dislocation and injury.

Most martial arts require a high degree of flexibility and this can be obtained through the proper training.

Agility

This is not a true component of physical fitness. It is actually a component of motor fitness but is included here because it is important to martial art practice. Agility can contain elements of strength, speed, flexibility and coordination, allowing the martial artist quickly to adopt a position, stop, then change direction and quickly move again. It is also necessary to the fast and accurate movement of body parts in relation to one another, or external objects.

Agility is developed by improving strength, power and flexibility and by practising martial art techniques.

Body Composition

Though perhaps not a component of physical fitness, body composition certainly has an effect on physical performance.

It is expressed as a proportion of fat to lean tissue in the body.

Fat is stored just below the skin and too much makes it more difficult to move with speed and agility. Both stamina and local muscular endurance are affected through the increase in weight brought about by excess fat. Fat reduces heat loss from the body and this can have an effect during extended training.

Its only advantage is the ability to absorb impact shock, cushioning deeper-lying structures from injury.

The proportion of fat to lean tissue can be altered by a combination of increased energy expenditure through exercise with controlled nutrition.

To summarise, there is a whole range of fitness, from low to extremely high levels. Within the overall term 'fitness' are a number of components some of which are interrelated. To improve any specific aspect of fitness, you must apply the right kind of stress by means of a carefully designed training programme.

It is difficult to define the components of fitness needed for martial arts practice and therebye generate an overall training programme because each has its own requirements. You must look at your own discipline and try to analyse its various components.

General Characteristics of Martial Art Practice

As their name indicates, the martial arts are the techniques of the military. Any system of military fighting, whether it be firing a rifle or neutralising a sentry with a knife, is a martial art. There are both armed and unarmed martial arts and some which are a combination of the two. For the purposes of this book, the arts referred to are the so-called traditional martial arts of China, Korea, Okinawa and Japan, plus those fighting and training systems derived from them.

All the martial arts involve fast movements, either in the way of limb speed, whole-body speed, or both. The martial artist has to close distance quickly to press home an attack and also to move in the right direction to avoid getting thumped. A technique applied with the arms or legs must be as fast and as accurate as possible if it is to succeed.

The martial artist has to react quickly to a situation – perhaps identifying an attack and formulating the correct response to it in a fraction of a second. In some schools of Southern kung fu, the participants fight at less than one arm's distance apart, with techniques often travelling a couple of inches and no more. This requires anticipation, recognition and response to avoid being clobbered.

Some martial arts require flexibility in certain joints. The aikido prac-titioner for example, needs to be able to tolerate the twisting and bending forces applied to wrist and elbow joints during training. The taekwondo athlete needs flexible hips and a good knee lift to raise the foot quickly into position for a high kick. He/she must be able to spring high into the air to deliver one of the many flying kicks for which that martial art is particularly well regarded.

Karateka require the ability to hold low and awkward stances for long periods of time. They also need good coordination of body movement for delivering high energy punches and strikes.

All martial art training involves a level of continuous activity which rises periodically to explosive peaks, according to the type of training. Repetition plays a large part in all martial art training and it therefore follows that certain muscle groups not used much in everyday life may have to be trained up until they are fit enough to cope.

Let's now look at the principal characteristics of individual martial arts.

Aikido

This is a Japanese martial art normally practised in pairs. Participants take it in turns to apply techniques to each other and typically these involve seizing the opponent's outstretched arm or leg and twisting it. The traditional aikido man does not initiate attacks but rather responds to them.

The attack must be quickly recognised and a complicated response adapted to deal with it. The attacker's strength is turned against him and his force is redirected in a way suitable to the defender. Because of this, great muscular strength is not required. No high kicks are practised and when strikes are used, comparison with other martial arts shows them to be relatively slow moving and of low energy content. Nevertheless there is a need both for flexibility and a range of movement.

The self-defence oriented forms of aikido are more strenuous and involve a greater degree of strength, particularly in the shoulders, arms and stomach muscles. Most strenuous are the sports forms in which two attackers go for a single defender. This requires a constant high level of performance with rapidly occurring peaks of activity.

Full Contact

Full contact is a hybrid striking system developed from karate, taekwondo and the hard schools of kung fu. It includes no grappling or wrestling techniques and has the same fitness requirements as boxing, plus an added flexibility requirement to allow strong kicks to the head. Power development is an important element of fitness training for full contact. Participants wear boxing gloves and padded boots to reduce the risk of laceration.

Training is performed singly, using such aids as a punching bag and mirror. Pair-form practice is used both to build up responses to attack by means of scheduled attacks and responses

and as a form of free sparring, using unprogrammed attacks. Techniques must be delivered quickly often over long periods of time, so endurance is important.

Hapkido

Hapkido is a Korean development of aikido, involving a number of high kicks and powerful strikes in addition to the holds and throws. Korean martial arts appear to be heavily influenced by the Northern kung fu systems and the latter are noted for their expansive movements and large repertoire of high kicks. The fitness requirements for aikido practice are thus supplemented by the need to have good legs, capable of delivering fast, high kicks.

The hapkido practitioner practises impact techniques on his own and grappling techniques with a partner. The system is both responsive to attack and, through its kicks and strikes, capable of initiating strong attacks.

Jiu Jitsu

Jiu jitsu is the forerunner of modern Olympic judo and the main Japanese martial art development from which aikido split off. It has the same fitness requirements as judo, endurance and strength being key elements. Impact techniques are used but typically they are low powered strikes aimed at vulnerable targets.

Except for a small amount of prearranged performance work (called kata) and solitary practice with striking techniques, jiu jitsu is normally practised with at least one partner. During periods of strenuous training, one person will face a line of attackers who launch themselves at him one at a

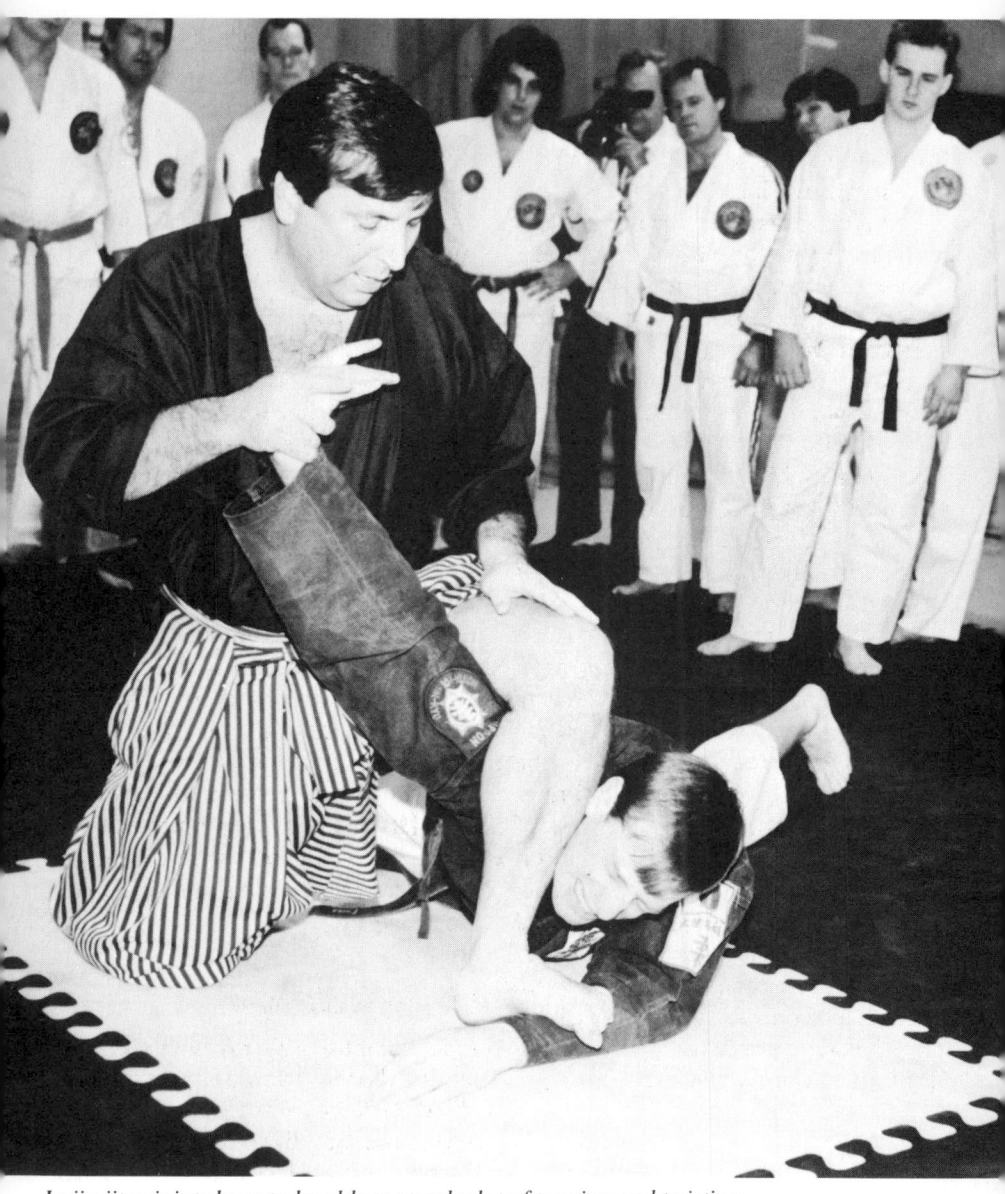

In jiu jitsu joints have to be able to stand a lot of tugging and twisting

time. When the whole line has been dealt with, someone else takes on the defender's role.

Typically jiu jitsu training is very strenuous and the arm joints have got to be able to withstand all the tugging and twisting they have to undergo. A lot of techniques come from the stomach, hips and legs, with the attacker coming in underneath the opponent's centre of gravity and levering him over.

Karate

Karate is originally an Okinawan martial art that was introduced to the Japanese mainland at the turn of the twentieth century and there adapted to make it suitable for teaching to large classes. Karate practice is split fairly evenly into solitary and pair-form training and the art itself is almost entirely impact based.

Developing fast, powerful muscles is an important part of karate training. Karate competition depends upon the controlled delivery of very fast techniques.

Kicks are practised in all styles and those applied to the head and upper body require flexibility in the hips.

In some schools there is emphasis upon the development of strength. Training routines which pit one muscle against the other, or which hold the muscles in a state of prolonged hard contraction are still widely practised in traditional schools.

Solitary training involves delivery of fast but often not particularly powerful punches and kicks to the empty air – ie 'unloaded' techniques. According to the Medical Officer of the Martial Arts Commission, poor training of this nature can and does cause long-term damage to elbow and knee joints. Pair form practice uses exchange of pre-agreed techniques. The exception is in free sparring, where each participant can use any technique approved in the rules.

Kendo

Kendo is the art of Japanese swordfighting. Its practitioners man-handle the practice sword, or *shinai* for several hours of training. *Suburi*, or 'cutting the air' is a form of wrist, elbow, shoulder and arm training. No grappling techniques are employed.

Kendo sparring involves long periods of frenetic activity in heavy armour. Fitness requirements are endurance combined with fast, explosive movements.

Kung fu

There is an entire spectrum of activities within the generic title of kung fu. Though schools may mix unarmed and weapon training, there are few grappling techniques except in one small school. The so-called 'soft' styles use meditation and relaxation to achieve the necessary power.

The 'hard' styles of kung fu are similar to karate in that they use a great deal of obvious muscle power. Different schools place different emphasis on techniques and the Mantis school, for example, trains the arms until they become insensitive to pain. The *wing chun kuen* schools use a wooden construction called a *mok yan jong* ('wooden man') to practise power development on.

In the southern hard systems, hip flexibility is not so important because at the close distances they spar from, lifting your foot off the ground to kick is sheer folly.

Shorinji Kempo

This Japanese martial art based system of *shorinji kempo* is most closely allied to Korean hapkido. It uses an admixture of joint-locks, holds and throws with punches and kicks. Impact techniques rely more on accuracy than brute strength.

The striking techniques are usually practised in a solitary manner, as with karate but grappling involves pair-form sparring.

Tang Soo Do

Tang soo do is a Korean martial art with close similarities to karate. Apart from a greater number of high kicks in its syllabus, it requires similar standards of fitness.

Taekwondo

Taekwondo is a Korean martial art which is also similar to karate except for a greater number of high kicks. The Olympic recognised form uses full contact kicks to the head, face and body, so there is a strong need for hip flexibility. Taekwondo competitions can extend over several rounds and stamina training is necessary to stand the pace.

Thai Boxing

The same comments apply to *Thai boxing* as apply to full contact. The two are very similar.

Assessing Fitness

Methods for assessing the components of physical fitness have been available for many years European students of Physical Education have studied them since the early 1930's but it is only recently that assessments, or 'fitness tests' as they are often called, have grown in popularity. Assessments are now regularly used in schools, sports centres, health centres and institutes of further education. BUPA also offers a range of physical fitness assessments.

Some health centres, sports and leisure centres offer a limited range of assessments and the charge for this is sometimes hidden within the enrollment fee for a particular course. The cost of an assessment generally indicates its accuracy and comprehensiveness. Currently a full BUPA Assessment can cost around £100, whilst the less comprehensive ones available in centres cost as little as £10. The full assessment requires expensive and sophisticated equipment, hence no doubt the increased charge.

Why bother with assessments at all? If anyone trains, they must obviously get fitter and feel that they are getting fitter in the process. This is true especially when you start from a very low level of fitness. Soon you realise that running is becoming easier and it is possible to run further and faster. This is an assessment of running performance and the fact that running is getting easier is a subjective view, a feeling which cannot be precisely measured. Being able to run further and faster is an objective assessment because we can precisely measure both time and distance.

Another form of objective assessment could be the monitoring of the heart rate using an instrument called a 'sports tester'. The run must be attempted twice at about the same pace and take about the same time to complete the distance. If the second run is completed with a lower heart rate, then we can say that the performer's aerobic endurance has improved. Providing that all measurements are accurately made, objective assessments give the best information.

Assessing Aerobic Endurance

Measure a distance of one and a half miles and run it as quickly as you can. Compare your performance with a reference chart such as that provided by the National Coaching Foundation (see table 2). It is better to run at an even pace for most of the distance and this can only be determined by trial and error. Run too fast early on in the run and fatigue will hold you back, producing a relatively slow time. Run too slowly and you will again turn in a slow time.

Motivation can also distort this type of assessment. You may find it hard to put in that last spurt when you are already tired. On the positive side, all this test needs to administer is an accu-

Table 2

Age (years)	very poor	poor	fair	good	very good	excellent	superb
Women							
17-29	19.48+	17.24+	14.24+	12.18+	9.54+	9.00+	8.06+
30-34	20.24+	18.00+	15.00+	12.36+	10.12+	9.18+	8.24+
35-39	21.00+	18.36+	15.36+	12.54+	10.30+	9.36+	8.42+
40-44	21.36+	19.12+	16.12+	13.12+	10.48+	9.54+	9.00+
45-49	22.12+	19.48+	16.48+	13.30+	11.06+	10.30+	9.36+
over 50	22.48+	20.24+	17.24+	13.48+	11.24+	10.30+	9.36+
Men							
17-29	16:30+	14:30+	12:00+	10:15+	8:15+	7:30+	6:45+
30-34	17:00+	15:00+	12:30+	10:30+	8:30+	7:45+	7:00+
35-39	17:30+	15:30+	13:00+	10:45+	8:45+	8:00+	7:15+
40-44	18:00+	16:00+	13:30+	11:00+	9:00+	8:15+	7:30+
45-49	18:30+	16:30+	14:00+	11:15+	9:15+	8:30+	7:45+
over 50	19:00+	17:00+	14:30+	11:30+	9:30+	8:45+	8:00+

rate mile and a half measurement and a stopwatch.

It is not necessary to use the mile and a half distance. Any distance which needs more than five minutes to run it will suffice, as long as that same distance over the same course is used each time.

Another way to measure aerobic endurance is to use the Harvard Step Test. This involves stepping up and down on a bench, the height of which is 20″ for males and 16″ for females. The stepping rate is 30 times a minute, controlled by a metronome set to 120 beats per minute. Each time the metronome beats, a foot strikes the surface of the bench or floor. The legs must be straightened completely when stepping up onto the bench. Wear light clothing because you will become quite warm during this test.

Duration of this assessment is five minutes, after which you sit on the bench and rest. An assistant counts your pulse rate, using the index and middle finger on the radial artery of the wrist, or on the carotid artery at the side of the neck. (Don't use too much pressure!). As a check, you can also count the beats. The first beat felt at the start of each recording period is counted as zero. The times given in the table relate to minutes after stepping has ceased.

Timing of pulse counts during recovery:

1 minute – 1.5 minutes =			beats
2 minutes – 2.5 minutes =			beats
3 minutes – 3.5 minutes =			beats
Total pulse counts	=		beats

From this a physical fitness index ('PFI') is calculated using the formula:

$$PFI = \frac{\text{Duration of exercise (in seconds)} \times 100}{2 \times \text{total pulse counts}}$$

The results can be compared with values taken from assessing 8000 American college students (see Table 3).

Opposite: *Assess your aerobic endurance with a one and a half mile run*

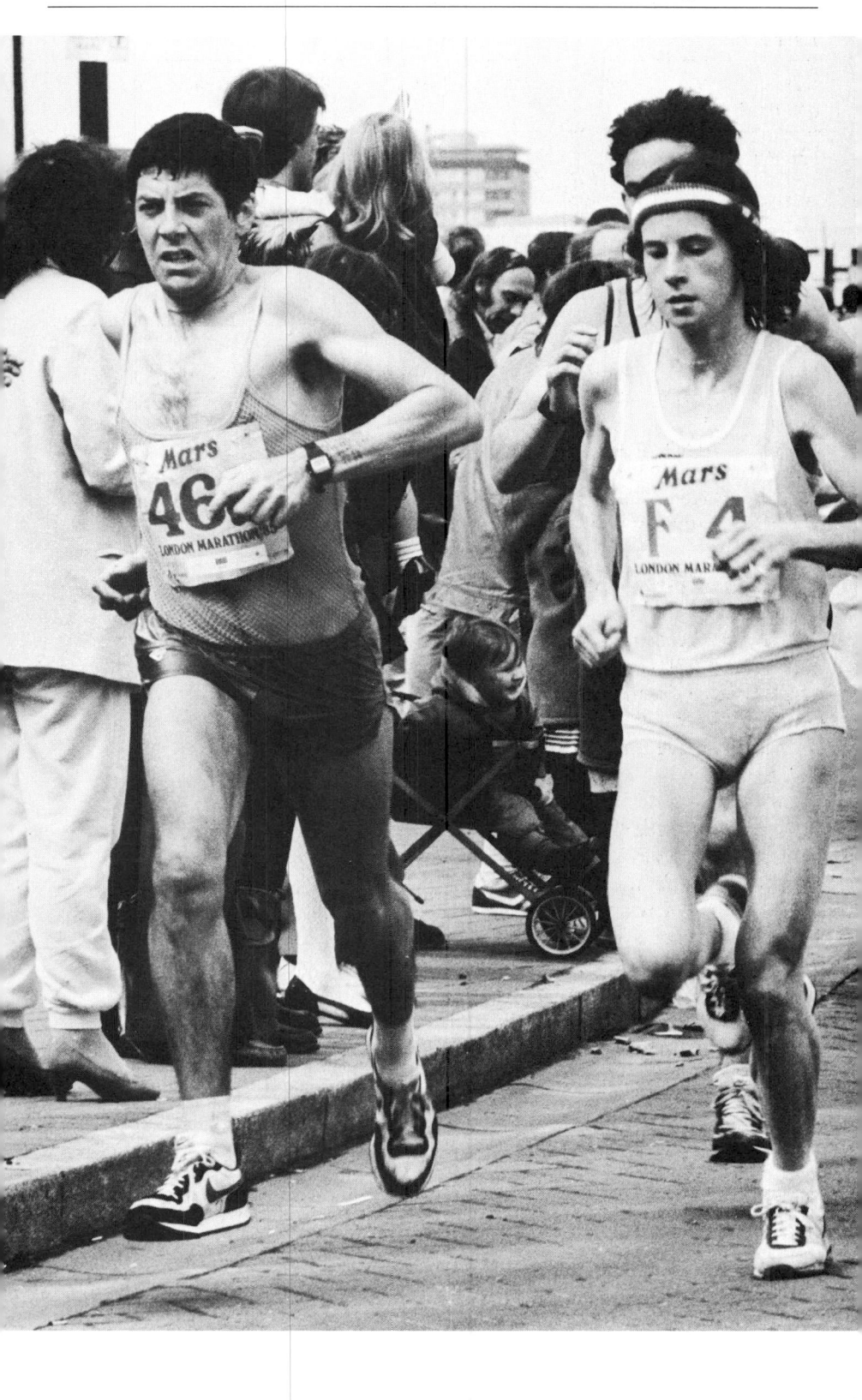

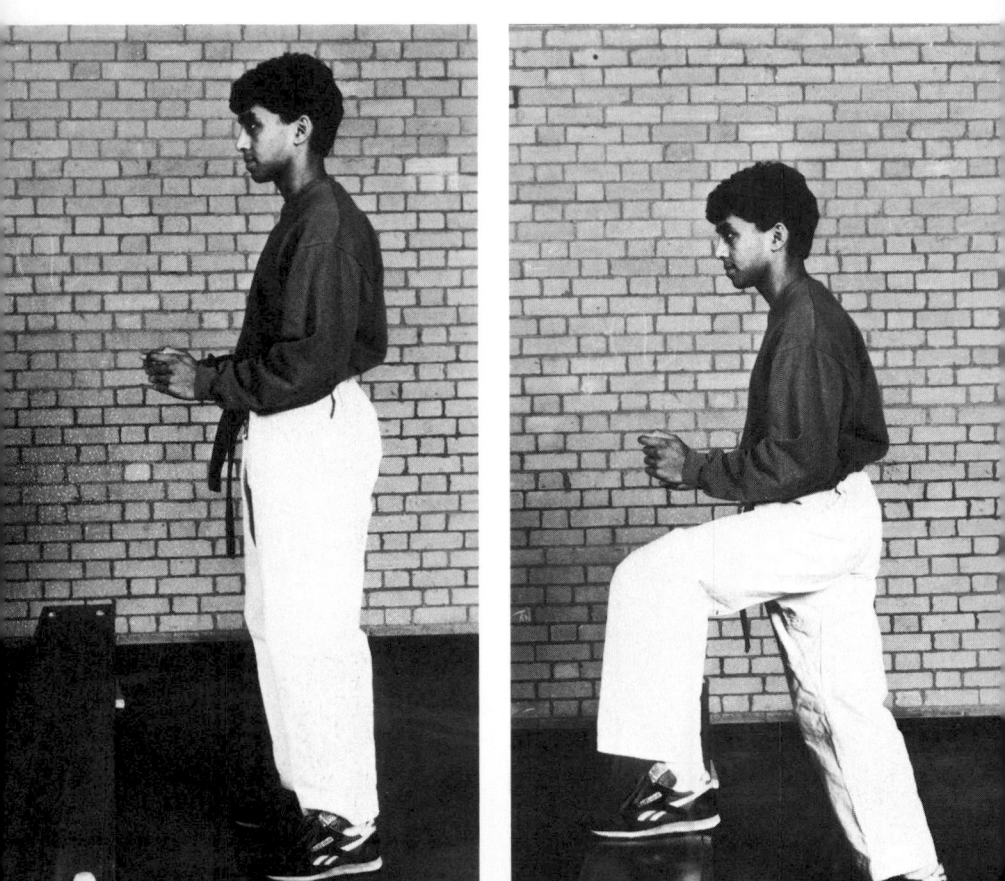

The Harvard Step Test is another way of assessing your aerobic ensurance

Table 3

Below 55	–	Poor
55 to 61	–	Low average
65 to 79	–	Average
80 to 89	–	Good
Above 90	–	Excellent

It is essential to time the test accurately for best results.

The disadvantage of the Harvard Step Test is that in its pure form, it is only suitable for performers with well established aerobic endurance. Performers with poor endurance will almost certainly fail to complete the five minutes because of fatigue. Although the calculation can take into account periods of stepping less than five minutes, this makes the test more difficult to administer accurately. Another disadvantage is that the pulse may not recover uniformly on each occasion; it can be affected by such factors as anxiety.

The advantages of the test are that it can be easily administered to large groups of performers and the equipment and expertise required are minimal.

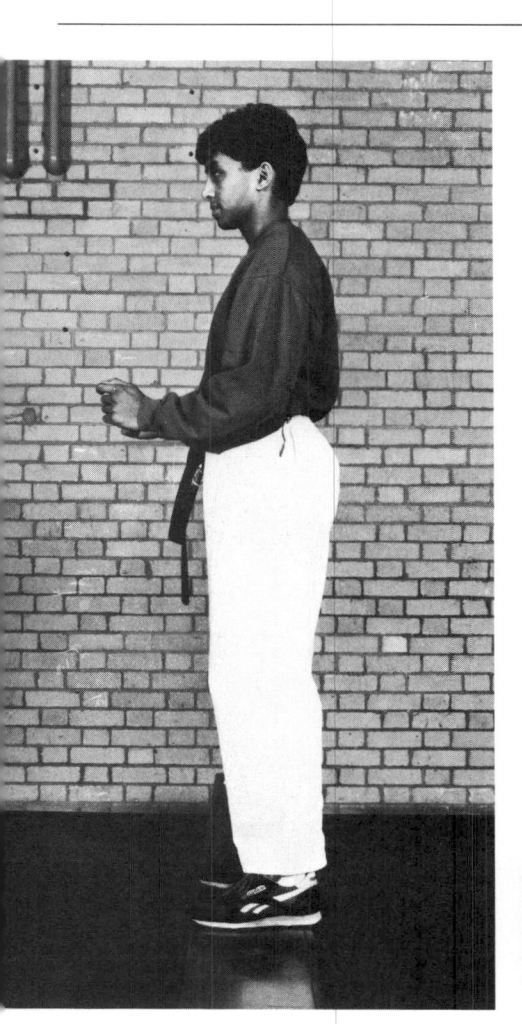

For performers with low aerobic endurance, a lower bench height and slower stepping rates may be used as long as when each performer is re-assessed, those same conditions are repeated exactly. The same procedure can be adopted for testing children.

An alternative to the Harvard Test is the Fitech Step Test. This is a commercial test especially suitable for performers with low aerobic endurance. Fitech also provides a series of progressive programmes for aerobic endurance in the same package as the test.

Other tests include the Cycle Ergometer and Treadmill Assess-ments. You either cycle on a stationary ergometer or run on a treadmill, the latter being a wide conveyor belt which can be inclined. The advantage of these is that the assessor has complete control over the rate of cycling and the load set on the cycle, the speed of the treadmill and the angle of inclination.

Because you remain comparatively still during the assessment, you can be hooked up to heart rate recorders and equipment which analyses expired air. Unlike the step tests which use recovery pulse rates, these recordings can be made before, during and after the exercise.

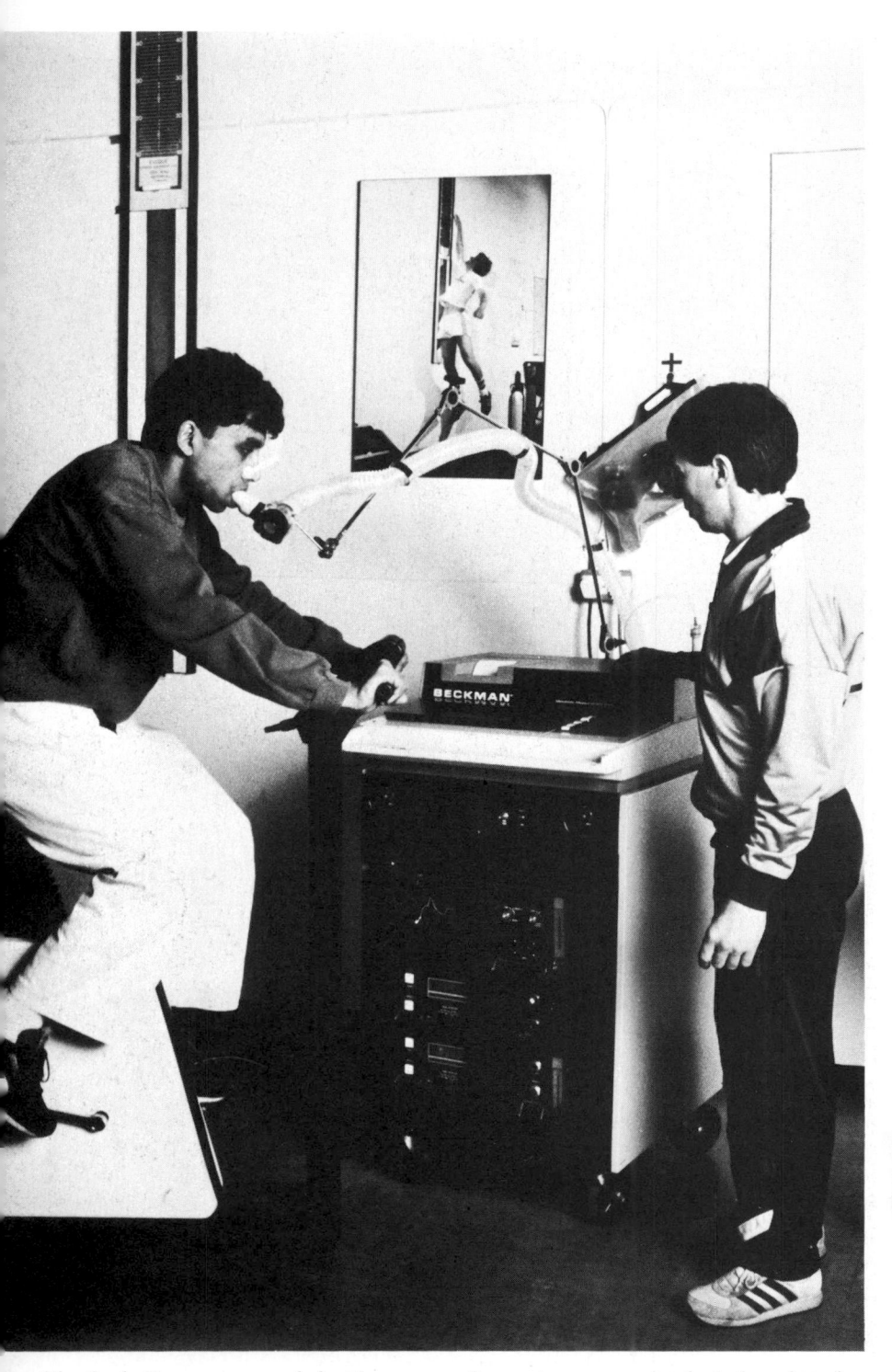

The Cycle Ergometer coupled with a means of assessing oxygen uptake is thought to be the best predictor of aerobic endurance

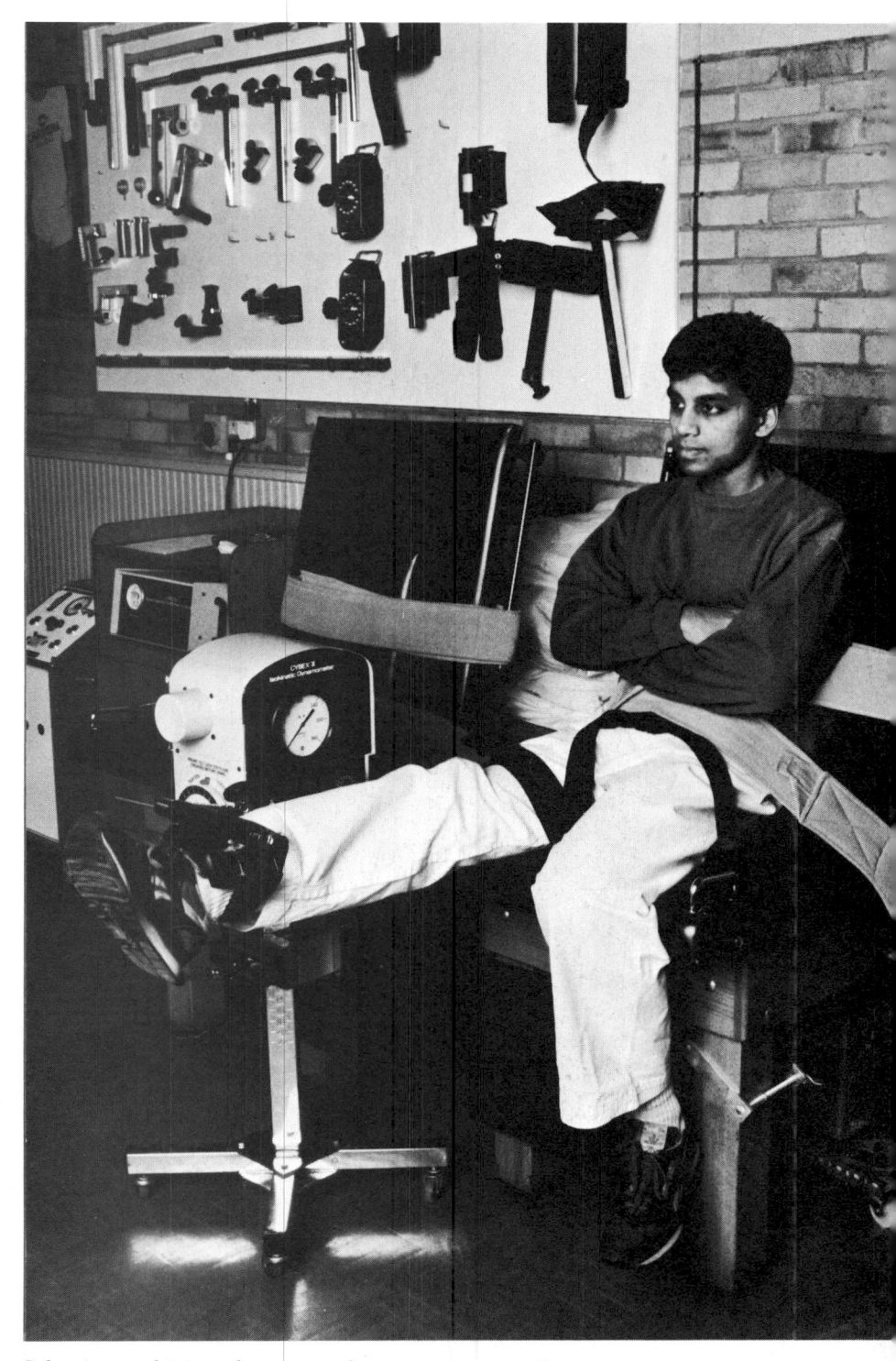

Cybex is a sophisticated apparatus for measuring strength

Information collected during the exercise gives a precise picture of how you are responding. One measurement of particular interest is that of the greatest amount of oxygen you can take out of inspired air and use for the production of energy. This is thought to be the best predictor of aerobic endurance.

Unfortunately, to provide these assessments requires expensive equipment and expert analysis of the results obtained. This can be costly.

Assessing Strength

You might consider that assessment of strength is quite simple. It is only necessary to determine how much force a muscle, or group of muscles, can generate in a single maximum contraction.

The traditional assessment machines for this are called 'dynamometers' and 'tensiometers' but since these measure contraction against a spring, the contraction is mainly isometric, ie, the muscles develop tension but there is little skeletal movement. This is quite different to most movements used in martial arts, where contraction produces skeletal movement.

Although dynamometers and tensiometers give an indication of muscular strength, they are not the best form of assessment for moving, or isotonic strength. Moreover they are expensive to purchase and are therefore found only in some fitness assessment centres.

Possibly the most effective machines for measuring strength are of the isokinetic type such as CYBEX. The latter is capable of measuring the force generated through an entire range of movement

and so would seem to be the best alternative except that it is hideously expensive.

A less expensive but good form of strength assessment can be found in the weight training room. A careful record of loads lifted will give an indication of the strength capabilities of the various muscle groups. It is possible also to get an indication of the maximum strength of a muscle group by gradually increasing weight until only one contraction is possible.

Though you may be the strongest martial artist in the world, you may not be the most successful because many other factors are involved in good performance. Therefore the measurement of maximum strength, although very interesting, may not be worth all the effort involved.

Assessing Muscular Endurance

Muscular endurance is more important than muscular strength. It is the ability of the muscle to contract time and time again. It is simpler to measure because muscle groups can be isolated and worked to exhaustion, or to a maximum number of contractions in a set period of time. They must be exercised without rest to give a true indication of their endurance capabilities.

Some of the activities which can be used are the maximum number of:

a. Press-ups keeping the body perfectly straight, with chest to the floor and complete extension of the elbow. Record the maximum number.

b. Dips, where the body is supported by both arms and lowered until there is a right angle at the elbow.

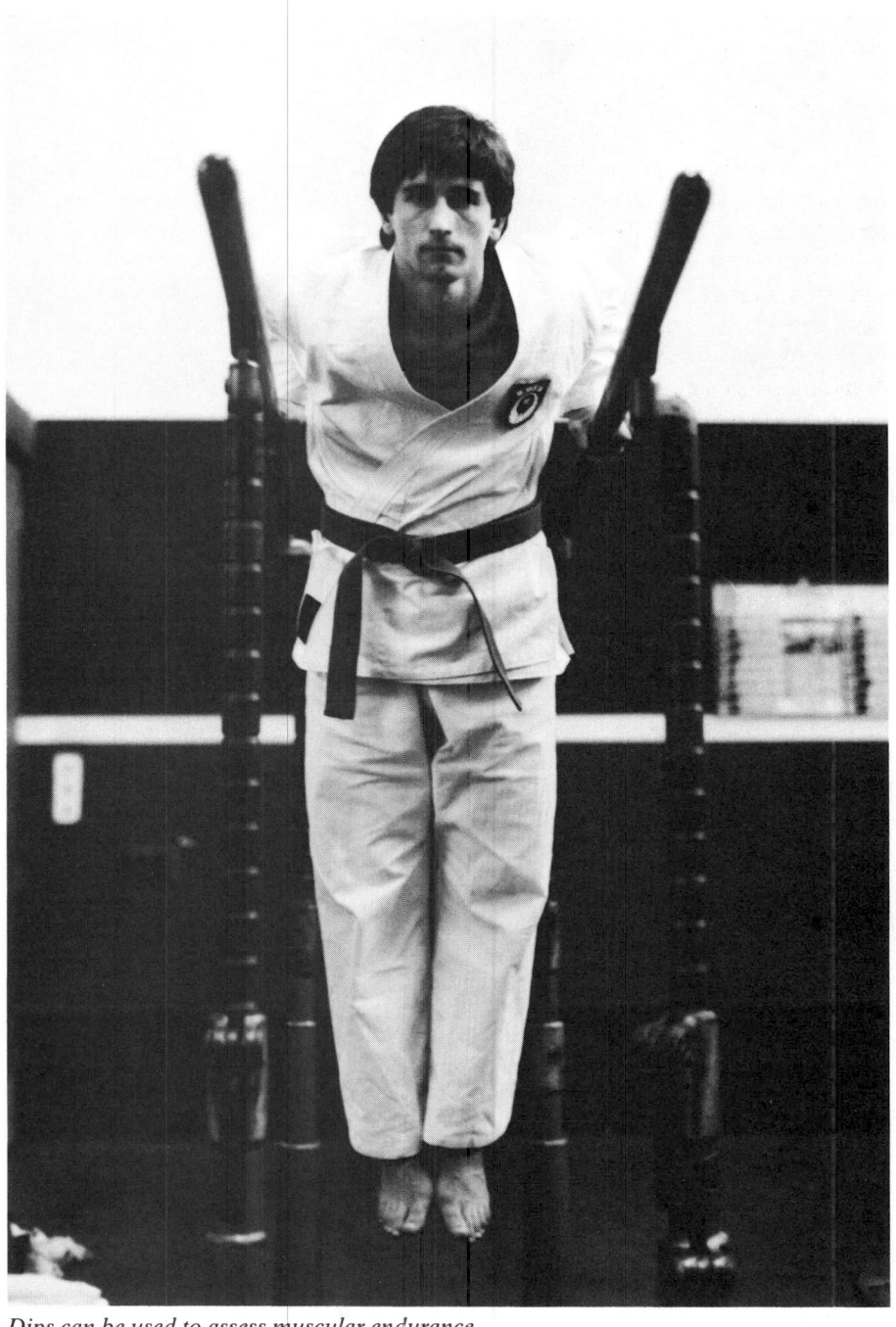

Dips can be used to assess muscular endurance

Extend the elbow until the arm is absolutely straight to complete each dip. Record the maximum number.

c. Sit-ups, performing as many as you can in 60 seconds. Bend knees to a 90° angle, clasp hands behind your neck and keep the chin away

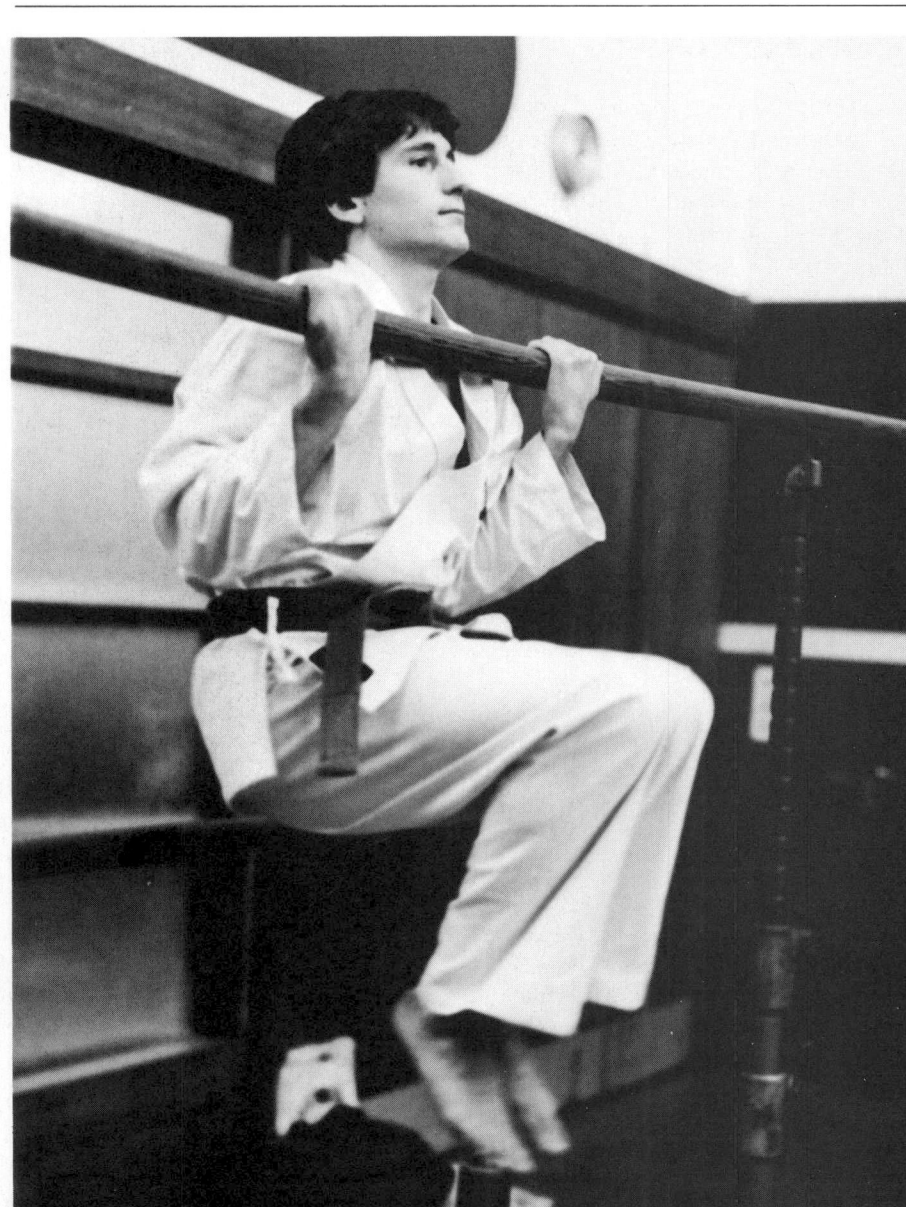

Pull-ups are an alternative exercise for assessing muscular endurance

from your chest. Touch elbows to knees to complete each sit-up.

d. Pull-ups, hanging from a bar and pulling up with the arms until the chin is above the bar. Then lower right down to full extension. Record the maximum number.

You can also assess muscular endurance through weight training. Perform the exercise with a certain weight until fatigued and record the result. If muscular endurance is improving, the number of repetitions will increase.

Assessing Power

There are two very simple methods for assessing leg power known as the 'Vertical-' and 'Horizontal Jump Test'. The results obtained are rarely converted into power values but are simply left as distances recorded in centimetres and metres respectively.

To perform the Vertical Jump Test, stand close and side-on to a wall and make a mark on it with a piece of chalk at maximum reach. Bend your knees and jump upwards as high as possible, making a second mark on the wall at the highest reach. Try this a number of times, using previous marks as targets to exceed. Measure the vertical distance between the maximum reach and the maximum jump reach marks.

A problem with this assessment arises because jump reach can be improved by a long and carefully co-ordinated arm swing which owes nothing to leg power.

To improve administration of the test, use a sliding scale attached to the wall, adjusting the zero to maximum reach. Chalk your fingers and tap the scale at the highest point of jump reach reading off the vertical distance from zero to chalk mark.

You can administer the Vertical Jump Test in yet another way by making a strong wooden box. In the centre of the upper surface is a hole in which is fitted a jamming cleat, its jaws flush with the top of the box. These cleats can be bought at marine suppliers. The cleat is drilled and a string attached, which when pulled, releases the jamming action.

Pass a thin rope through the cleat and tie it to your waist or belt. Adjust the rope so it passes vertically down from the belt to the cleat without any slack. Measure the rope from flush

The Vertical Jump Test is used to assess leg power

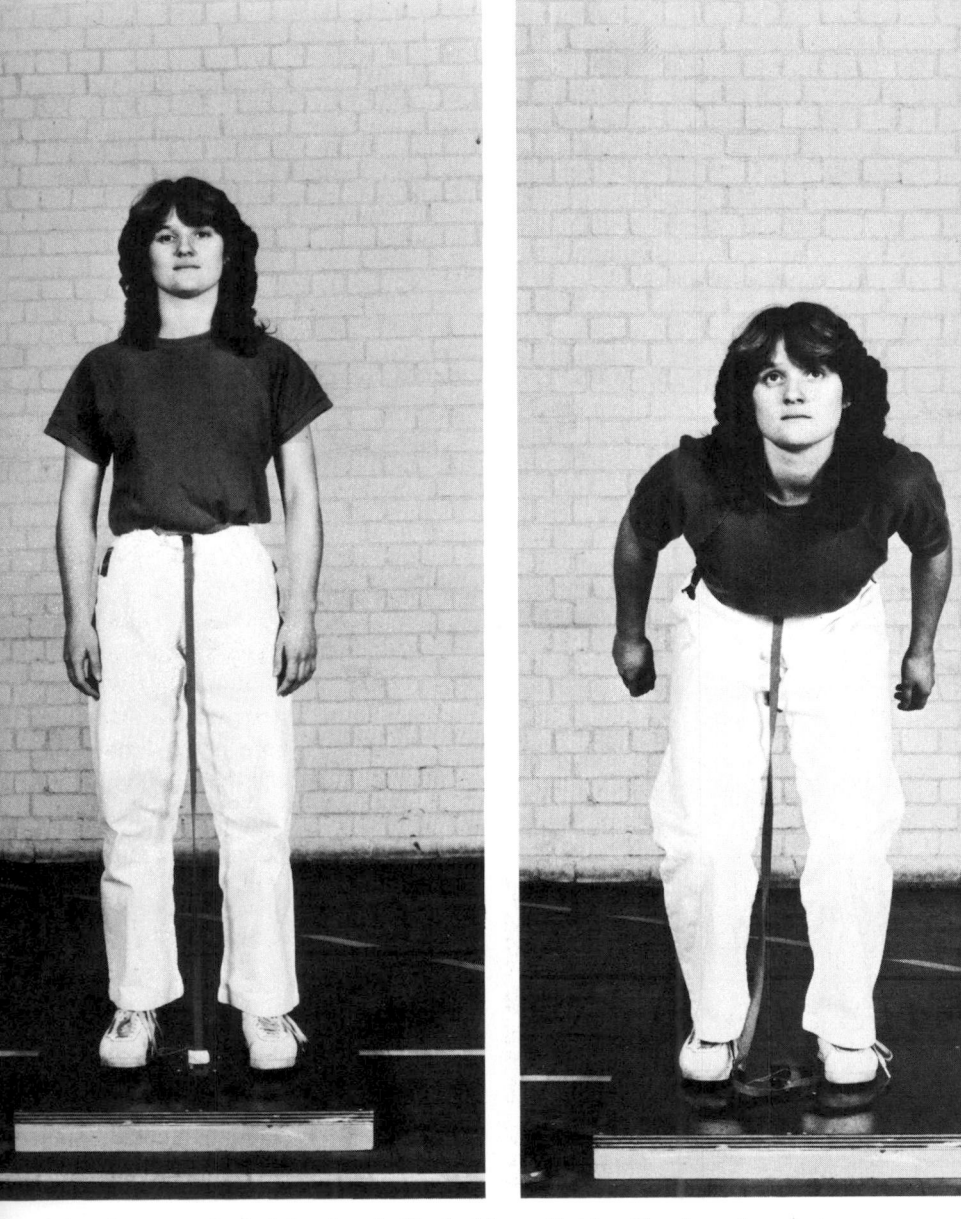

Another way of administering the Vertical Jump Test is with a jamming cleat

with the box top to its point of attachment and then jump vertically and as high as possible. Land as close to the take-off position as possible.

The cleat allows rope to run freely through it and the extra length can be measured, giving the height of the jump. Try a number of jumps and measure the rope after the last one. Since this test does not rely on arm movement, it gives a better indication of leg power.

To try the Horizontal Jump Test, stand with your toes touching a line.

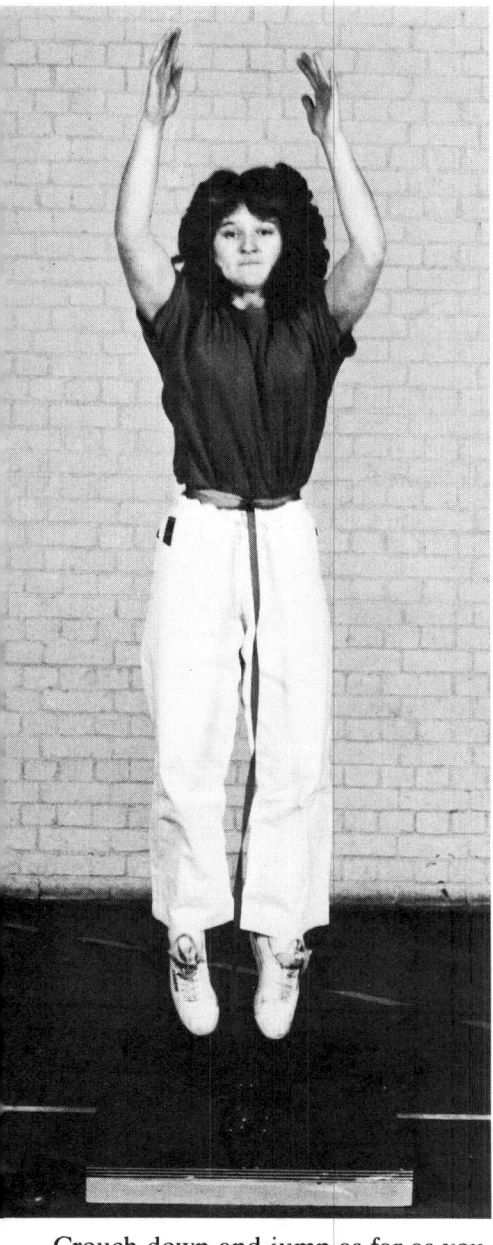

Crouch down and jump as far as you can, using an arm swing to assist. Remain wherever you land and mark the floor just behind the heel closest to the start line. Allow three jumps and record the furthest distance reached.

You can extend this distance by improving your technique but if your technique remains the same, then any increase can be attributed to improvement in leg power.

Arms and shoulder power can also be assessed through such as the 'medicine ball throw'. Lie on your back and extend your arms above your head. Throw a medicine ball as far as you can but keep your back and head firmly pressed to the floor. Measure the distance from the soles of the feet to where the ball lands. Make a number of attempts and record the farthest throw.

This test also responds to improvement in technique as well as power. The point at which the ball is released is critical. For comparative testing, the weight of the medicine ball must remain the same.

An alternative test with the medicine ball has you with your back to a wall, holding the ball against your chest. Push the ball out as far as possible, extending your arms fully and horizontally from the body. Keep your head in contact with the wall. As before, make a number of attempts and record the furthest distance from wall to landing point.

The jump board can also be used to measure upper body muscle power. Attach the rope to your neck but don't fix it too tightly. Put your hands a shoulder width apart and take the slack out of the rope. Mark it level with the board, then drop down and do an explosive push-up. Record the best attempt.

Sprint assessments are another method of assessing power. Use a distance of 20/50 metres and sprint from a standing start, measuring and recording time with a stopwatch. It is difficult to time the shorter sprints so take extra care, or use the electronic timing facilities available at some athletic tracks or fitness assessment centres.

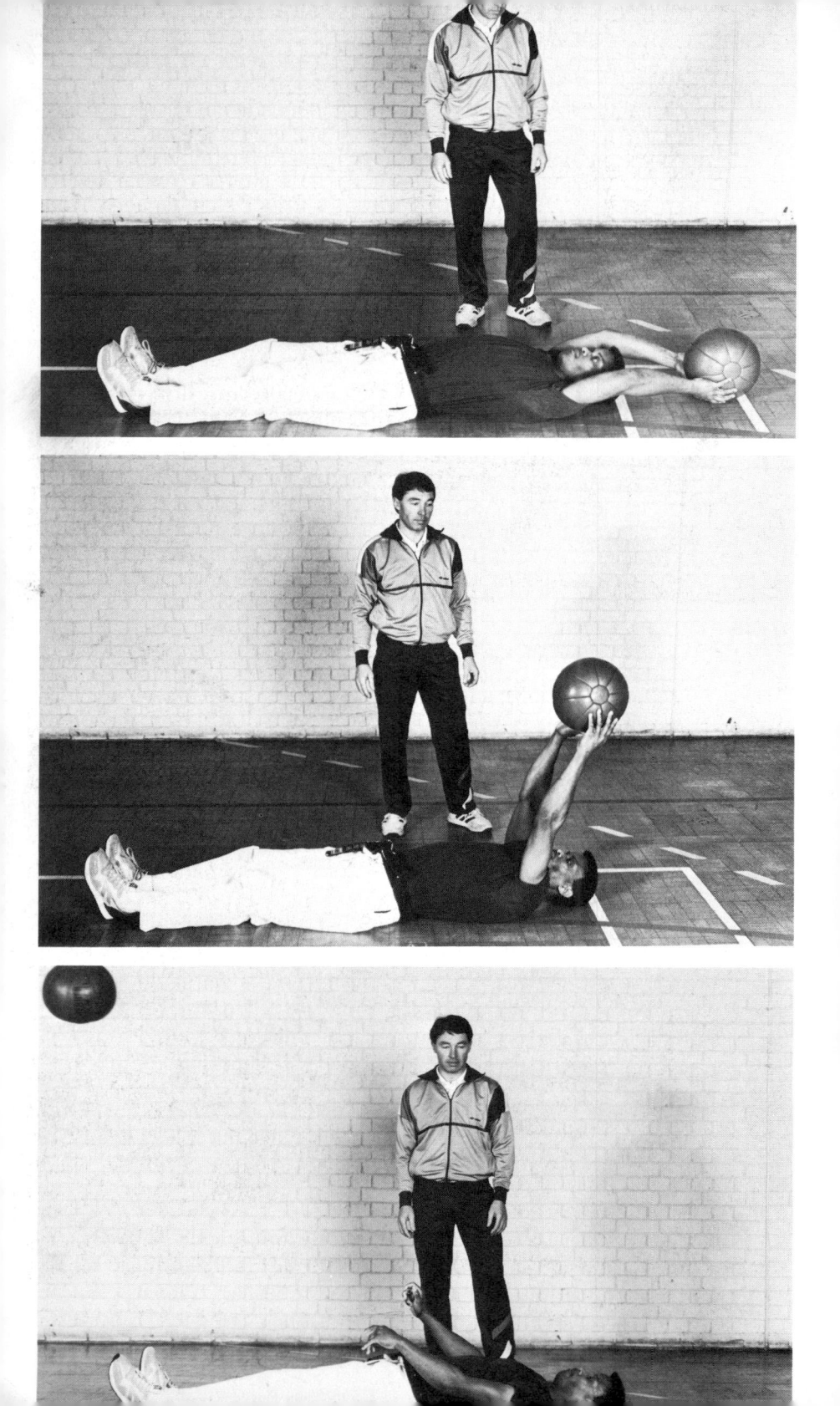

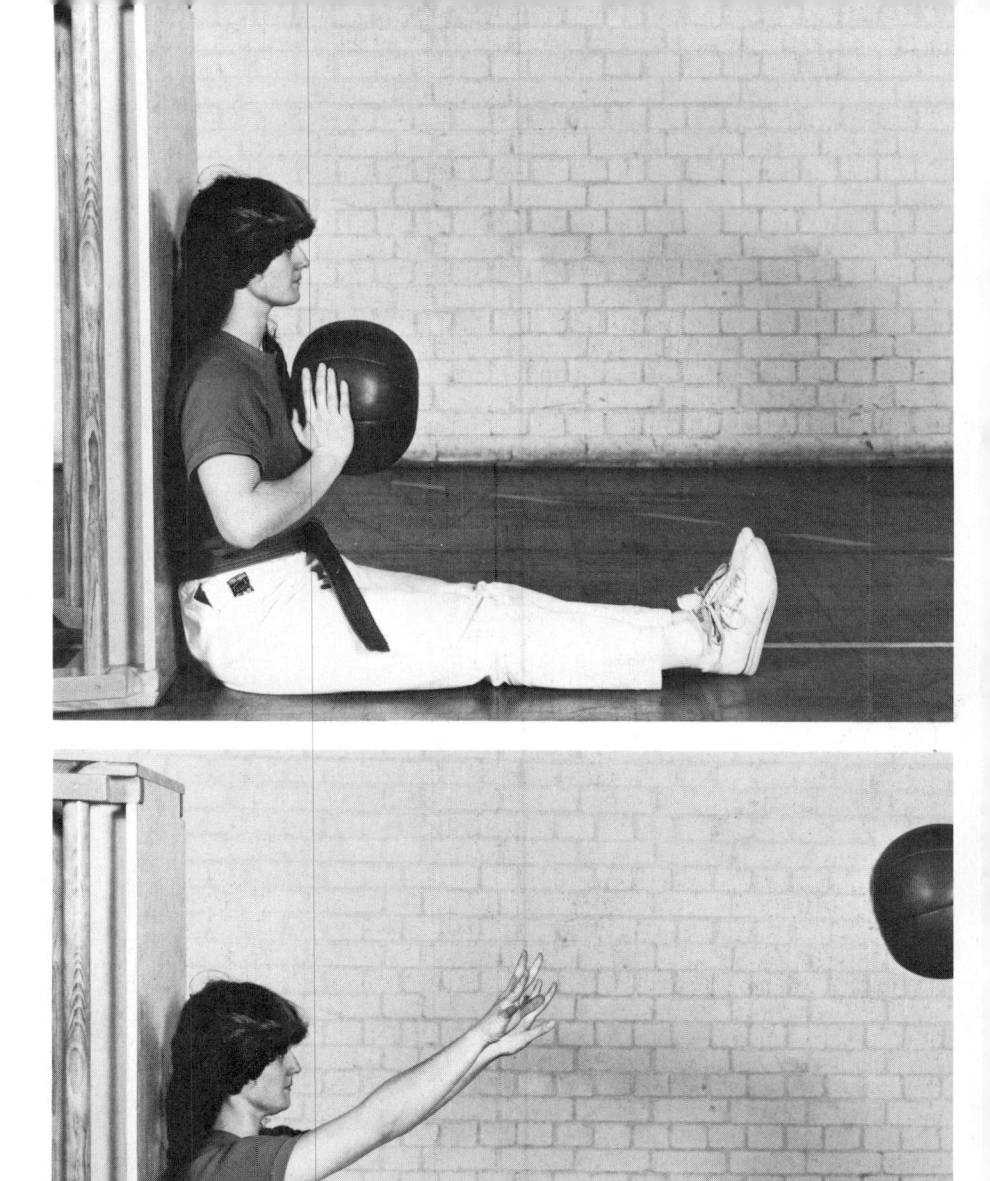

Opposite and above: *These are two ways of assessing arm and shoulder power using a medicine ball.*

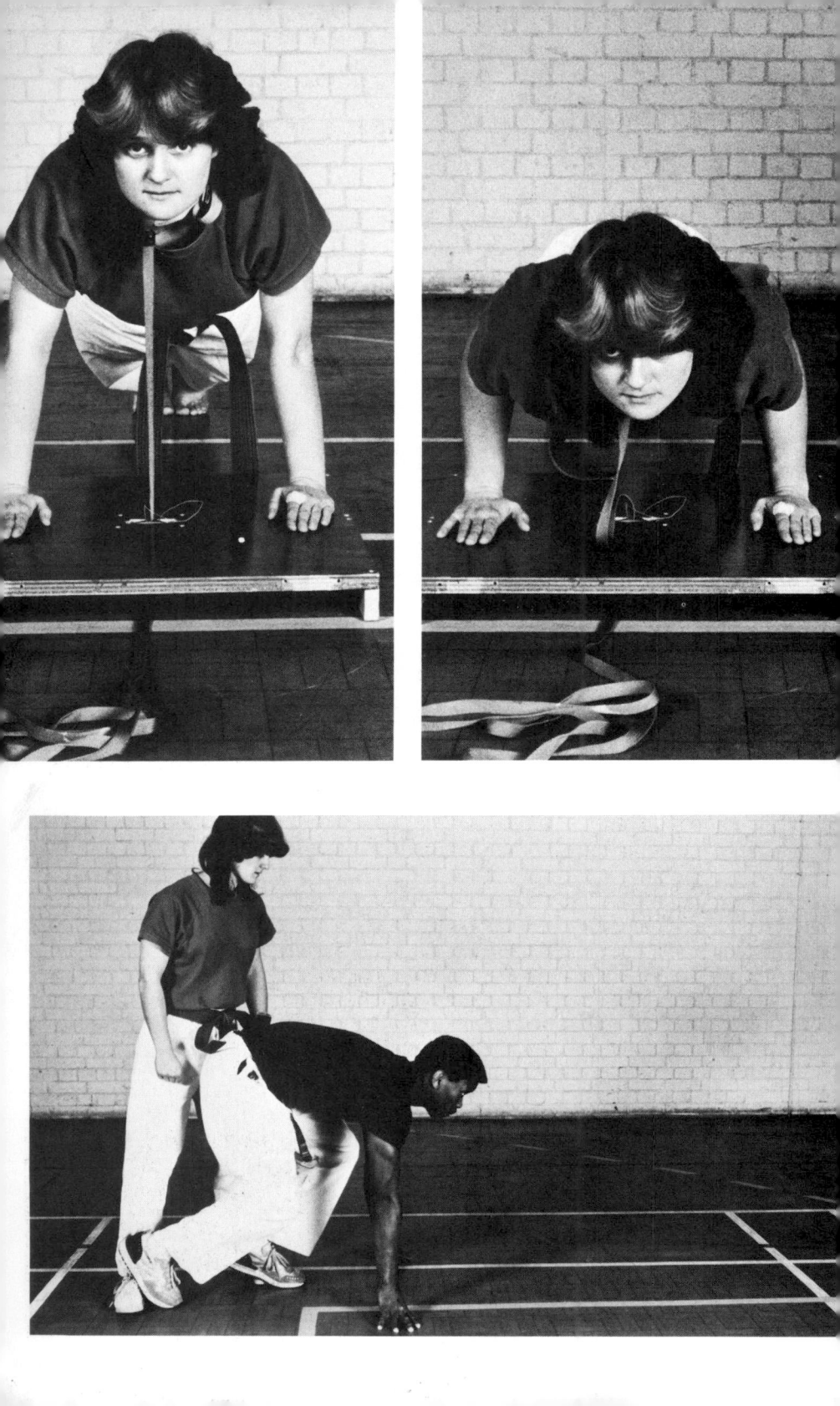

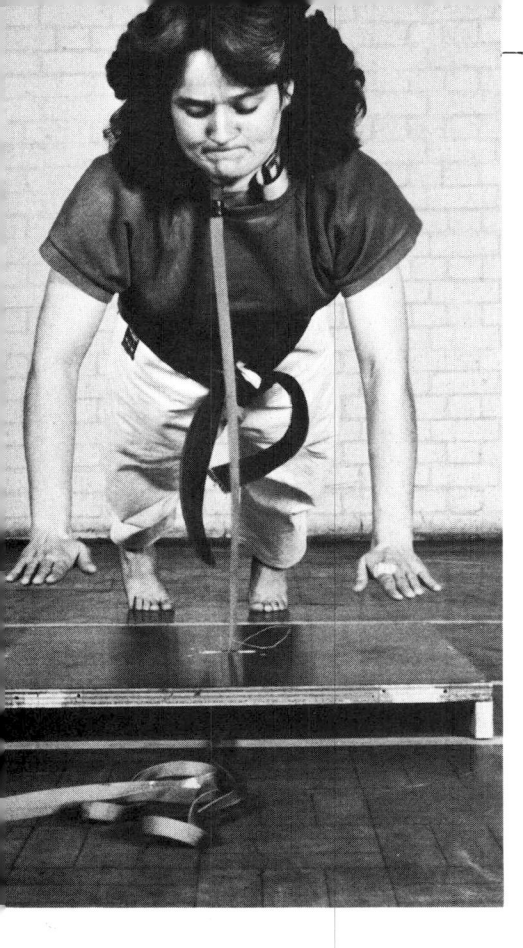

Upper body muscle power can also be assessed with a jump board and jamming cleat

Sprint 20/50 metres against the stopwatch to assess leg power

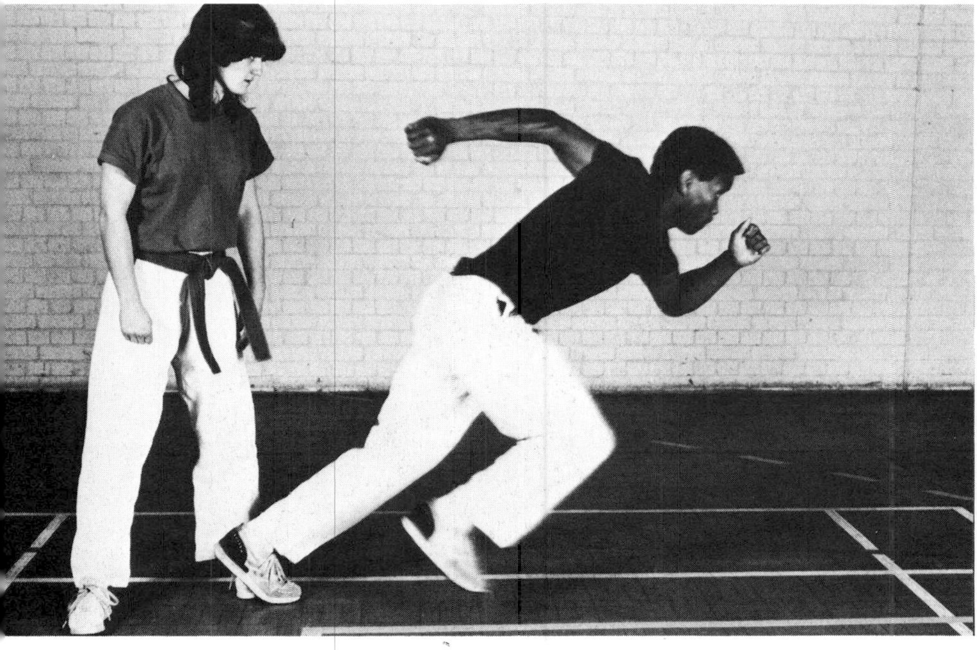

Assessing Flexibility

The best known assessment for hip and lower back flexibility is the 'Sit and Reach Test'. Sit on the floor and reach as far past your feet as possible whilst keeping your legs straight and your feet vertical. Try three stretches before going for maximum and hold the stretch for at least three seconds whilst measurements are taken by your assistant. If you fail to reach your feet, a negative score is recorded.

To make assessment easier, make a wooden box with a rule attached to the top. Put the soles of your feet against the side of the box so the rule projects towards you. A slider fits onto the rule and this is pushed along by your finger tips as you stretch.

There are many other ways of assessing flexibility. One of the simplest is to sit down and spread your legs as wide as you can while an assistant measures the distance between your heels.

Do realise that having good flexibility in one part of the body does not mean that all the other parts are as flexible.

Assessing Agility

Agility can be assessed by a run over a short distance, during which you have to change direction. The standard test is a 20 yard run, repeated five times and involving four changes in direction. You must step over the line at the end of each sprint before turning and sprinting off the other way. The length of sprint can be reduced if required. The assessment requires very accurate timing.

Assess flexibility with the 'sit and reach test'

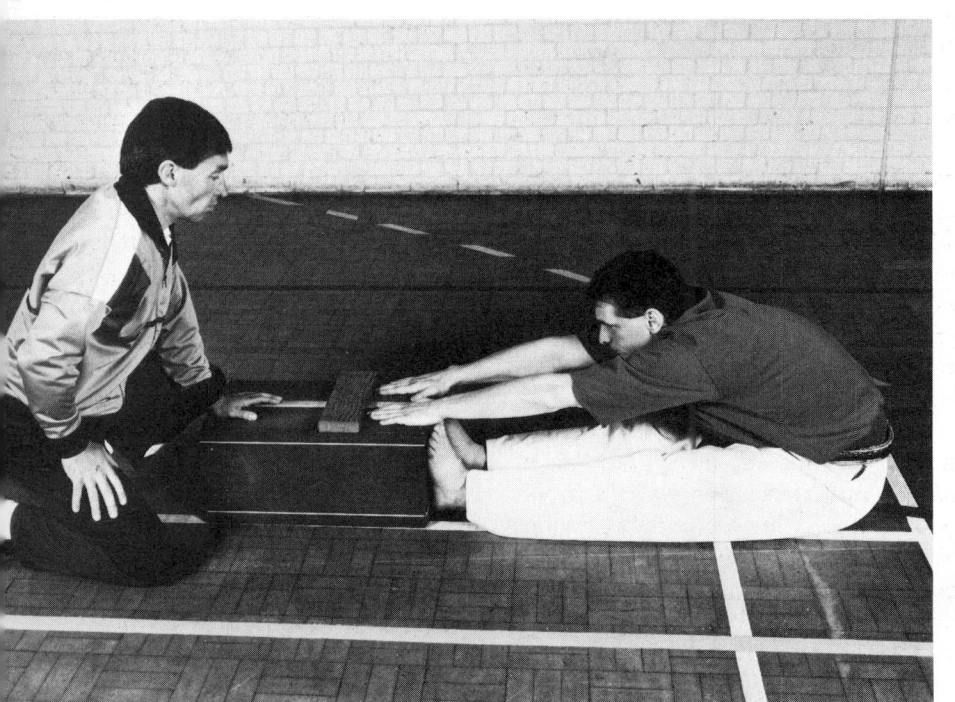

Assessing Body Composition

For a majority of people, height/ weight tables give a reasonable guide to body composition. If you are overweight then chances are this is due to subcutaneous fat but if you are a muscular athlete, then excess weight can be put down to larger muscles. These tables are therefore unsuitable for martial artists involved in serious training.

A skinfold caliper is used to measure the thickness of subcutaneous fat at various sites on the body. The values are then used to calculate percentage of fat stored in the body. The most accurate calipers are precision made from metal but cheaper plastic ones are also available at a price the club can afford.

You will have to decide whether the time and effort taken in collecting and processing measurements is worth it. In most cases it probably will not be, unless you want to check whether a specific student is under-achieving because of excess body fat. The weight of fat carried can tax the muscles and use up additional energy which would otherwise be employed more advantageously. If this becomes evident, then a weight-reducing programme is indicated and the calipers can be used to measure whether fat is being shed.

You can make some general assessments without calipers. Look in a large enough mirror and if you think you look fat, then you probably are. Try on some of the clothes you wore a couple of years ago and if you haven't been training and they are tight, then you have increased your body fat.

If you decide you are too fat, increase the amount of aerobic exercise you do each week and gradually reduce fat and sugar intake.

Using Fitness Assessments

If this chapter has got you thinking about using assessments, pause for a moment and consider the following:

- What assessments do you think will be useful?
- Why have you chosen them?
- Who will be assessed?
- Will they accept the idea of assessment?
- Do you have time to administer the assessments?
- How will you use the results?
- Would the time be better spent doing something else?

If you still think assessments are a good idea, then you may find that introducing them into a programme will motivate many martial artists to train harder. Do time the assessments in the programme so they highlight improvements. If the martial artists are beginning a period of aerobic endurance training, it is preferable to do the step assessment beforehand and again towards the end of training.

If a martial artist lacks flexibility where it is needed, assess him/her before the start of a flexibility programme. Do a second assessment after a couple of weeks into the programme when improvement can be expected to show up.

It is not really appropriate to compare assessments of one martial artist with another, though when you have a large number of records at your disposal, you may be able to identify some of the fitness components essential for excellence. Use assessments to

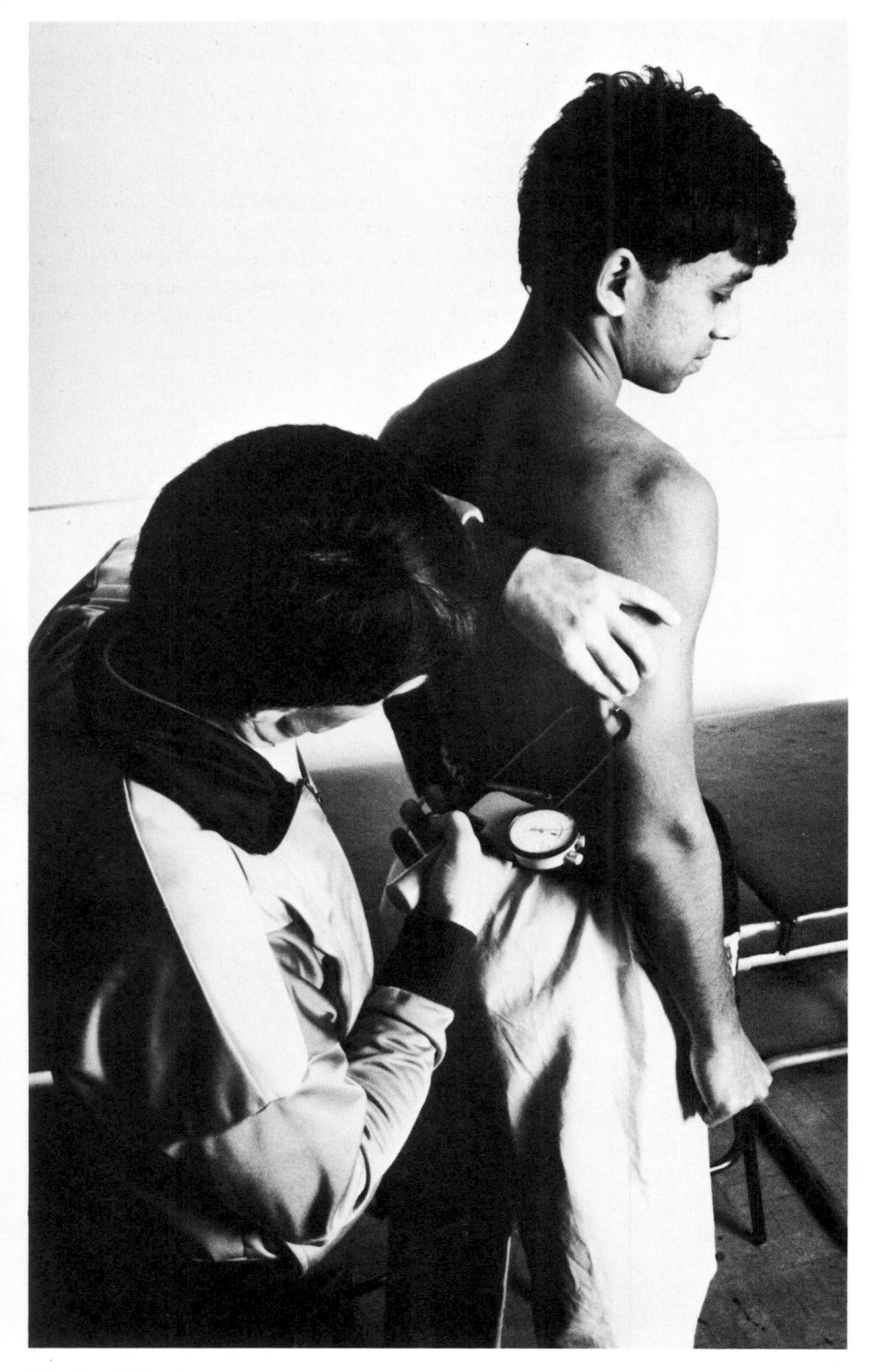

The skin fold caliper is used to measure body fat

confirm suspected weaknesses in a martial artist's fitness.

A comparison with norms, such as those provided by the step assessment give an indication of fitness level compared to other groups of people. It is preferable to compare a martial artist with data taken from within that discipline, if it is available.

It is also useful to compare assessments taken throughout a martial artist's career. A complete record can indicate the changes taking place in a martial artist as a result of training, gradings and competitions. Assessments are therefore useful to both the martial artist and coach.

Finally, if you decide to use fitness assessments as part of a training programme, it is very important that they are carefully selected and precisely administered on each occasion so that information collected is strictly comparable.

Fit for Life

Although this book concentrates on aspects of training for the martial arts, it is important to stress that physical considerations go beyond this and address questions about health-related fitness. At the moment there is concern about the growing number of people suffering from the disease *AIDS*. Unfortunately being fit does not cure, or even protect you from this disease.

The greatest killer in the Western world since the last war is cardiovascular disease. This can attack in the form of a stroke arising out of interference to the oxygen supply of the brain, or a heart attack caused by interference with the supply of oxygen to the heart muscle. One of the causes of both is a build-up of fatty deposits on the insides of those blood vessels carrying oxygenated blood.

The coronary artery supplies the heart muscle with oxygenated blood and if this is narrowed by fatty deposits, the heart may be starved of sufficient oxygen to sustain a high rate of activity, producing a severe chest pain known as *angina*. Worse still, blood platelets may build up on areas of fatty deposit, producing a clot which can jam in an already narrowed artery. This causes a heart attack and a portion of heart muscle will actually die.

Even when the heart attack is non-fatal, the results can be severely debilitating.

A number of risk factors relating to heart disease have been identified. Some are controllable and others are not. Uncontrollable factors are age, sex (males suffer more heart disease than females) and heredity – if your parent(s) had it, you stand an increased chance of suffering from it too. Controllable factors are smoking, obesity, nutrition, exercise, stress, high blood pressure and alcohol consumption. If you are serious about improving your performance of the martial arts, then you will have *ALREADY* adopted a life style which avoids many of the risk factors.

Don't smoke.

Smoking not only increases the risk of heart disease, it also causes lung cancer. It artificially increases the heart rate by about ten beats per minute and it reduces the oxygen carrying capacity of the blood. These two effects put additional stress on the cardiovascular system causing early onset of fatigue during training, especially in activities requiring aerobic endurance. In the short term, smoking will reduce your potential level of fitness. In the long term it may kill you.

Obesity (carrying too much fat), nutrition and exercise are closely linked. Obesity is a result of too much food consumption, too little exercise, or a combination of the two. Martial artists who expend considerable amounts of energy during training require a considerable energy intake. They can eat large quantities of food without putting on additional fat

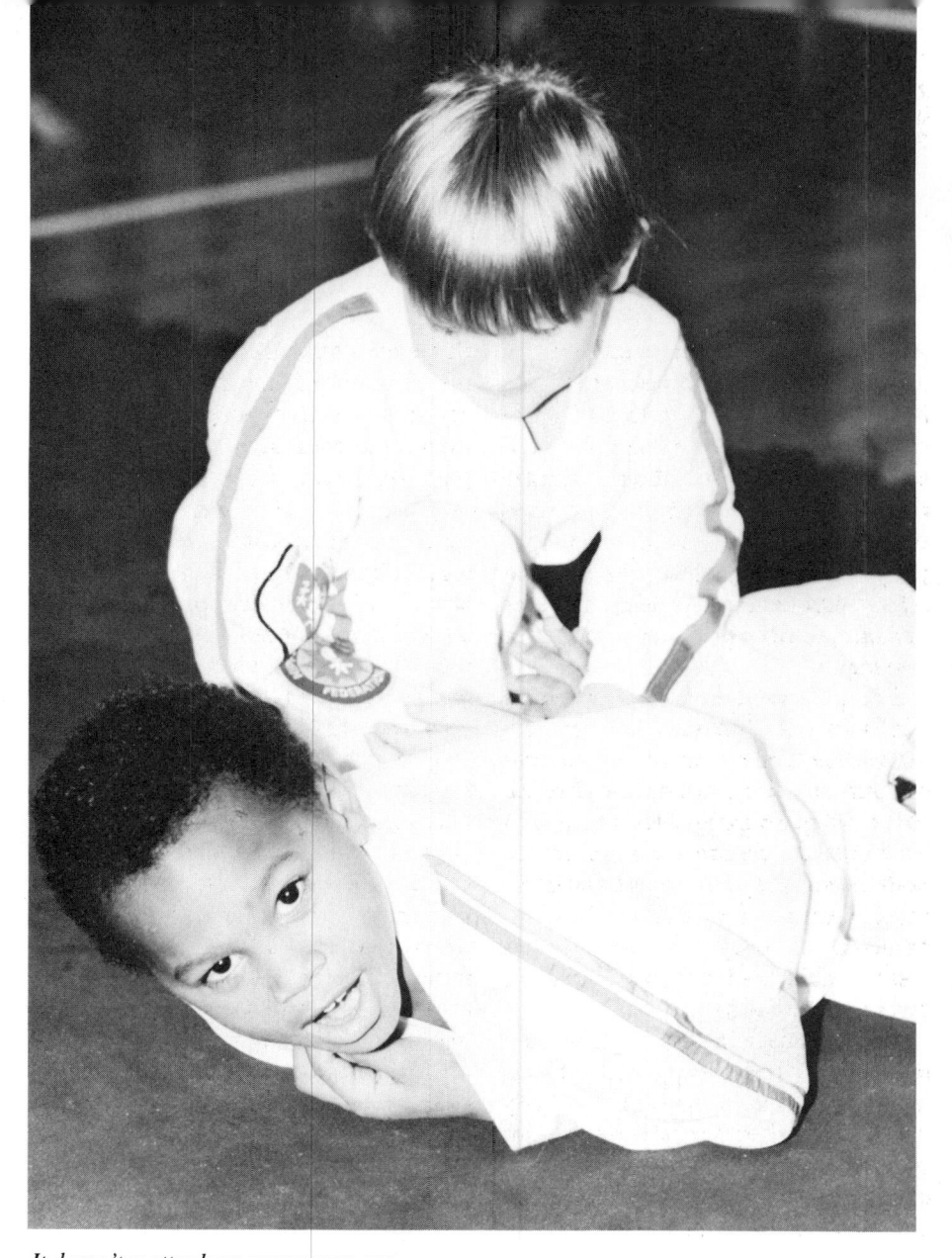

It doesn't matter how young you are...

because the food they take in is burned off in exercise.

If body weight is constant, don't worry but if it is gradually increasing over an extended period of time, consider your life style. Increase exercise, reduce food intake, or do both.

It is preferable to get your energy from complex carbohydrates such as are found in rice and pasta rather than from simple carbohydrates and fats. Although a link between a high intake of animal fats and the build up of fatty deposits in the blood vessels has not been conclusively proven, it is probably best to play safe and cut your animal fat intake.

Alcohol in small amounts may

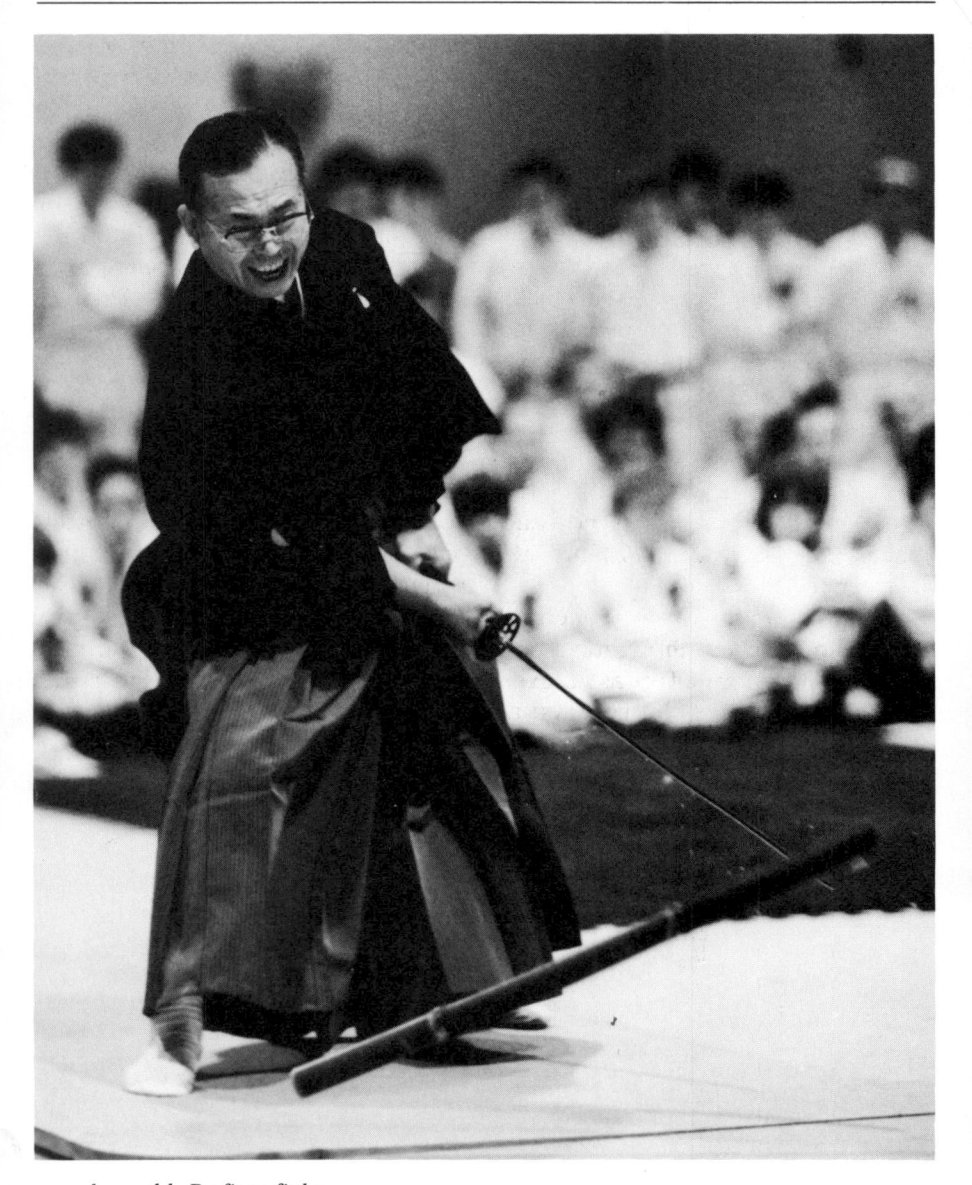

...or how old. Be fit to fight

actually reduce the risk of an early death through heart disease. A high intake may cause obesity and liver problems, so moderation is the key.

Without doubt if you are fitter, you will be a better performer. Exercise contributes towards the quality of life. Good aerobic endurance, muscular endurance, strength and flexibility is valuable at any time in life.

The training process removes you from the stresses of the day into another world, where concentration is directed away from mundane, day-to-day problems. It provides a form of active relaxation of real benefit to the person who would otherwise be under stress all the time. Relaxation persists even after training is over and may extend into a night of good sleep. It has been suggested that people who exercise regularly will have less absences from work and perform better in the work place.

A lifestyle of physical activity should allow a person who has entered old age to enjoy this part of their life. It may seem a blessing to remain active during these years but it is a blessing that can be worked for through exercise and good nutrition.

In the short- and mid-term, it may be important to be a better martial artist but remember that life goes on after martial arts practice has tapered off. Physical exercise may not add years to life but it will certainly add life to years.

Whilst exercise has a beneficial effect, approached thoughtlessly it can have as bad an effect as no exercise at all. Fatalities during physical exercise are often caused by trying to do too much too soon. Your exercise programme must be progressive, moving gradually from mild exercise to the more strenuous over a period of time.

Do not neglect warming up and cooling down exercises because they prepare the body for the increased activity of training, or for a return to normal activity levels. Perform stretching with great care and if you work with a partner, total cooperation is imperative.

If you suffer injury, hold off full training until the injury has recovered but carry on with selected aspects of your programme provided they don't put you at risk of making the injury worse.

If you know that a particular form of training puts you at the risk of injury, either now or in the future, then do make a value judgement to see whether the risk is worthwhile.

Nutrition and Fitness

Why do you eat what you eat? Is it because?

- It is the type of food you have always eaten since a child?
- It is prepared for you?
- It is quicker to prepare?
- You like it?
- It doesn't cost a lot?
- It is considered to be a healthy diet?
- It provides all the essential energy and nutritional requirements for a martial artist in training?

Whatever the reasons for a particular kind of diet, it is possible that you may be under-achieving in training and competition because you don't get enough of the right type of food. It doesn't matter how hard you train, the quality of your nutritional requirements remain the same, though you may need more quantity to off-set the additional energy burned during training.

What is a healthy diet? Recommendations from the DHSS lay down quantities and qualities sufficient to maintain the average person's body weight and health and it is suggested that increasing these values would not bring any additional benefits. (see Table 4)

Bear in mind that these requirements are for Mr and Ms Average whereas individuals will vary in their needs according to age, size, sex and level of activity. Pregnancy also affects the body's nutritional needs.

Food like fitness, consists of components. These are proteins, fats and carbohydrates, plus vitamins, minerals, water and fibre. The diet must be such as to mix all these in the correct relative quantities.

If we consider those components which provide energy, then we can get an indication of whether enough (or too much) is being taken in by measuring the change in body weight through training. If body fat is increasing, then too much is being eaten. Conversely, if you lose weight, more needs to be eaten.

Energy can be obtained from carbohydrates, fat, alcohol and even protein. Carbohydrate is stored as glycogen in the muscle and during prolonged and strenuous exercise, it is gradually used up, bringing on symptoms of fatigue. To reduce fatigue, the glycogen must be replaced by eating a high carbohydrate diet. Whilst piling all this stuff in, it is also useful to take in the necessary fibre, vitamins, protein and minerals. Wholemeal bread and pasta, brown rice, cereals, vegetables and some nuts fulfil this role.

Glycogen can be replaced by eating simple refined carbohydrates such as the sugar found in cakes and chocolates except that these foods sometimes also contain high levels of fat,

Table 4 Recommended intakes of nutrients

Age range years	Occupational category	Energy			Protein	Thiamin	Riboflavin	Nicotinic acid	Ascorbic acid	Vitamin A	Vitamin D	Calcium	Iron
										μg. retinol equiv	μg chole-calci-ferol		
		kcal	MJ	g		mg	mg	mg equiv	mg			mg	mg
Boys													
9 up to 12	..	2500	10·5	63	1·0	1·2	14	25	575	2·5	700	13
12 up to 15	..	2800	11·7	70	1·1	1·4	16	25	725	2·5	700	14
15 up to 18	..	3000	12·6	75	1·2	1·7	19	30	750	2·5	600	15
Girls													
9 up to 12	..	2300	9·6	58	0·9	1·2	13	25	575	2·5	700	13
12 up to 15	..	2300	9·6	58	0·9	1·4	16	25	725	2·5	700	14
15 up to 18	..	2300	9·6	58	0·9	1·4	16	30	750	2·5	600	15
Men													
18 up to 35	Sedentary	2700	11·3	68	1·1	1·7	18	30	750	2·5	500	10
	Moderately active	3000	12·6	75	1·2	1·7	18	30	750	2·5	500	10
	Very active	3600	15·1	90	1·4	1·7	18	30	750	2·5	500	10
35 up to 65	Sedentary	2600	10·9	65	1·0	1·7	18	30	750	2·5	500	10
	Moderately active	2900	12·1	73	1·2	1·7	18	30	750	2·5	500	10
	Very active	3600	15·1	90	1·4	1·7	18	30	750	2·5	500	10
65 up to 75	Assuming a	2350	9·8	59	0·9	1·7	18	30	750	2·5	500	10
75 and over	sedentary life	2100	8·8	55	0·8	1·7	18	30	750	2·5	500	10
Women													
18 up to 35	Most occupations	2200	9·2	55	0·9	1·3	15	30	750	2·5	500	12
	Very active	2500	10·5	63	1·0	1·3	15	30	750	2·5	500	12
55 up to 75	Assuming a	2050	8·6	51	0·8	1·3	15	30	750	2·5	500	10
75 and over	sedentary life	1900	8·0	48	0·7	1·3	15	30	750	2.5	500	10
Pregnancy 2nd and 3rd trimester	..	2400	10·0	60	1·0	1·6	18	60	750	10·0	1200	15
Lactation	..	2700	11·3	68	1·1	1·8	21	60	1200	10·0	1200	15

Department of Health and Social Security.
Recommended daily intakes of energy and nutrients for the UK, 1969

few or no vitamins and minerals and no fibre. Refined carbohydrates do provide energy and it is probably unwise to suddenly reduce them in the diet until enough complex carbohydrates are substituted. Monitor your

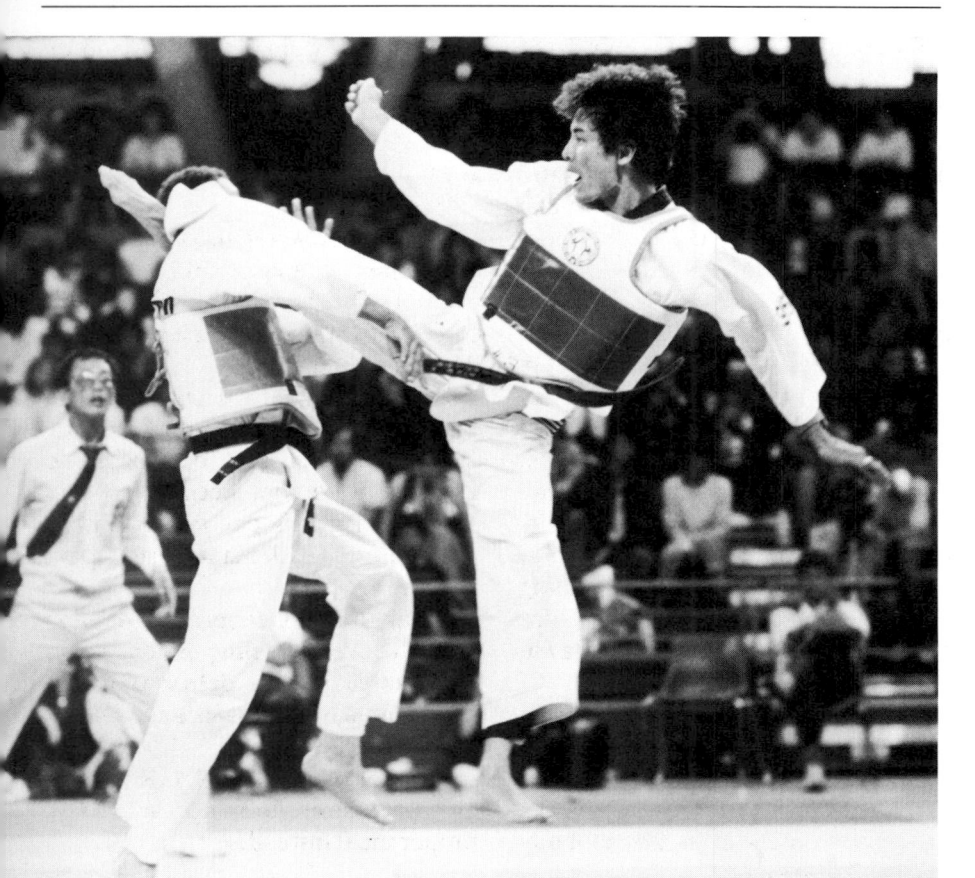

You need a balanced diet to supply the energy demands of training

body weight during the change in diet and adjust your food intake accordingly.

A small amount of fat is essential to proper body functioning but it is now considered that many people consume too much in their diet. An over-consumption of fat, especially that derived from animals is believed to be linked with the fatty deposits that build up on the walls of blood vessels. It is for this reason that fat intake should be reduced below 40% of the total energy intake and the complex carbohydrate consumption increased to at least 50%.

People probably eat too much protein and the surplus is broken down and excreted. It would appear that there is no need to increase the intake of animal protein even during the hardest stages of your programme. Since most animal protein also contains large amounts of fat, this is just as well. Eat less meat and then only of the lean variety.

If the diet is properly balanced, then the martial artist who consumes large quantities of the right kind of food to sustain energy requirements will also take in enough vitamins, minerals and fibre to facilitate normal body function and there is no need for any kind of nutritional supplement.

If you don't have a balanced diet

and want to change to one, then do so gradually. Try out different foods and progressively eat more of the type which provides complex carbohydrates, whilst cutting down on fatty foods and animal protein. Don't make your diet too difficult to maintain through lack of variety or cost because a sensible diet is a lifetime commitment.

Don't eat for the two hours preceding a competition, grading, or training session because training on a full stomach can prove uncomfortable. Eat a light, easily assimilated meal. Digestion requires a good blood supply which may deplete the supply to working muscles. Pace your eating habits to ensure that your muscles are recharged with glycogen on the day of competition or grading.

Drink fluids just before and during a hard event. Take between 4/600 millilitres at this time. This is especially important if you tend to sweat a lot because as little as 2% of body weight lost in fluid has been found to adversely affect performance. You can take around 150 millilitres of fluid every 15/20 minutes during exercise and this will prepare you for doing it in an event.

A change in weight recorded before and after exercise indicates the amount of fluid to be replenished. The object is to start and finish training at the same weight.

It is claimed that absorbtion of fluid is increased when the drink is cool. You can add sucrose or glucose to drinking water but keep below two and a half grams per 100 millilitres, otherwise you will actually slow fluid uptake.

Drink fluids to rehydrate your body after the event. Feeling thirsty always lags behind actual dehydration, so drink enough to produce a light straw coloured urine.

Alcohol does not replenish muscle glycogen after training, so eat a proper meal instead.

Fitness and Drugs

There is no proper definition of the word 'drug'. The definition given in a general dictionary says that a drug is any natural or synthetic chemical substance used in the treatment, prevention or diagnosis of disease. This is actually a bad definition because some drugs have nothing whatsoever to do with disease. The medical dictionary tells us that a drug is 'any medicinal substance, or a narcotic'. Quite why narcotics have been singled out and not other classes of drug is not clear.

This lack of a proper definition has meant that martial artists may have unwittingly offended against the drug control regulations imposed by governing bodies. Is a cup of strong coffee taken before a match or grading a drug? Is the long-acting cold cure you took to temporarily ward off the symptoms of 'flu enough to get you banned for life? Will your asthma inhaler produce a positive drug test? Does a woman's contraceptive pill contain steroids of a type which could trigger a drug test?

The International Olympic Committee has tried to tackle this problem by defining whole categories of drugs from the way in which they act upon the body. Less important but for guidance only, are lists of scheduled drugs within each category. As drug companies develop new products, the latter schedules must be constantly updated. There are five categories of forbidden drugs, the first of which is the psychomotor stimulants.

Psychomotor stimulants increase alertness and reduce the effects of fatigue. If you are tired after an early drive to a competition or grading venue, a psychomotor stimulant will pep you up. The fatigue so miraculously swept away is not banished; it remains on the sidelines until the effect of the stimulant wears off, after which it returns with a vengeance.

Psychomotor stimulants were used in the second World War as a means of extending the emergency capabilities of pilots on long missions. They can lead to heart failure when taken in high dosages.

Sympathomimetic amines are drugs of the amine group which mimic the effects of the sympathetic nervous system. The latter gees up the body ready for fight or flight, diverting blood supply to the muscles and readying the body for a strong response. They will temporarily suppress the effects of injury, allowing the body to carry on responding, even when quite severely damaged. It is the action of the sympathetic nervous system that allows the mortally wounded animal to keep going long enough to escape its attackers.

Before a grading or competition, the sympathetic nervous system is already winding the body up tighter than a guitar string, so quite why anyone should consider taking a sympathomimetic amine is a mystery! Administration of such a drug to an already aggressive martial artist can produce a dangerous lack of control.

Miscellaneous central nervous system stimulants is the name given to a category of various drugs whose components may be widely different from each other but which produce a similar effect. They raise the sensation of awareness without necessarily linking it to improved muscular coordination. They can also reduce nervousness and increase confidence. In fact in some cases, they have a similar effect to that well-known drug, ethyl alcohol. High dosages can actually ruin performance.

Narcotic analgesics are powerful pain inhibitors and the most potent appear to work by stimulating the so-called 'pleasure centres' in the brain, so pain messages are blanked out by a stronger signal. They are highly addictive and a susceptible martial artist may need only one dose to become hooked.

Anabolic steroids reduce recovery time after rigorous training. In theory, martial arts practice relies upon application of scientific, rather than brute force principles so the advantages of such drugs to the top performer are limited.

Their application is all the more limited when you consider that high doses of anabolic steroids can produce cancers and a reduction in the sex drive.

In some cases, one or more of the above classes of drug may be mixed together into a single preparation and if you are in any doubts, refer your enquiry to the Chief Medical Officer of your governing body. In any case, do not take any pills or potions handed to you by your coach unless you know exactly what they are for and whether they are acceptable to the governing body.

Drugs have been used in the martial arts for millennia. Those beautiful little red, white-spotted mushrooms that the fairies and elves of childrens' books sit on are *Amanita muscaria*. This was much prized by the Vikings who called it 'berserker' because of its effect upon them. The trick was to take it at the right time before landfall, otherwise uncontrolled fighting broke out on the longship itself. The Vikings also learned how to modify the dosage, so they didn't get the urge to burn and pillage hopelessly confused with the desire to rape.

Drugs should not be used in martial art because they give an artificial and unfair advantage to one performer. The person taking drugs doesn't win on their own merit and they therefore undermine everything that modern day martial arts practice stands for. Using drugs is akin to slipping a horseshoe inside the fist mitt, or kicking your partner somewhere nasty when the examiner isn't looking.

It is just plain cheating!

Not only is it that but it is also dangerous. The whole rationale for practising the martial arts is not to bash other people but to improve one's health. Taking potent drugs does not improve health and can actually cause death – the state of ultimate unhealthiness.

Because of the tiny minority of people masquerading as martial artists who do take drugs, your governing bodies have introduced drug testing. People caught by the tests can expect to be dealt with very severely and pleas of "Sorry sir, I won't do it again!" will fall on deaf ears.

At any stage during training, in a squad session, before a grading, after a selection or just about as you are going into the finals, the tournament doctor may ask you to follow him to the Testing Station. If you refuse to cooperate, your governing body will take the view that you have committed a serious offence against their drug policy and discipline you accordingly.

Some governing bodies will require you to sign a consent form before allowing you into a selection programme or championship. Read this carefully and answer truthfully any questions there may be relating to medication you are taking. Remember, a false declaration can cost you your martial arts career!

The following questions may be asked:

Are you taking any drugs at the moment? (Includes headache pills, cold cures, contraceptive pills and hay fever treatment).

Are you suffering from any of the following:
  asthma;
  migraine;
  epilepsy;
  diabetes;
  pregnancy;
  nervous disorders.

When taking the drug test proper, you will be asked to undress to your underwear and be ushered into a toilet. Female martial artists may request that a female nurse or orderly be present and this wish will be granted at the discretion of the governing body. You must pee into a sterile container which has been chosen by you.

When you have done, hand the container to the doctor. He/she will divide the sample into two and then ask you to sign a further form. This will request you to re-state whether you have taken any medication – for asthma, for a cold, for contraception – anything within the last 48 hours. Don't be in a hurry. Read it carefully and ask the medical officer for advice on any point you are unsure of.

The urine sample will be analysed in a laboratory approved by the governing body and the results notified to the governing body medical officer concerned. If you consider that the results of your drug test are incorrect, then you may apply to have the second sample analysed in the presence of a governing body approved person.

Fitness and Biorhythms

The concept of biorhythms fits in well with traditional martial arts practice, much of which is based upon Buddhist and Taoist philosophies. These postulate the existence of a form of energy which can be generated through certain activities and harnessed to improve vitality and power. This *chi* (the Japanese synonym for this Chinese term is *ki*) energy flows through the body along certain pathways known as 'meridians' and depending upon the time of day, some meridians are actively transporting *chi* whilst others are latent.

This rhythmic flow of energy is a comparison of the human being with the universe, where events take place in a constant and predictable cycle, or rhythm. The seasons come and go, autumn follows summer and night follows day. In everything there is a rhythm of activity that is constant and unchanging.

Modern science does not consider *chi* though it does recognise the rhythmic behaviour of the human body and its effects upon fitness. Most people believe that, barring fevers, the human body temperature is constant but in fact it is not. It oscillates above and below the constant according to a very precise rhythm. At set times of the 24 hour day the body increases and decreases the level of ions in body fluids.

A rhythmic interplay of hormones from the ovaries and pituitary makes menstruation a regular problem for many women martial artists but more of that later.

Each rhythm has its own inherent periodicity; that is, the oscillation occurs at a rate which is independent of other rhythms. This natural periodicity is however suppressed by the division of the day into light and dark periods. If anything occurs which interferes with this regular cycle, the martial artist quickly feels out of sorts and unable to train properly.

Just one night without sleep can disrupt the daily rhythms of the human body for several days afterwards. This may not be much of a problem for the average student but for someone going for a grading examination or a selection, the effects can be quite serious. One coach felt that his team should be tough, so when they went on an intercontinental trip, he sent them by the longest route, timing their arrival to the day before the competition. As a result, his team never got anywhere and he is no longer the coach. The new coach allowed his team to recuperate and adjust properly to the new day cycle with the result that the same team came second at the World Karate Championships.

Individual martial artists will operate to their own body clocks and they should heed the signals and not be tempted to stay up that extra hour or skip a scheduled meal. Synchronising with your body rhythms will help you to give your best performance on the day of competition or grading.

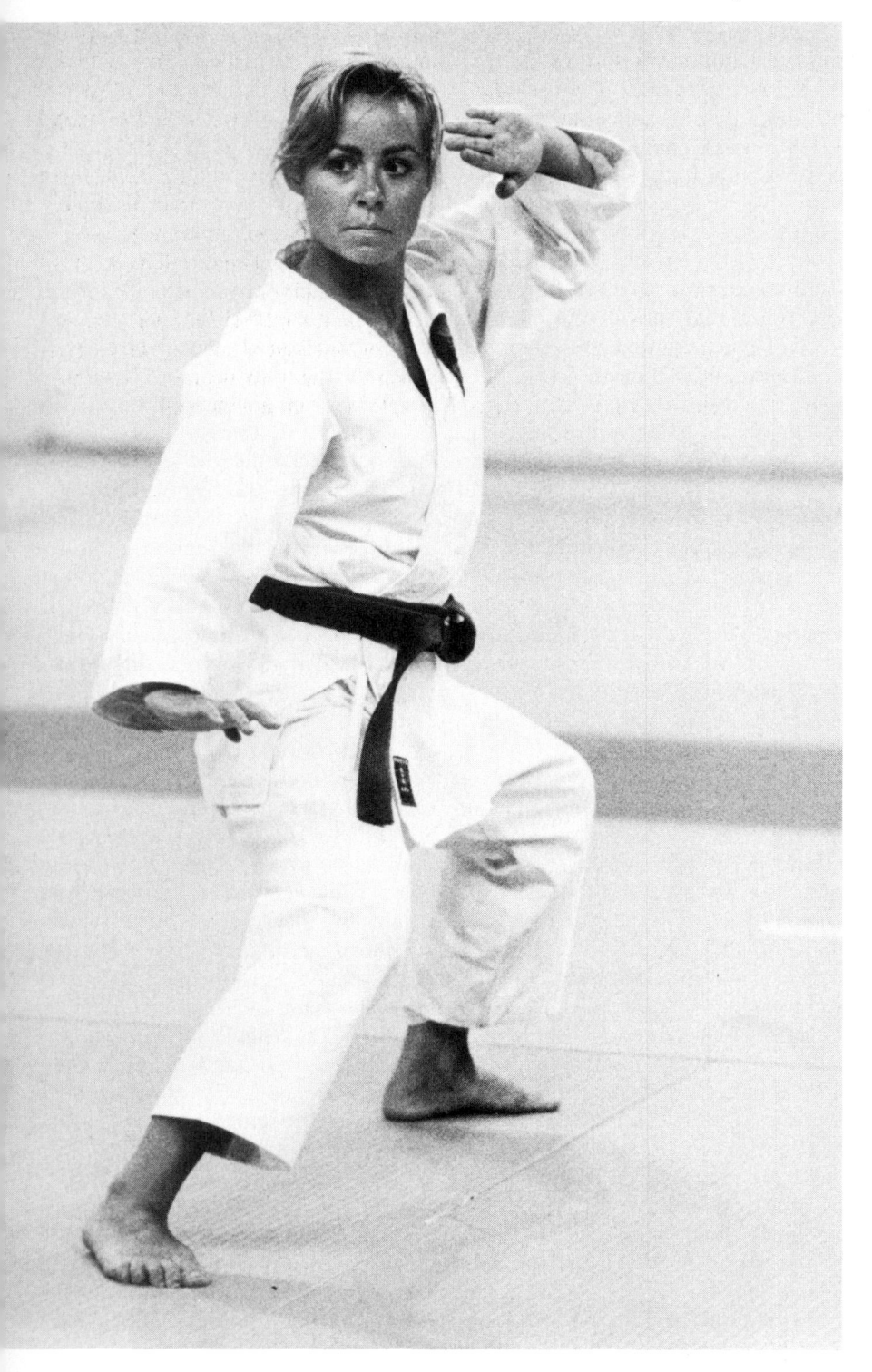

The female martial artist is more susceptible to biorhythms than the male

Maintaining a regular eating pattern is very important and it is better to eat four small meals at regular times throughout the day than one or two large meals. After eating, larger quantities of blood are diverted from the muscles to the viscera where they aid in the digestive process. The body will not perform to its maximum after food, so meal times must be adjusted to suit training requirements.

The effects of menstruation vary. In some women it passes without fuss. In others it produces all kinds of undesirable symptoms. The martial artist may complain of headaches, backaches, feeling swollen and heavy or all of these. She may also become very aggressive and her coordination suffer. Martial artists taking oral contraceptives may wish to seek their doctors' advice either about taking the next course of pills immediately after the first concludes, or attempting to modify their cycle. Either will change the time of onset of menstruation and prevent the customary adverse symptoms from developing.

Fitness and the Training Environment

In the traditional Japanese training hall – the *dojo* everything was kept simple. There were no showers and no heating for the old masters believed that the temperature of the dojo should be ambient. Training was often out of doors and typhoons were regarded as an excellent training environment to learn stable stances. The traditional teachers reasoned that since fighting did not always take place on a perfectly level floor, then training should take place on uneven surfaces such as the edges of cliffs.

Bearing in mind that the martial arts are actually fighting systems, these severe conditions make some sense. Their purpose was not merely to strengthen the body but also to increase resolve and fortitude. The students taught by this system were not today's average martial arts student. Any attempt to impose those conditions on a large class nowadays would lead to a sudden drop in class numbers because the majority of people practising the martial arts want to do so in a 'fun' way.

It is for this latter class of person that a description of what constitutes a modern adequate training environment is offered.

The average student will appreciate training in a comfortable environment and temperature is a major factor. In all the martial arts, training starts slowly and builds through the session, so what is cold at the outset becomes comfortable, or even too hot by the end. In winter, the training hall should be heated sufficiently to banish chill from the air. Whatever the source of heat, the air should not be dried out, or polluted with either exhaust fumes or tobacco smoke. One window at least, should always be open to provide a through-flow of fresh air. A considerable amount of water vapour is given off by the active body and if this cannot be taken away, it condenses on cool surfaces and will eventually lead to a smelly training hall.

One of the most important parts of the training environment is the floor surface. Martial arts such as aikido, jiu jitsu, hapkido and shorinji kempo require a padded floor because students are thrown violently to the ground during the course of normal training. The mats should grip the floor so they don't move about and separate and their upper surfaces be smooth enough to allow fast foot movements. During the execution of certain throws, the weightbearing foot must be able to pivot easily. Any resistance from the mats can damage ankles and knees.

Mats should be thick enough to mute the force of landing but should not be so resilient as to make moving around difficult. They must be large enough to accommodate the numbers training and the coach must check to see they don't come apart during training.

Activities such as karate, kendo, taekwondo, tang soo do, full contact and kung fu do not need mats for ordinary training, though they are better to do warm up exercises on. During the course of an average karate session, the student is not likely to get dumped forcefully on the floor, though accidents do of course happen. Consequently, the floor can be of sprung wooden construction, or have a layer of resilient synthetic rubber covering it.

Whatever the martial art, no training should take place on a solid floor. Tile, parquet, or stone floors can become slick with perspiration and cause a nasty fall. There have been a number of cases where martial artists have fallen backwards onto a hard floor and sustained serious head injuries.

The floor area must be kept clear at all times. The Martial Arts Commission has set certain limits on the numbers of people who can train in one area and these limits must be adhered to. For example, each person practising karate, kendo, kung fu, hapkido, full contact, taekwondo and tang soo do requires at least one and a half square metres of space. The other martial arts need at least two square metres per person. To find out how

Mats are essential for certain forms of safe training

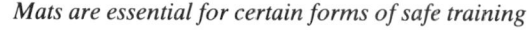

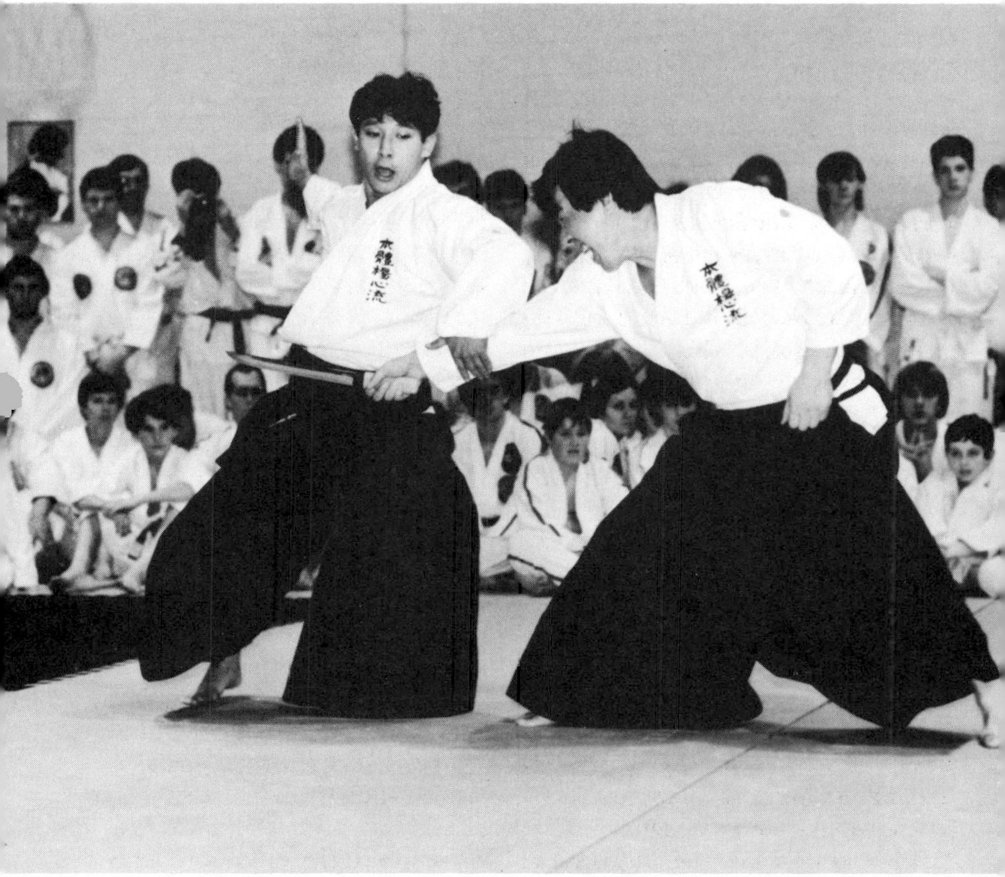

many people can safely train at one time in a facility, determine its floor area and divide by half. Then divide this figure by one and a half, or two square metres to roughly estimate safe numbers.

Larger classes should be divided into two and whilst one half practises, the other sits cross-legged at the side of the facility and learns by observation.

Mirrors are very handy to have in the training hall. They reveal deficiencies in posture and technique. Unfortunately they are also a source of danger because they can so easily shatter, showering the training hall with razor-like slivers of glass. The aware coach will keep students away from this danger area.

Glass doors and low windows are similar danger areas. The training area must be moved away from glass doors. There is one case on record where a martial artist lost the use of his right hand after being thrown through a glass door. Windows must be kept covered with a light grill. The area immediately surrounding the training area must also be kept clear of hazard. Training bags should not be allowed to clutter the floor. Chairs should be moved back.

There is a case on file where a martial artist fractured his arm through falling against the edge of a supporting pillar. All pillars and radiators must be adequately padded. Where this cannot be done, it is the coach's responsibility to keep students away from potential danger areas.

Light fittings should be high enough to permit proper training. A bamboo *shinai* or a six foot staff needs a lot of head room because the last thing you want is a shower of sparks and flying glass as a fluorescent fitting explodes.

The training environment must have adequate fire escape facilities and elementary fire-control equipment such as an asbestos blanket should be readily available. A working telephone should also be in easy reach and the address and location of the nearest 24 hour Casualty Unit known. A first aid kit must be on hand during every training period. This need not be comprehensive but it should contain such items as a kitchen towel or tissues (for staunching a haemorrhage), scissors strong enough to cut through a martial arts uniform, a triangular bandage, eye-pad, some sticking plasters and a blanket.

Though not a part of Fitness and the Training Environment, it is nevertheless convenient to mention at this point the need to take sensible precautions when training anywhere. You will at some stage train with another martial artist and however careful you both are, the likelihood of injury cannot be ruled out. Risk is highest with less experienced martial artists and is never entirely absent from any form of training. Therefore it makes sense to insure yourself against claims of injury arising from your alleged carelessness.

It is a regrettable fact that litigation between martial artists is on the increase, so protect yourself by taking out and keeping a current Martial Arts Commission licence. These are issued through approved associations of clubs and they incorporate a specially written policy indemnifying the martial artist. As an additional bonus, the insurance cover includes personal accident benefits payable either as a capital sum, or as weekly payments – whether or not you happen to be employed.

The Martial Arts Commission licence with its incorporated insurance is as vital to your safe training as a suitable training environment.

We started this section with a description of traditional martial art concepts and it is appropriate to conclude it with the same. Regardless of how seriously we study our martial arts, let us remember that they are mental as well as physical disciplines. The place of training is to be treated with the same respect that we show to the teacher and to each other. Each time you enter or leave the training hall, stop and face the senior person present and perform a proper salutation. If no-one is present, face the centre of the training hall and make your salutation.

It is that depth of feeling and awareness which separates martial artists from the followers of other physical disciplines.

Preparing for Fitness

All martial arts training requires motivation to start and even more motivation to continue. Being mentally prepared is essential if you intend training hard enough and for long enough to improve fitness. The longer and more severe training is, the more drop-outs will occur. Therefore when you set up your training programme, consider the mental side as well as the physical.

People drop out of training for a variety of reasons, boredom being perhaps the most common. Long, grinding sessions with few achievements in the form of self-felt improvement or success in a grading or competition will demotivate all but the most determined martial artist. Even if you don't give up at this stage, boredom will result in a lower work rate and reduction in concentration, leading perhaps to mistakes creeping in.

Over-motivation is just as bad because if you are mad keen, you may plan too hard a programme or set such a high exercise rate that your body cannot adapt to it. 'Overtraining' happens when demands exceed the body's capabilities and you feel jaded and later on, bored. The physical stress can make you more susceptible to injury which takes longer to clear up.

The overtrained martial artist is burnt out and likely to catch any virus going the rounds. Training sessions are approached with a "Here we go again," attitude. Work-rate drops and training in this manner may actually become counter-productive.

Various skills and procedures can be used to keep your training effectiveness up to the optimum mark. One of the best skills is goal setting, a technique taken from business and industry.

Top class martial artists have to be very single-minded to achieve the highest levels of ability. This single-mindedness, the ability to ignore immediate rewards of socialising for the longer term reward of elite performance in competitions or gradings is very rare. That is why so few ever make it to the top.

The path to this long term goal can be smoothed by setting smaller, short term targets along the way. By this means you can keep aware of your progress. Goal setting is also useful because it helps you focus on what you want to achieve and diverts attention away from problems and performance failure.

Goal setting starts with a dream – of mounting the winner's rostrum in a world championships, of becoming the national coach of your association. What you must do is translate the dream into a goal which you feel you can attain. If you are a novice martial artist and fix your sights on becoming a black belt, the effort and expertise needed look as if they will take forever and a day. You look up and see the mountain of effort looming over you and wonder how in the world you are ever going to climb it. By saying to yourself "I will take a series of small steps – steps I can easily manage," you reduce the size of the task to measurable proportions.

Look at your training syllabus and make a plan of how you will tackle each section – even making the plan can improve your motivation.

It doesn't matter that you will have to learn all those complicated techniques to reach black belt because you only need to learn a couple for your next grading. You will gain motivation as you pass each milestone and before you know it, you have crested the mountain and achieved your aim.

If your dream isn't that important to you, then motivation will be lacking and at some stage along the way you will say "That's it, I've got far enough." Sad though it is, this is the natural selection process in action, sieving out those people who aren't committed enough to their goal.

Martial arts are already structured in such a way as to help with the setting of goals and intermediate targets. The grading system provides a built-in series of progressive steps towards the black belt grades. As you become more advanced and gradings are further apart or targets more complex, goal setting becomes ever more important because you may not be aware that you are still progressing.

If you want to set goals effectively, consider the following points.

First of all, set a positive goal. Do not emphasize the negative side of performance – such as "I must stop being tense during basic practice" – because this will merely focus your attention on what it shouldn't be focussed on, leading to increased worry and a worse problem. Secondly, you should state your goals in terms of behaviour which is preferably observable and/or measurable. A clear state-

ment of what you need to do focusses the mind and helps you to see whether you are achieving what you aim for.

Thirdly, goals must be agreed between yourself and your instructor or team coach. If you are personally committed to the goal, then you are likely to work harder for longer to achieve it.

All sorts of goals covering every aspect of performance can be set. The following are a few examples:

- You suffer from a lack of flexibility, so your goal is to spend ten minutes on stretching exercises after each session. Or you decide to increase hip flexibility by three centimetres over the next three months.
- You don't have enough knowledge, so your goal is learn the techniques you require for your grading by the end of the month.
- You lack power, so your goal is to improve your personal best by lifting an additional five kilos in the Power clean weightlifting exercise.
- You lack stamina, so your goal is to be able to spend four two minute rounds on the punchbag, each round including at least 25 hard combination attacks.
- You feel unhappy about free sparring practice so your goal is to practise with at least four higher grades during each training session.
- You want to do better in competition, so your goal is to place in at least two competitions entered in the next twelve months.
- You suffer from nerves during practice, so your goal is to practise relaxation techniques for at least ten minutes each day.

In all the above examples, you have had to identify a crucial weakness in order to define the correct goal to aim for. If you're not sure what your weaknesses are, try and get a reliable third party analysis. Once you have decided what your goal is, next identify the blocks which may hinder you from reaching it. Then set down a plan which identifies the steps needed to achieve your goal.

Short term targets, each consisting of manageable tasks, must be hard enough to stretch you but not impossible. There is no substitute here for a good coach, if only to rationalise any setbacks and put them into perspective. You may be able to do this for yourself but the support and guidance of a coach or more experienced performer is a big advantage for anyone undergoing long term training.

Goal setting need not be quite as structured and formal as outlined here. A structured approach does however leave less to chance and is the most productive way of tackling the job for all except the most experienced coaches. Goal setting is a skill within itself and as with any skill, it takes time and effort from both coach and student if it is to be effective.

How do you deal with overtraining and maintain your enthusiasm? Avoiding boredom seems to be the key. Change schedules regularly and have the odd 'fun' session to stimulate interest and round out training. Training should never degenerate into a social chat but support from a tightly knit group may well help you through a slump and encourage regular attendance by what amounts to social pressure.

Whilst your commitment to the aims and methods of your training is very useful, a coach may still benefit your practice by imposing sessions, practice or ideas, especially when you are worried or uncertain about something – such as forthcoming grading. If you recognise your coach as the authority on your type of training, then in the short term this will take decision pressures off you. In the long term however, you must realise that if you are to mature in martial arts practice, the decisions must be made by you. Always be prepared though, to consider the advice of your coach or more senior grade.

You will find that as you train over the long term, you will experience 'plateaus', when you don't seem to be making much progress towards your next target. Some think this problem is entirely mental and resort to tricks to overcome it. A weight lifter may get stuck at a certain weight which becomes built into a barrier. The coach or colleagues may swap the weights for slightly heavier ones without the lifter realising it until after the lift has been successful. This certainly does work in a restricted number of cases.

It is simpler and perhaps more effective to drop the problem exercise and switch to another, returning later on to the original. Often the previous block is removed by this method. Alternatively you may have to re-assess the situation and set new targets which by-pass the blockage or use a more gradual progression. This obviously cannot happen all the time but occasionally target reassessment will avoid a localised blockage degenerating into a major problem blighting overall progress. In fact

Opposite: *The martial arts grading syllabus provides accessible goals and maintains motivation*

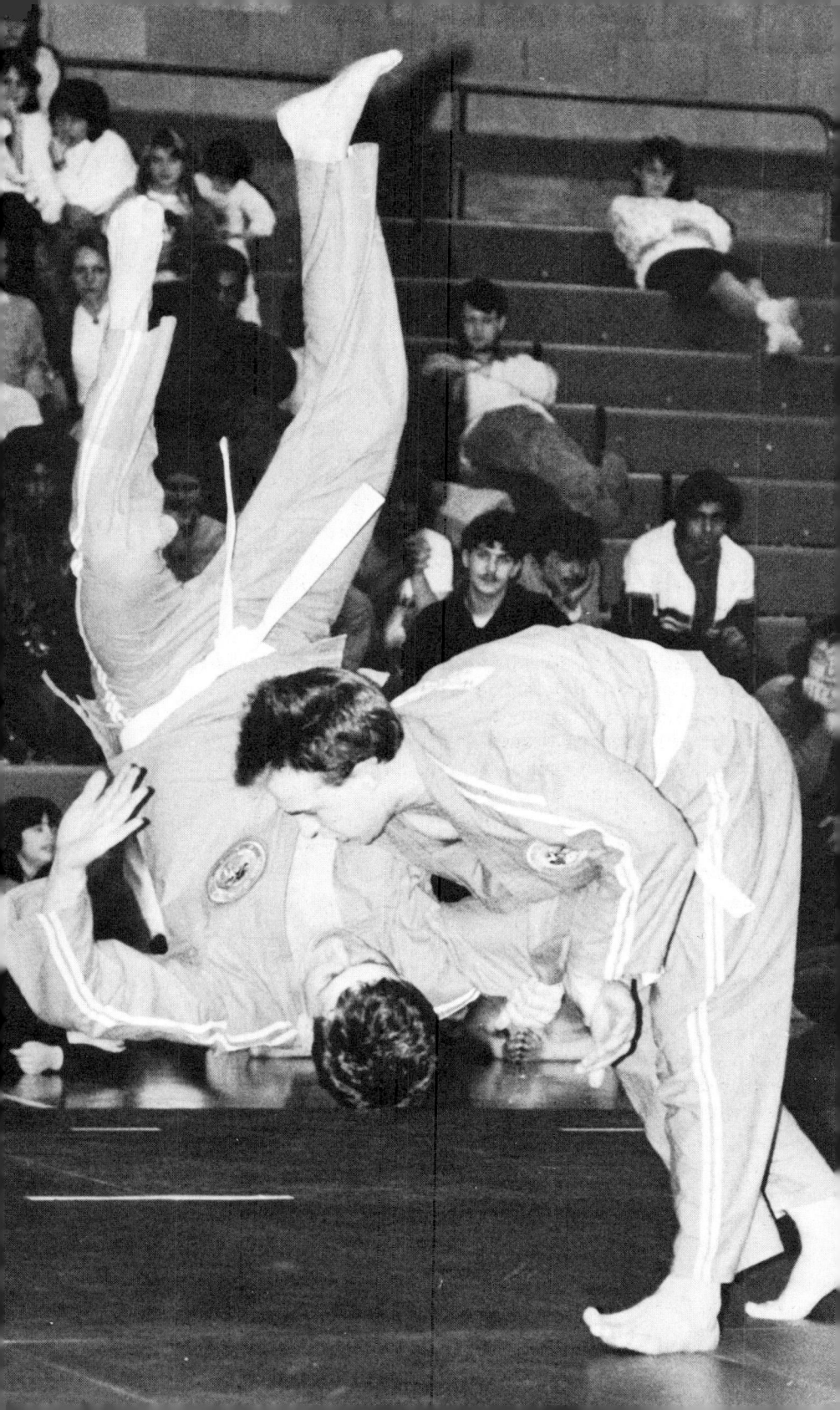

small problems often grow out of all proportion and this is where the rationalisation of a coach or senior grade can help.

If you are properly prepared, you should go in for a grading or competition feeling on top form. Nerves may affect you but overall, you feel like you could demolish a house. Hard training should therefore be seen as a confidence builder as well as a means of physical preparation. Martial artists should come to feel that their preparation has been thorough and certainly better than anyone else's. Believing that your training has been beneficial can have a measurable effect on your performance.

As you approach the grading or competition, you taper off the training load. This may be difficult to accept but you must ensure your fitness is kept for the event and not left on the training floor. Your preparation will be helped by training drills which increasingly reproduce the demands of the event. This is true both for mental and physical fitness, helping you to come to terms with the demands of the event. This is important if needless pre-event anxieties are to be avoided.

Sometimes martial artists develop a liking for one particular aspect of training. This is fine until performance in that type of training eclipses performance in the overall activity itself. If you enjoy weight training and spend more and more time on it, then the physical factors needed for your development in martial art may move out of balance. You may find you prefer sparring and concentrate on doing well in it to the exclusion of all other aspects of your martial art. Again, if you do this, your martial art practice will become unbalanced.

To summarise some points on the mental approach to fitness:

- Training must be realistic and you must accept that you are capable of the work demands and that the training will actually help you to achieve your aims.
- Training must be progressive, stretching your limits but keeping to attainable targets.
- Training must be varied to maintain interest but practice of the same drills must be maintained long enough to develop the optimal fitness factors required.
- Training progress must be monitored to show improvement and provide feedback.

To help you identify goals, here are some questions to help you visualise the situation.

A. What is it you want to achieve? Is it something you'd like to be better at, or something you'd like to change?

B. Why do you want to achieve it now?

C. State what you want to achieve:
    –Is what you want to achieve positive?
    –Do you know what you need to achieve it?
    –Can you achieve it with those factors under your control?

D. What will it take to achieve this?

E. How long have you wanted to achieve this?

F. What have you been doing (if anything) to achieve it?

G. Did you ever get near to achieving it? If yes, describe how you managed to do it.

H. Have you ever missed achieving it? If yes, describe what caused your failure.

I. How did you feel and what did you think when you nearly reached your goal and when you were furthest from it?

J. Why do you think you failed to achieve it?

K. What do you think you must actually do, in terms of knowledge application and technique, to achieve it?

–What extra things do you need to know?
–What additional skills do you need to learn?
–What risks do you have to take?
–What social support do you need?
–What fitness improvements do you need to make?

L. Restate the goal within the above criteria and make up a plan listing each step to be taken.

Planning your Training Programme

In many books dealing with Exercise Physiology, you will find a section called 'Principles of Training'. This sets out the principles to be considered if a training programme is going to be successful. Those principles listed below apply to suitable training for all the components of physical fitness, except for body composition.

Regularity

As a serious martial artist you will know that regular training is essential. Yet many practitioners fail to make the progress they are capable of because they miss too many training sessions. Sometimes they blame the training programme for their lack of progress but it is usually the discipline of the martial artist that is at fault. If you keep a regular training diary, as indeed you should, this may well show where the fault lies.

Training must be regular.

Overload

To improve performance, you must overload the tissues of your body during training. The demands which training places upon the heart, lungs, muscles, ligaments and tendons etc, must exceed those you require for normal daily life or this improvement will not take place. Some people argue that in preparation for gradings or competition, intensity of training should exceed that expected in the grading or competition itself. If this is not the case, then the martial artist may get injured through being insufficiently fit for that grading or competition.

Training must overload.

Progression

Excessive or early overloading may cause injury, so any training programme must be progressive. Novices must realise that body tissues need weeks and months to adapt to training requirements. Therefore you must carefully plan a progressive programme and as improvement is seen and felt, continuously revise your programme and set new goals.

Training must be progressive.

Specificity

It is obvious that a flexibility programme is not intended to improve aerobic endurance. If you want to improve that particular aspect of fitness, then you must select the appropriate type of training. Specificity actually goes much further than this and suggests that it is better to train the muscles in the same way they will be used during a grading or competition. However, because of the need to overload, this may not always prove possible. Therefore select those activities which will bring about the desired improvements, without putting you at risk through injury.

Training must be specific.

Reversibility

What happens when you lay off training for a couple of weeks because of injury? Your fitness declines and this can actually be shown by means of a fitness assessment. Also, if you concentrate totally on developing your speed, your aerobic fitness level may decline. Fitness is not permanent and once you have reached a certain level, you must work to maintain it. If you reduce your training, your fitness will decline.

Training must be part of your life style.

Rest

Hard training sessions should be followed by lighter sessions, or by a complete rest. Body tissues must be given time to recover and regenerate. If you over-stress yourself with too much hard training and too little rest, you will run the risk of injury. Fit martial artists may be able to string together a number of days of hard training but these should always be followed by days of lighter training or rest.

Rest is *just as important* as training.

Warming Up

During martial art training, your body has to work harder than it does during the day. Therefore it is a good idea to gradually prepare your body for the demands that training will place upon it by a procedure known as 'warming up'. A proper warm up will reduce the risk of injury, especially where explosive movements are used and it can even assist your performance in a grading or competition.

The whole idea of warm up is to raise the body's activity level so the muscles contract more powerfully and stretch more effectively, thus allowing a greater range of movement at a joint. The heart and respiration rates are gradually increased in such a way as to minimise discomfort.

Do a thorough job of warming up so the whole body benefits. Try to develop a good sweat by working hard within your limits but don't overdo it, or you won't have enough energy left to launch flat-out into the grading or competition. Warm up at the right time, so there is no delay between the end of warm up and the beginning of competition.

Try to use exercises which are directly related to the techniques you will use in the competition or grading.

Training for Muscular Fitness

As with general fitness, muscular fitness consists of a number of factors which must be balanced according to the demands of your martial art. Let's begin by defining a few terms we will use.

'Endurance' is the ability of a muscle to work repeatedly. 'Strength' is the ability of a muscle to move once against great resistance. 'Power' is the ability of a muscle to move quickly against a resistance.

Many armchair experts consider that strength training can only be done at the expense of speed and flexibility. This view is not one shared by sprinters for example, who are not the slowest movers, yet who do use weight training as part of their training programme. In fact there is more disagreement between 'experts' in this field than in any other. When trying to find your way through the maze of contradiction, get the various experts to justify their opinions and then evaluate them. There may be no single correct answer but once you have the options available, you may be able to find out which one works best for you.

There are many different forms of muscle fitness training, some involving quite complex apparatus or regimes. For our purposes, we can consider the following:

Isometric

This means 'same length' and whilst the muscle is contracted, the limb it acts upon does not move. If you put the palms of your hands together and push inwards with each, you are working isometrically. During weight training, you may eventually reach the point where the weight you want to lift is simply too heavy. You heave and strain, your muscles bulge but the weight doesn't move. This is isometric work. Expressed another way, isometric contraction occurs when the force generated by the muscles is equal to or less than the load on them.

Isometric training is good for building static strength such as that needed to hold a particular low stance, but it is otherwise fairly limited. A disadvantage of isometric training is that it raises blood pressure and this can make for problems with the older or more unfit martial artist.

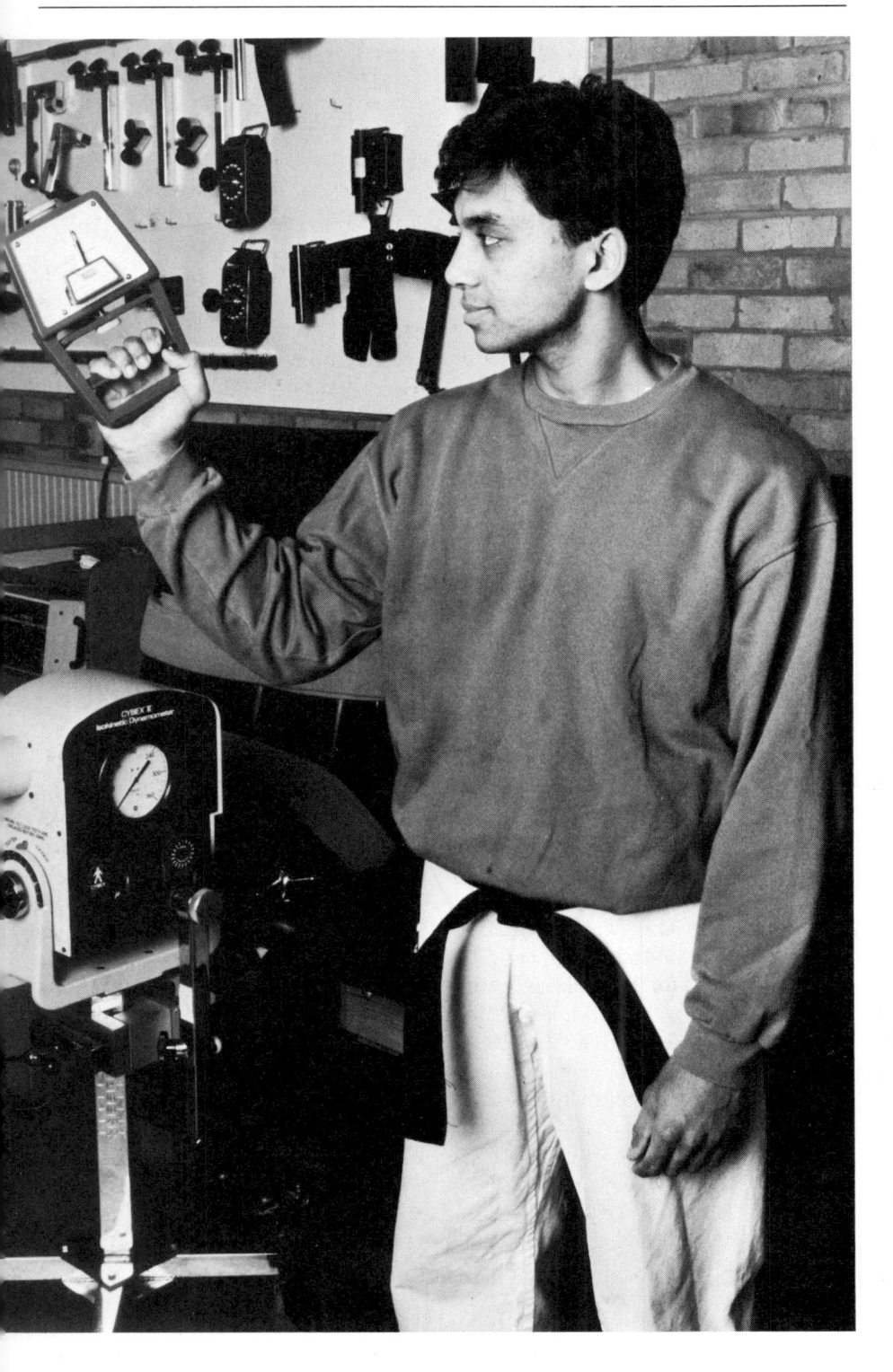

Testing the strength of your grip against a powerful spring connected to a moving pointer

Isotonic

Isotonic means 'same tone' and during isotonic training, the muscles move against a set resistance. It is the most common and simplest form of muscle fitness training. Press-ups, weight training, working on simple Multigym machines and repetitious technique work are all examples of isotonic training.

To increase strength, you must increase the resistance against which you are moving. When you walk upstairs carrying a heavy suitcase, you are using an isotonic training method because you are working your muscles against a load greater than normal body weight.

Expressed another way, isotonic contraction occurs when the force generated by muscles is greater than the load on them. It's not quite that simple though. As load increases, you may find yourself cheating by cutting down on the range of movement. When a class is doing press-ups for example, as the number of repetitions increases, so the exercise deteriorates into a short bobbing motion of the shoulders, depth of movement being gradually lost. This will eventually result in little or no training benefit. It will be no good, for example, in training to do techniques which need a fully extended arm – such as punching.

Another drawback occurs when using weights to increase resistance. You may decide to increase the strength of your technique by gripping a 20 kilo dumb-bell as you punch but this could tend to make you fall over as a result of the considerable momentum generated by the moving weight. If you do alter the technique to accommodate momentum, it will no longer match the movement you are trying to strengthen.

Ingenuity and thought is required to match suitable exercises to martial art techniques and some will require two or three different exercises to cater for all the muscles involved.

Olympic lifting movements require a lot of power and are ideal for general muscle fitness.

The *clean* is a fast lift of a bar-bell from the ground to the shoulders. The *jerk* is a fast lift from the shoulders to above the head and the *snatch* takes the bar from the floor directly above the head, without a deep squat. The *curl* takes the bar from in front of the thighs to just below the chin. The *dead lift* involves bending forward and raising the bar, returning the body to an upright position with arms hanging. The *good morning* places the bar across the back of the neck as you bend forwards. *Bench press* requires you to lie on your back and push the bar upwards.

To be effective in the martial arts, you need to perform fast strengthening exercises through the full range of joint movement and for this, hand held dumb-bells may be a better choice than work with the bar-bell. If you stick to the right sort of training, you will become faster and stronger but if you decide to go for the macho image and pump really heavy weights through limited range movements, you won't be much good for the martial arts though you may well be able to bust open cans of spinach with your bare hands!

Strength/power/endurance development is a matter of repetitions, loading and recovery time. Beginners need to complete a certain amount of strength work before they can go on to high quality power schedules, or endurance work to the point of exhaustion. So to start off, do three sets of ten repetitions. Develop this to

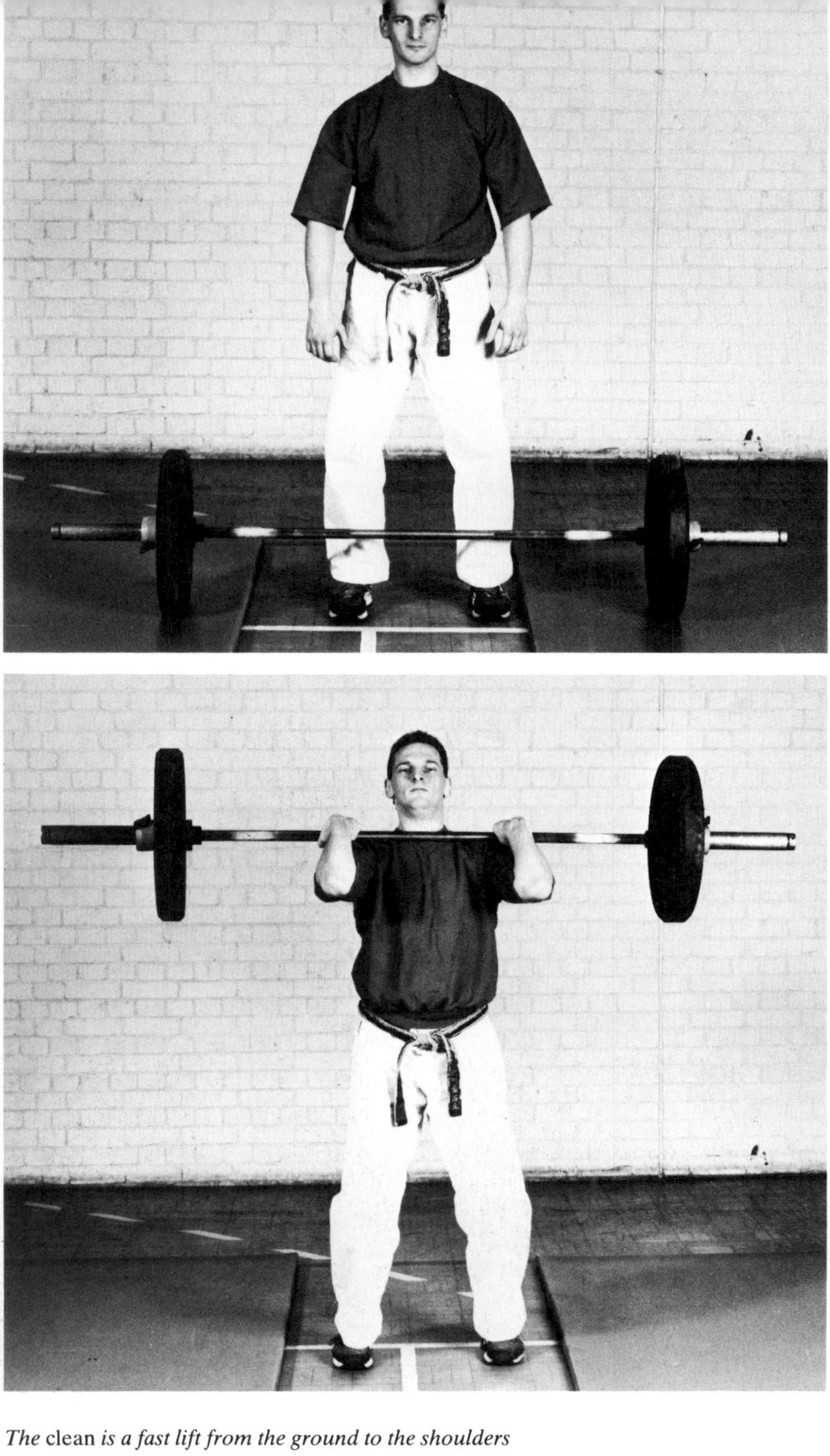

The clean *is a fast lift from the ground to the shoulders*

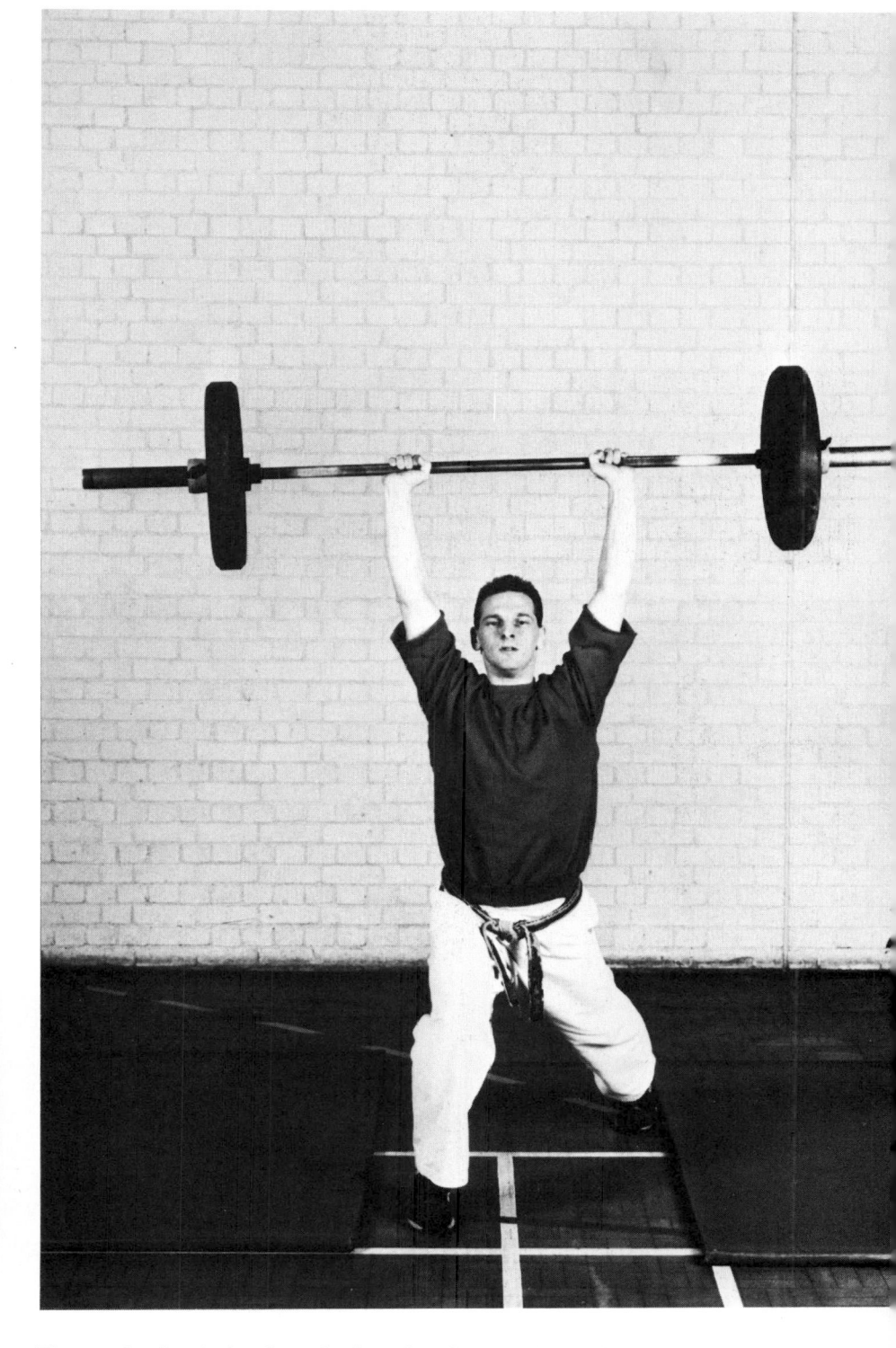

The snatch *takes the bar from the floor directly above the head*

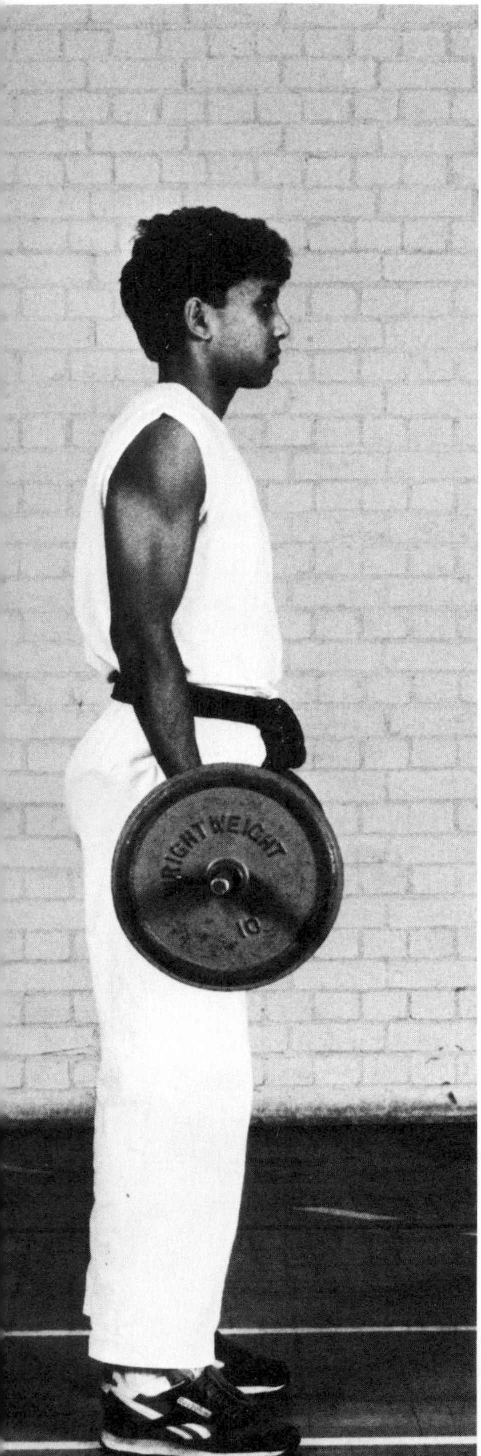
WRIGHTWEIGHT
10

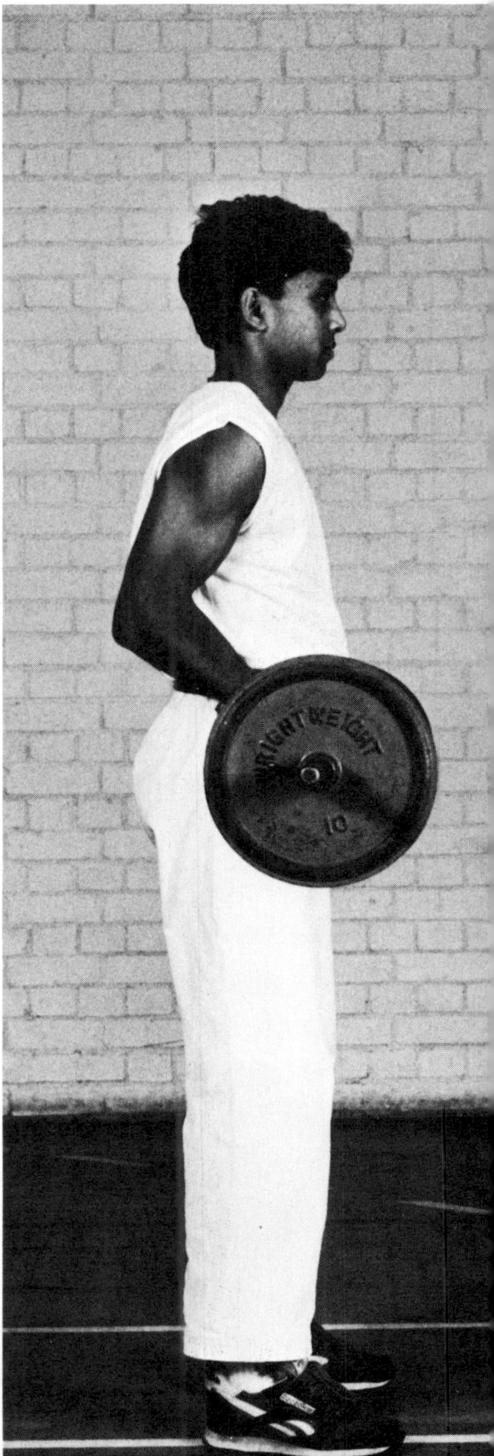
WRIGHTWEIGHT
10

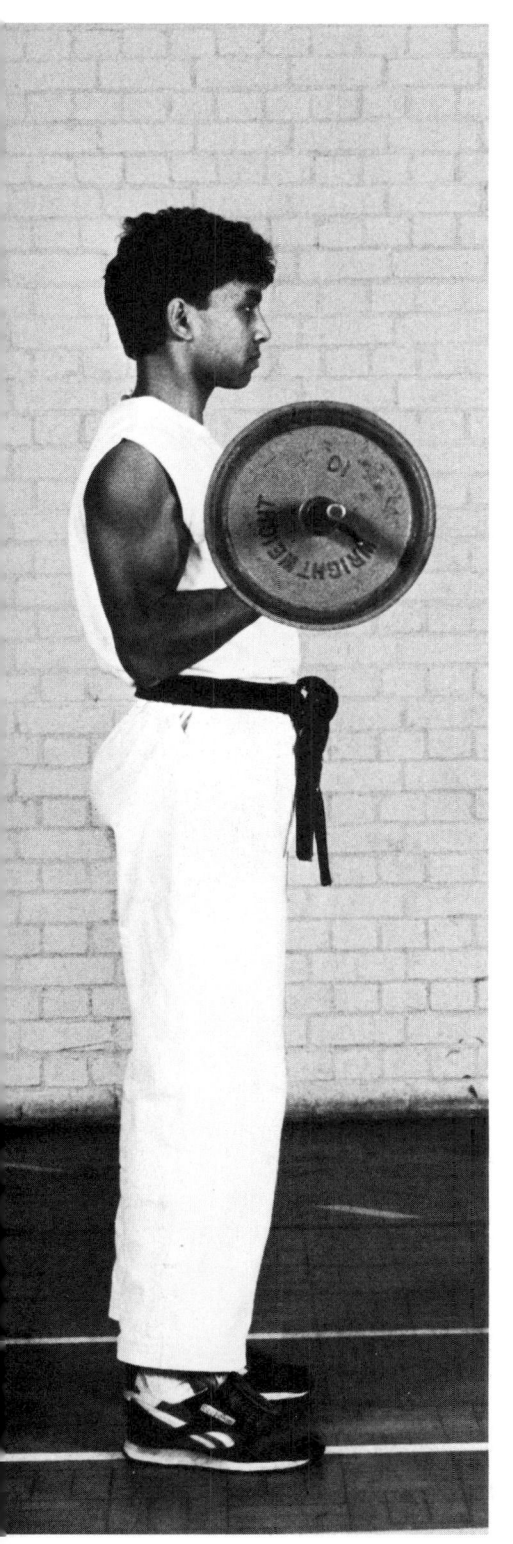

The curl *takes the bar from in front of the thighs to below the chin*

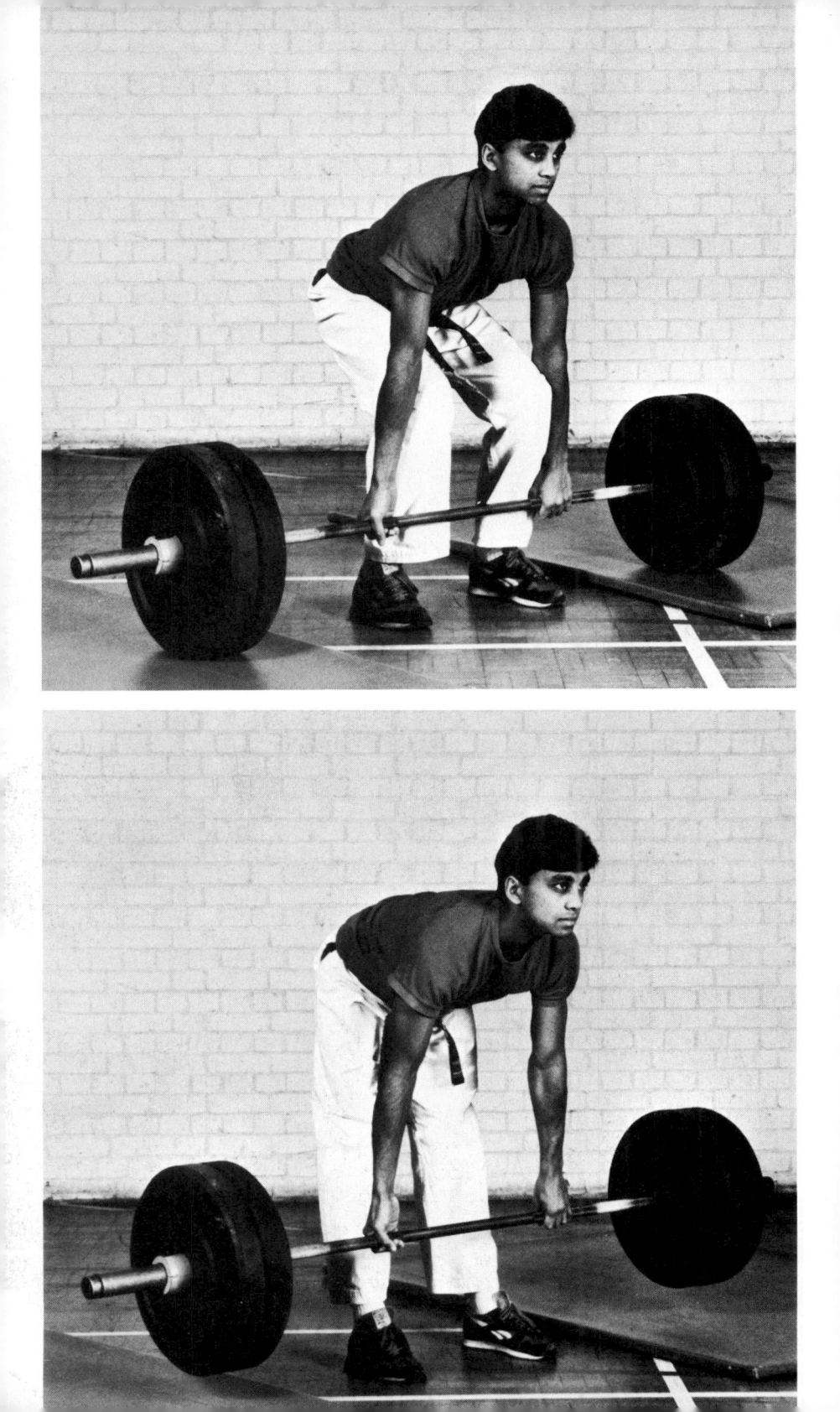

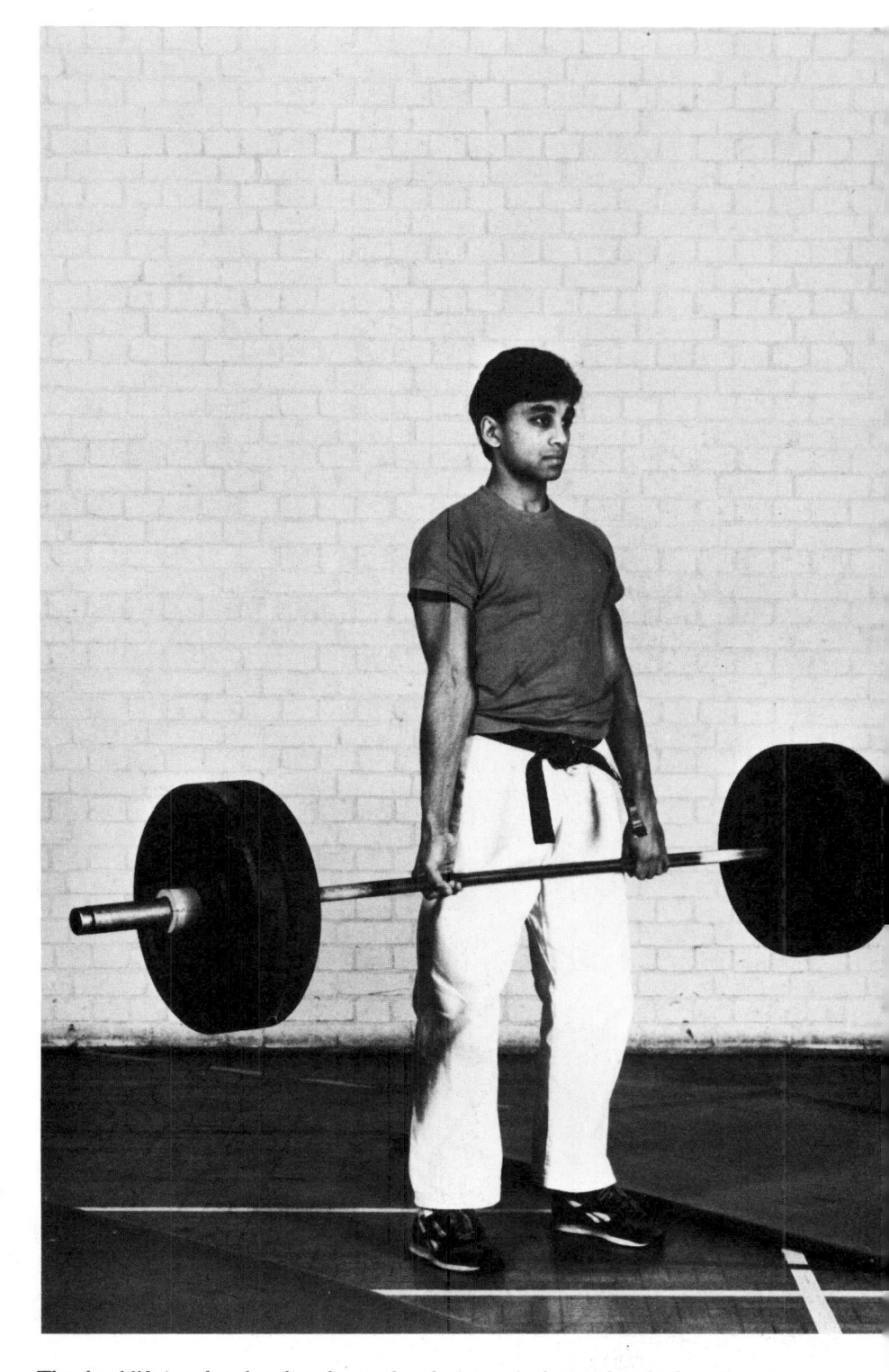

The dead lift *involves bending forward and raising the bar with arms hanging*

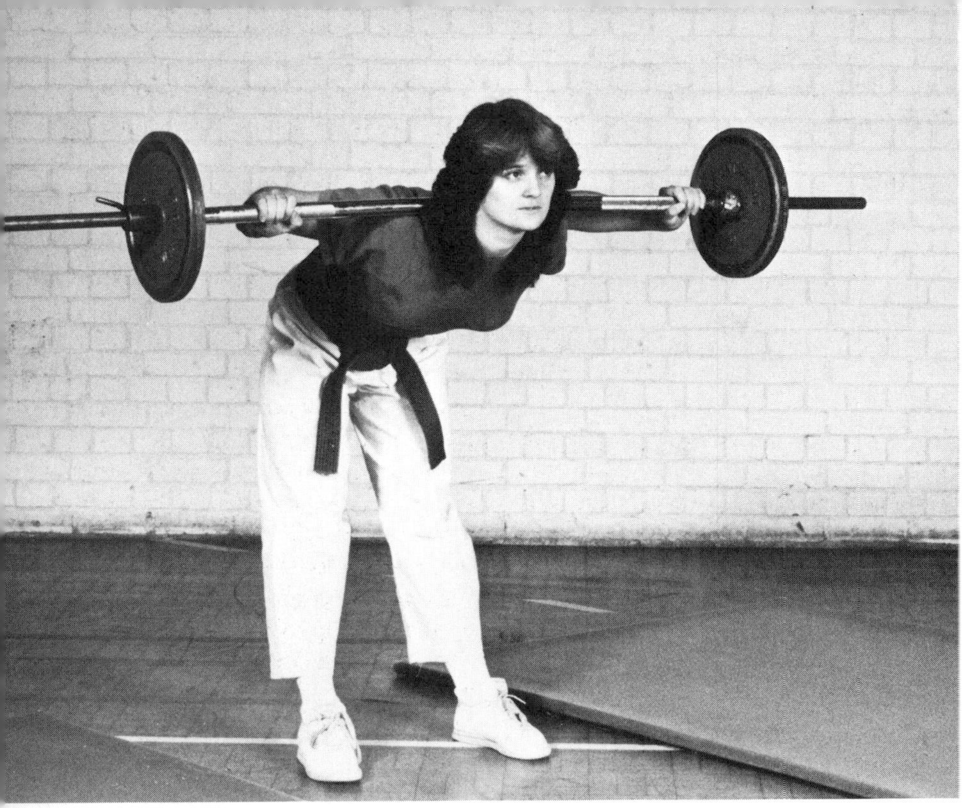

The good morning *places the bar across the back of the neck as you lean forward*

Bench press *requires you to lie on your back and push the weight upwards*

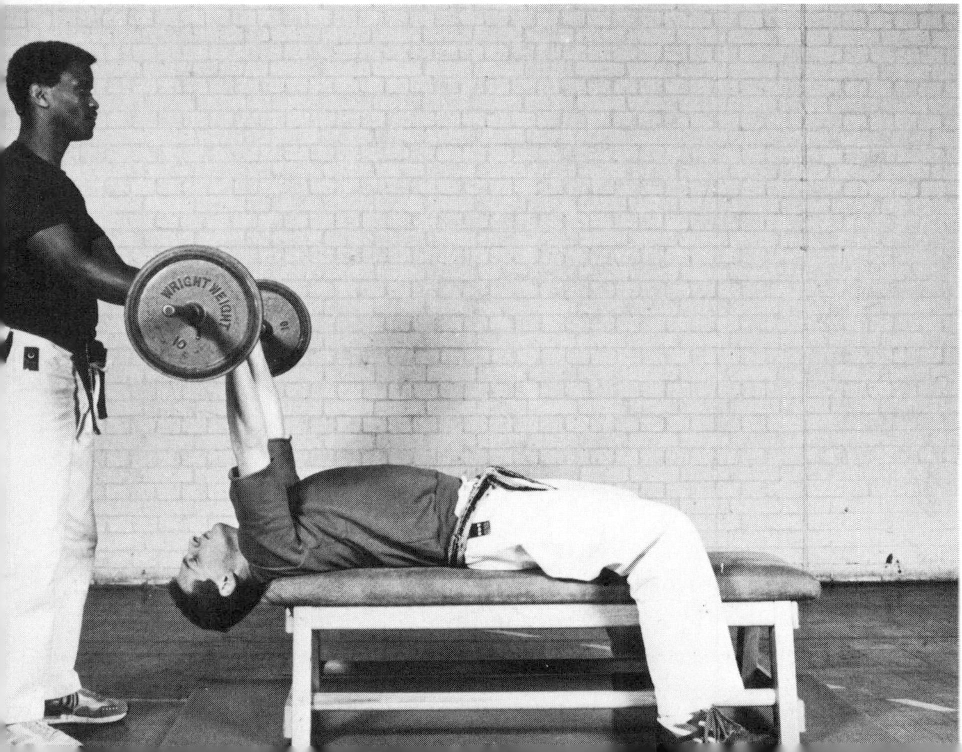

four or five sets of reducing repetitions going from ten-eight-four-two in what is called a 'pyramid'.

Base endurance work on moving the bar between two fixed points over a set period of time to prevent cheating. Power work can be based on squat jumps over an obstacle or alternatively, by slow lowering into squat position followed by explosive rapid extension. When doing the latter, get your partner to call off an irregular count. This will stop you from anticipating the extension. It also makes for harder work and develops concentration whilst tired.

Make sure your knee joints are capable of withstanding this type of exercise and if there is any doubt at all, use a half-squat instead.

Isokinetic

This means simply 'same speed' and refers to a form of training where resistance to muscle action can be set to increase the faster your muscles act. Expressed another way, isokinetic contractions occur when the force generated by muscles is just greater than the load applied throughout the range of movement. Isokinetic training has received a great deal of attention recently and equipment such as swim benches, certain kinds of weight units and the Cybex assessment/ rehabilitation apparatus are all examples of this mode of training.

Most of the apparatus required is expensive and suitable only for higher level performance. An exception is the cannibalised swim bench which provides a cheaper alternative. Using isokinetic equipment, you can get very close to replicating the movements of martial art training. The lack of momentum problems (if you stop moving, the resistance disappears) makes isokinetic training particularly good for rehabilitation. Another advantage is the way in which resistance varies at different parts of the

This output from a Cybex Isokinetic unit shows that the muscle is strongest in the middle of the movement. On this graph the higher the curve the greater the force. Notice also that the muscles are stronger for extension than flexion

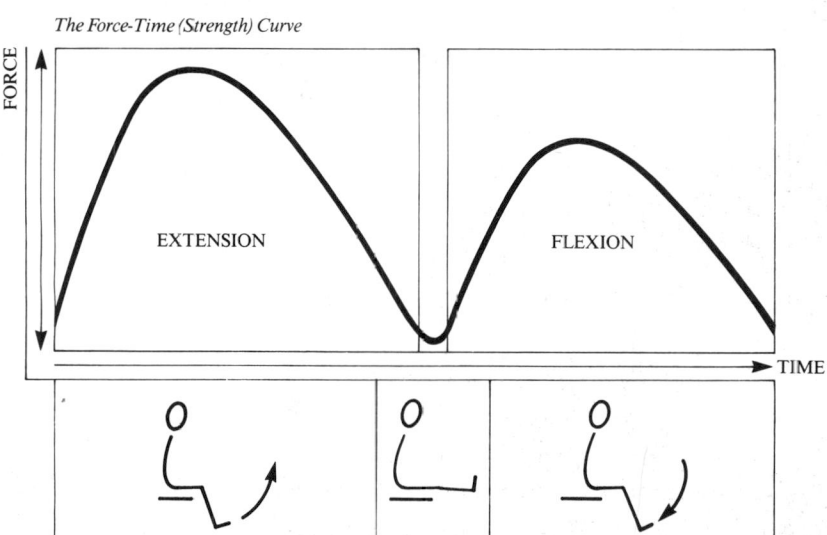

The Force-Time (Strength) Curve

movement to match the muscle's natural capabilities. Compare this with an isotonic exercise such as the two-handed curl.

Since muscles exert their maximum effective strength in the middle of their range of movement, then you must either get someone to assist you during the first part of the curl, or you have to settle for curling a weight less than your arm muscles can handle at their strongest mid way position. The first option requires a cooperative and knowledgeable partner and the second limits the effectiveness of the exercise because the muscles are not

Isokinetic training ensures that the muscle is always working to its maximum

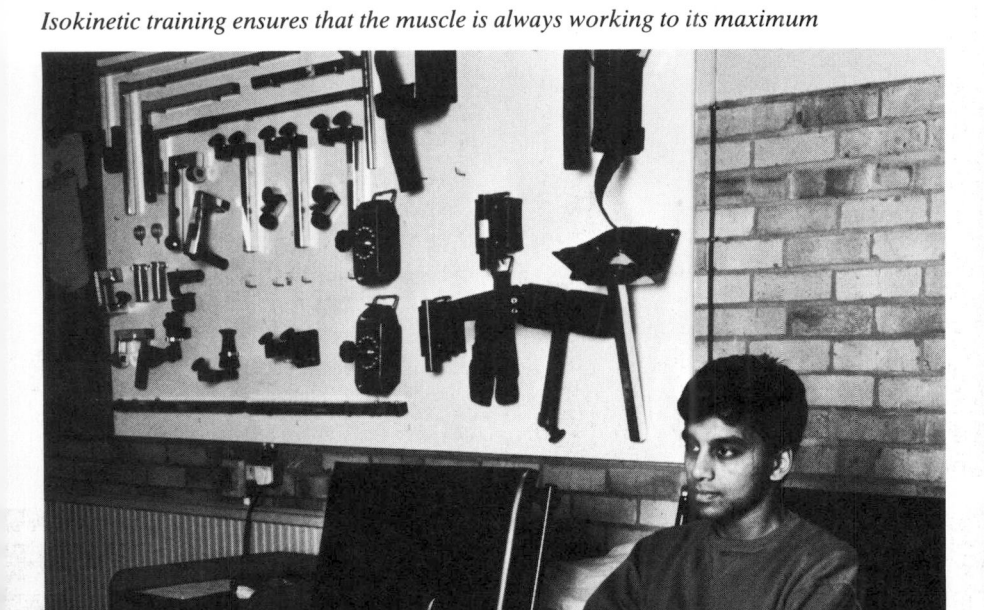

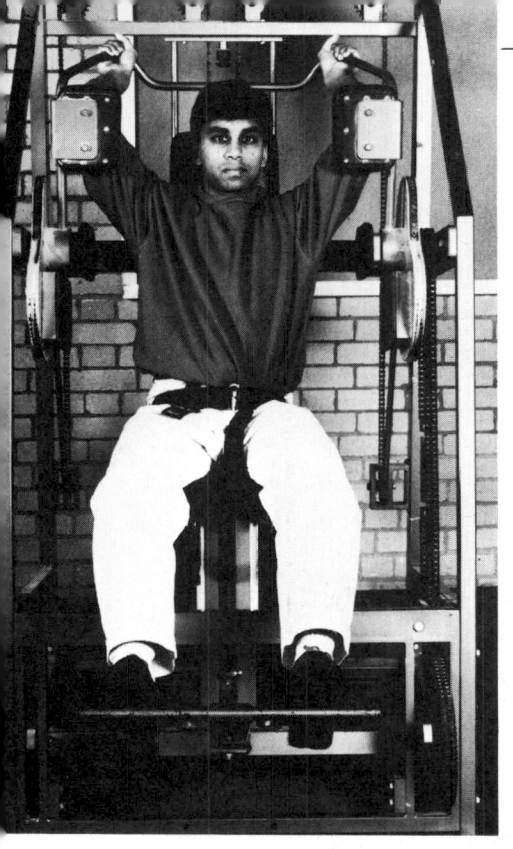

working as hard as they might be during a part of the full movement.

By comparison, isokinetic equipment ensures that the muscle is always working to its maximum, assuming of course that you don't cheat. The crucial decision you have to make is what speed setting to use. Low speeds produce greater strength gains and higher ones are more suitable for power and endurance work.

Dynamic Variable Resistance

A number of strength training equipment manufacturers have tried to cope with the strength/position variations inherent in muscle action by

Manufacturers of strength training equipment use the lever principle to keep the muscle working to its maximum

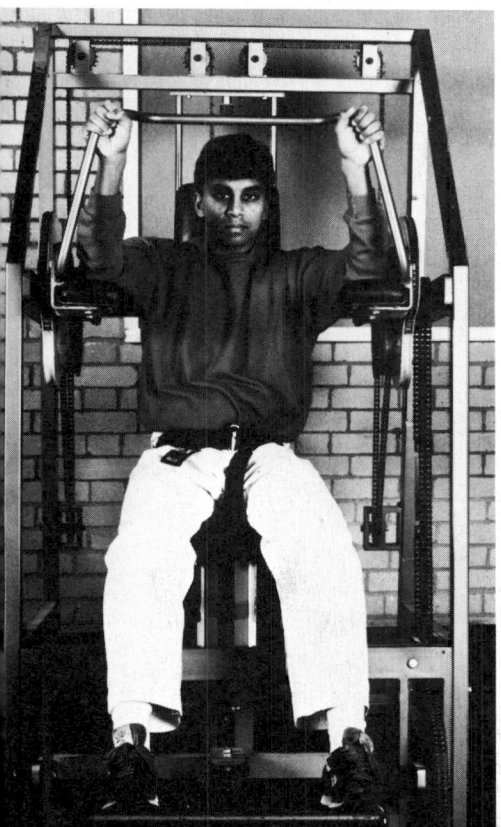

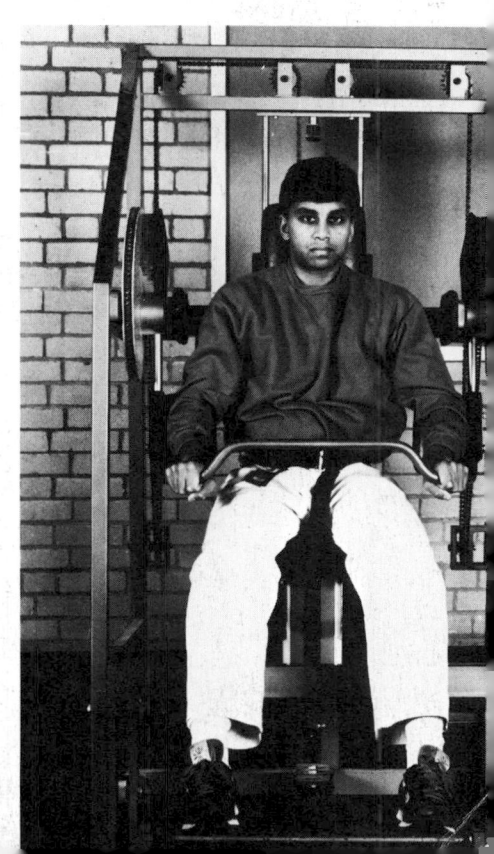

The D.V.R. Bench Press

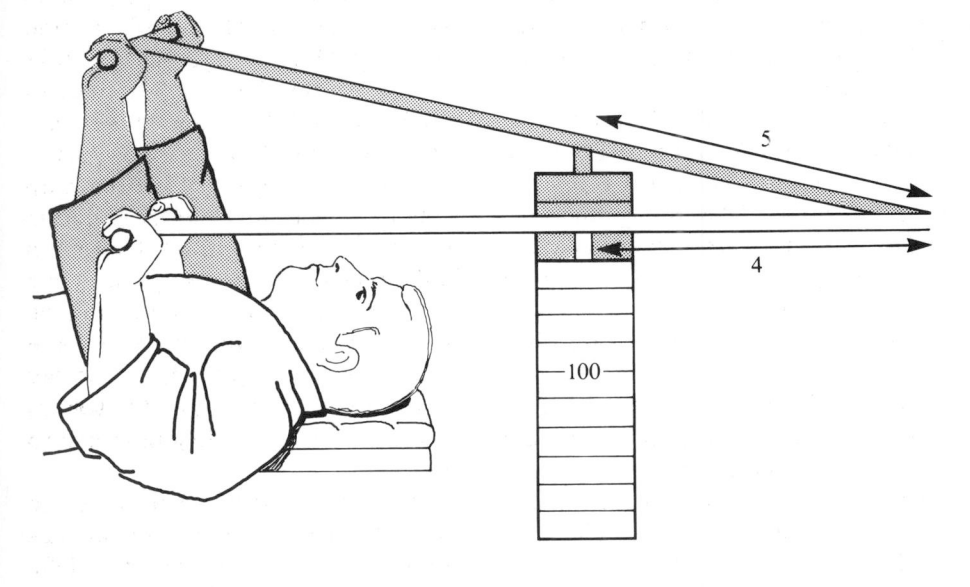

The load increases as the weight is raised because the distance from the weight to the
fulcrum is increased
i.e. at the bottom: load=100×4=400
    at the top: load=100×5=500

The 'Nautilus' Cam

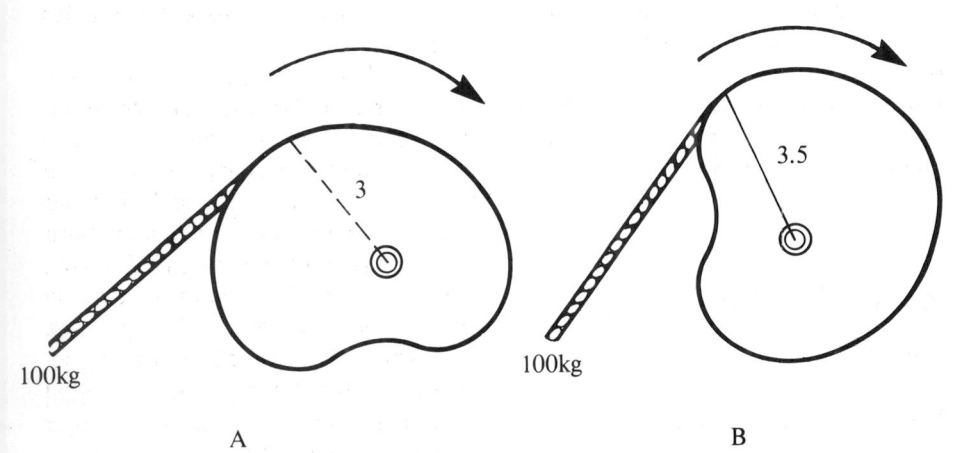

A   B

Note how the load is increased by changing the distance from the fulcrum (where the cam
is fixed) to the chain
i.e. in A load=100×3=300
    in B load=100×3.5=350

varying resistance in different parts of the movement. Their ideas are mainly based on the lever principle, where the loading equals weight times distance from the fulcrum.

When the martial artist holds a barbell in an extended position it will feel heavy because distance between the weight and the fulcrum is greater. The diagrams show how this principle is applied in the straight lever and cam-type machines.

Though these machines are effective in working your muscles more thoroughly, they are very expensive and take up a lot of space in the training hall. Also their load variation mechanisms are set to average values so unless you have them tailored to suit your own particular capabilities, they will always be a compromise. Even when all else is right, there remains the problem of matching the exercises for which they are suitable to the martial art techniques you want to strengthen.

Some trainers and coaches maintain that these machines are the best option available since they require less tuition and supervision than free weight training. However, little tuition means less return from training since mistakes will undoubtedly be made and remain uncorrected.

Body Weight Exercises

Body weight exercises can be manipulated to produce effective alternatives to weight training. Repetition of the exercise keyed to a count can be used to develop speed of movement. Certain exercises, such as switching quickly from left to right fighting stance, are good for developing endurance and incorporate a useful degree of agility. Hourglass jumps and split jumps – moving from a left forward to a right forward stance and return – are also good agility/endurance builders.

Patter stepping is a good warm-up exercise which develops both endurance and explosive power. Get into a half squat with your body erect and run on the spot whilst maintaining the posture. On the count, or in response to a visual signal, jump high into the air and resume running on the spot as soon as you land. 20/30 jumps make a set.

There are several alternatives to these. You can make repeated attacks from stance to the count, whilst moving forwards or backwards. You can also do single leg squats using a partner to help you keep balance, or explosive step-ups in which the steps are made by one leg. Both of the previous pair of exercises have a high power demand. Sprint starts from various positions and from blocks make for fast reactions and powerful legs.

Hard body weight exercises may need a particular approach to avoid having trouble with them. A good exercise in this category for the novice is termed *dips*. In this, you hold yourself up, arms extended and both hands gripping a pair of parallel bars. Lower your body weight forwards, so there is a good range of movement and your elbows flex. Work explosively on the effort phase and when you can't do any more, cheat by either getting a partner to help you lift, by lowering yourself back down slowly to a count of four before springing up, or by using the support of a platform to take some of the weight.

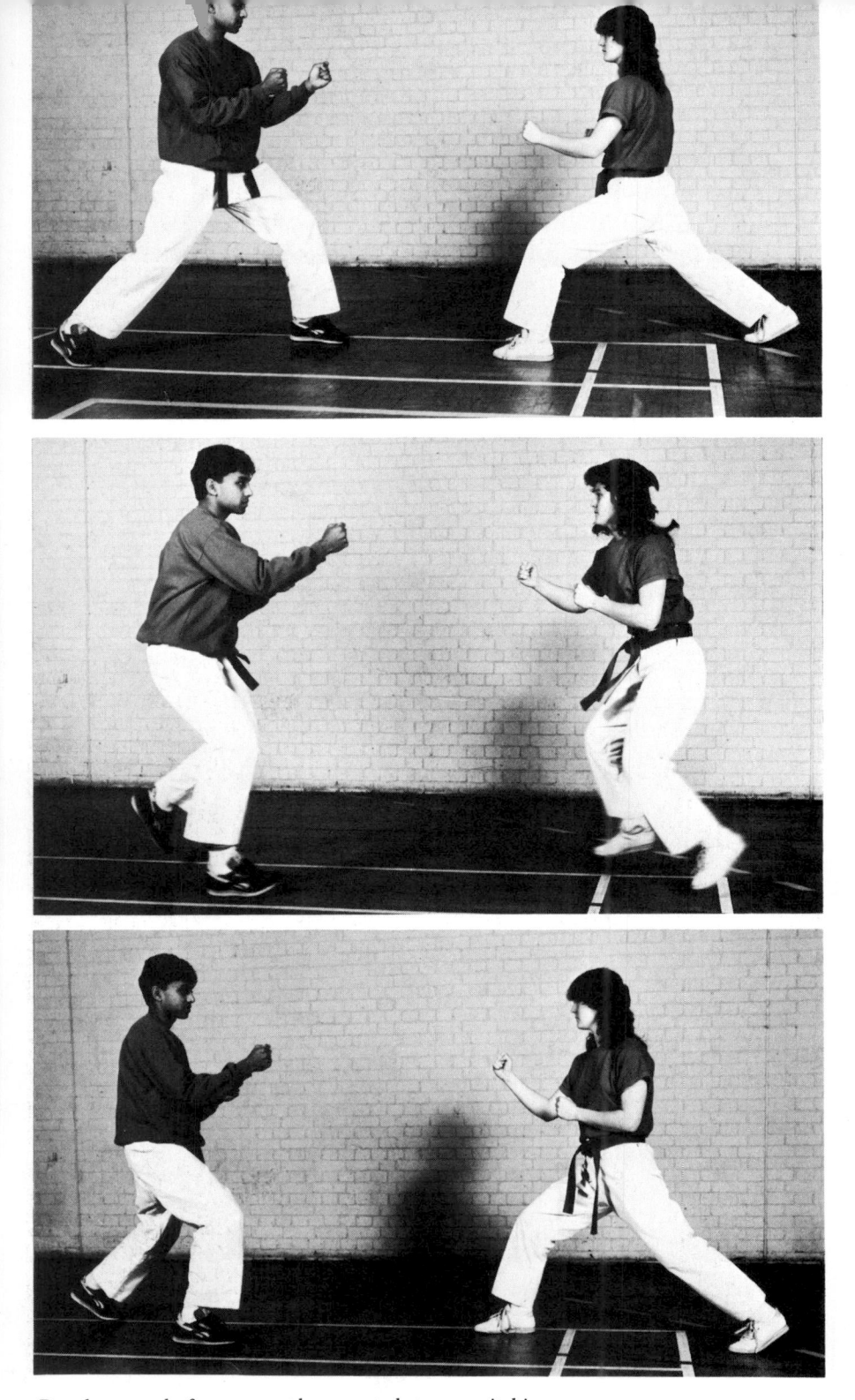

Develop speed of movement by repeated stance switching…

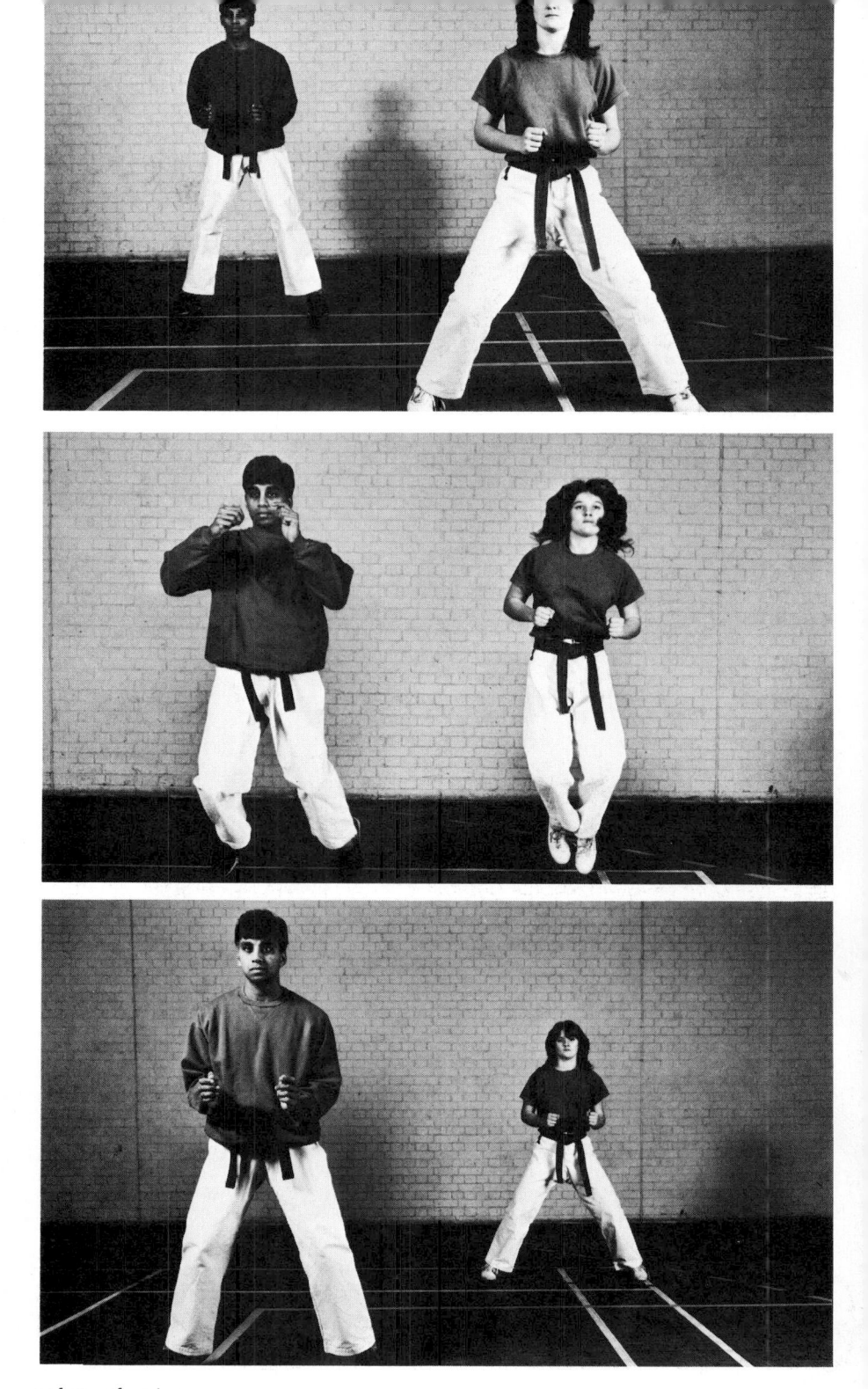

or hour glass jumps

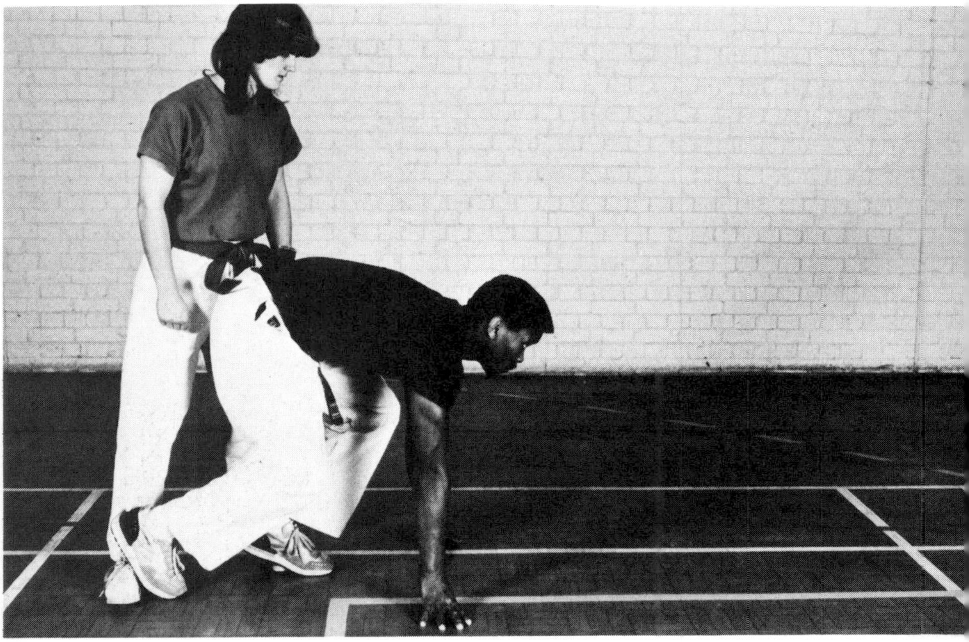

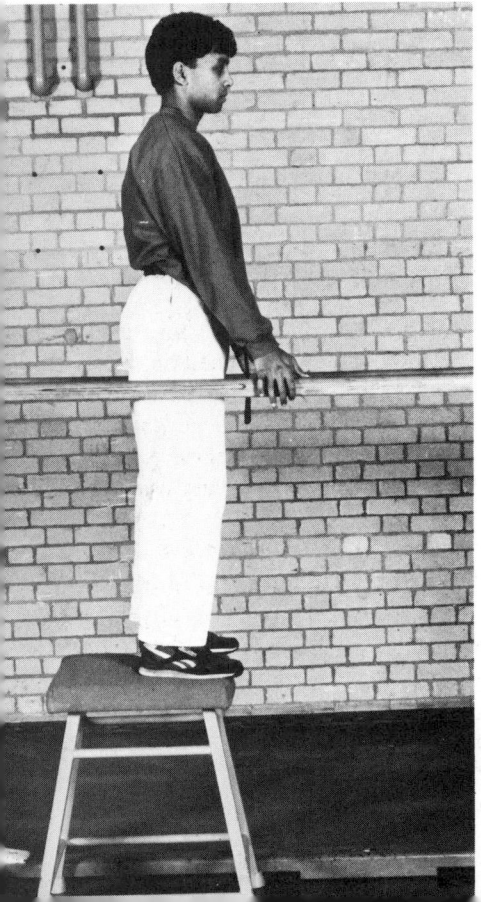
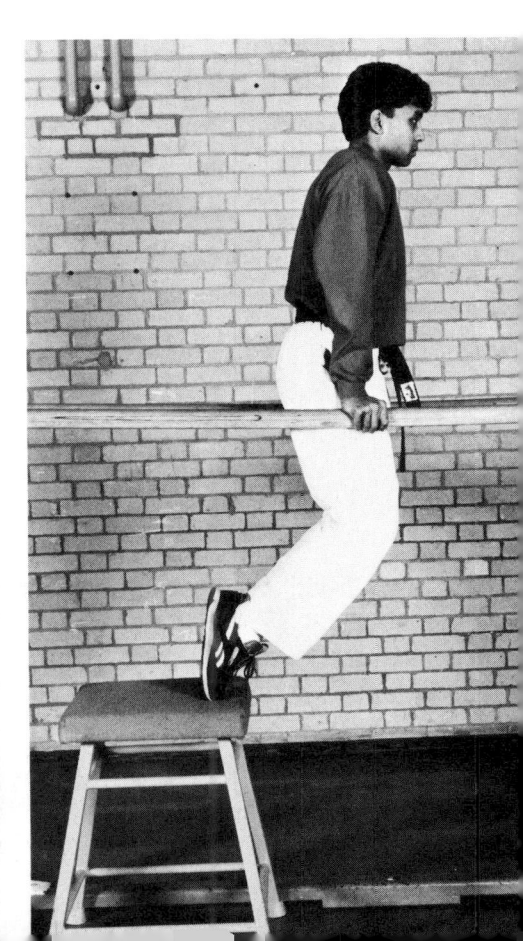

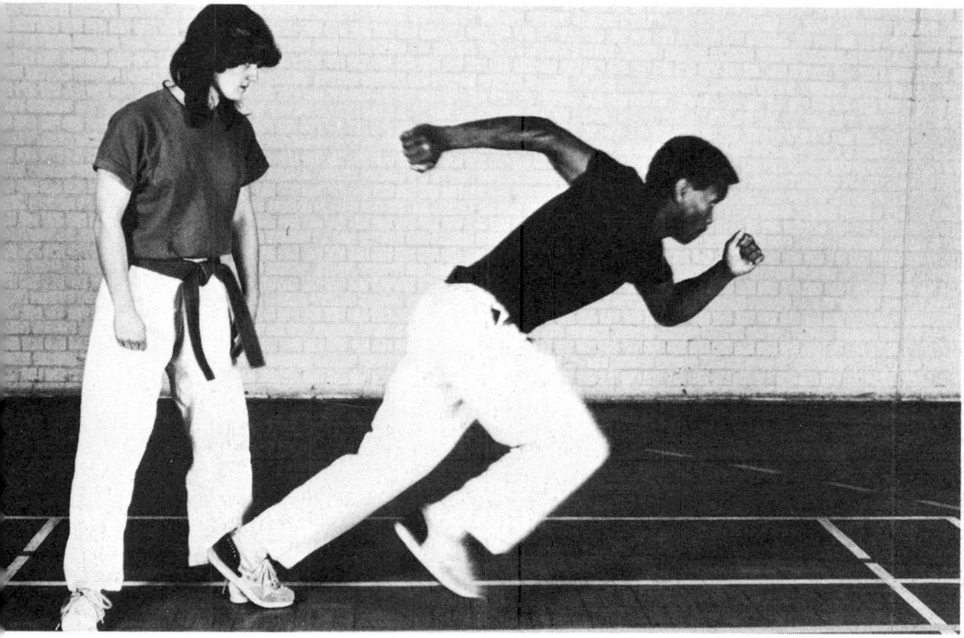

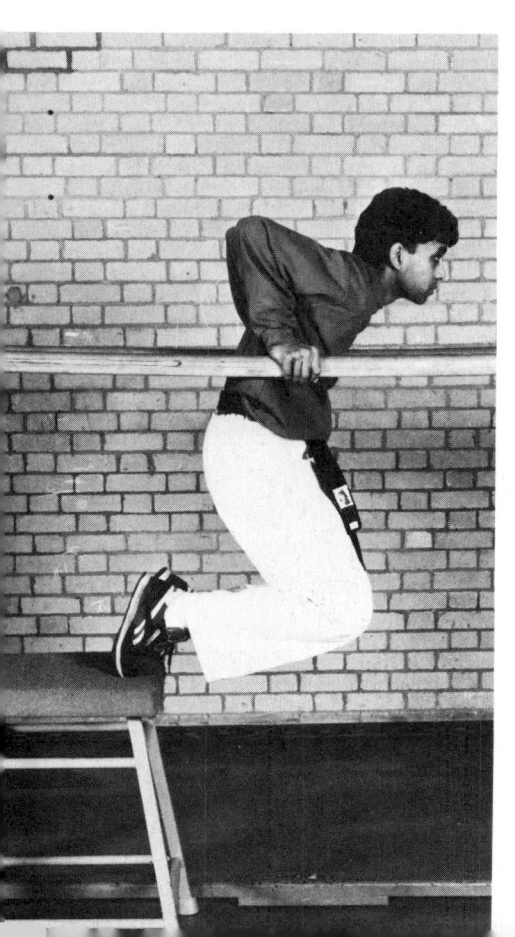

Above: *Sprint starts make for powerful legs*

Left: Dips *are a hard body weight exercise*

Plyometrics

Another alternative to using weights is *plyometrics*. This is used currently in track and field athletic training and is the subject of several recent books and articles. Its applicability to martial art training is at a very early stage of assessment, so you must experiment to find the regime best suited to the requirements of your martial art.

The underlying theory of plyometrics rests on the premise that when a muscle is pre-stretched immediately prior to a movement, it is primed or loaded with energy, making the subsequent muscle action more effective.

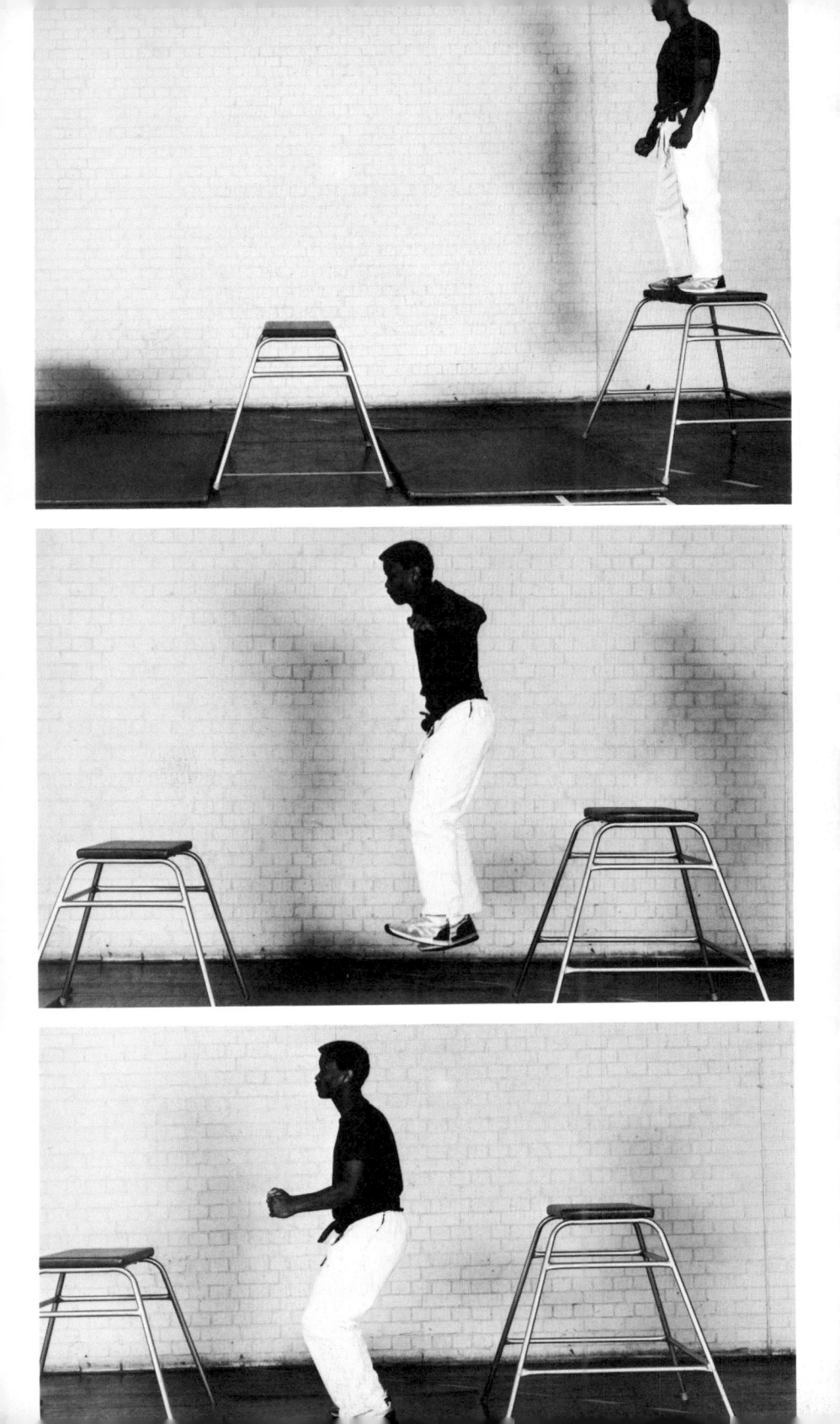

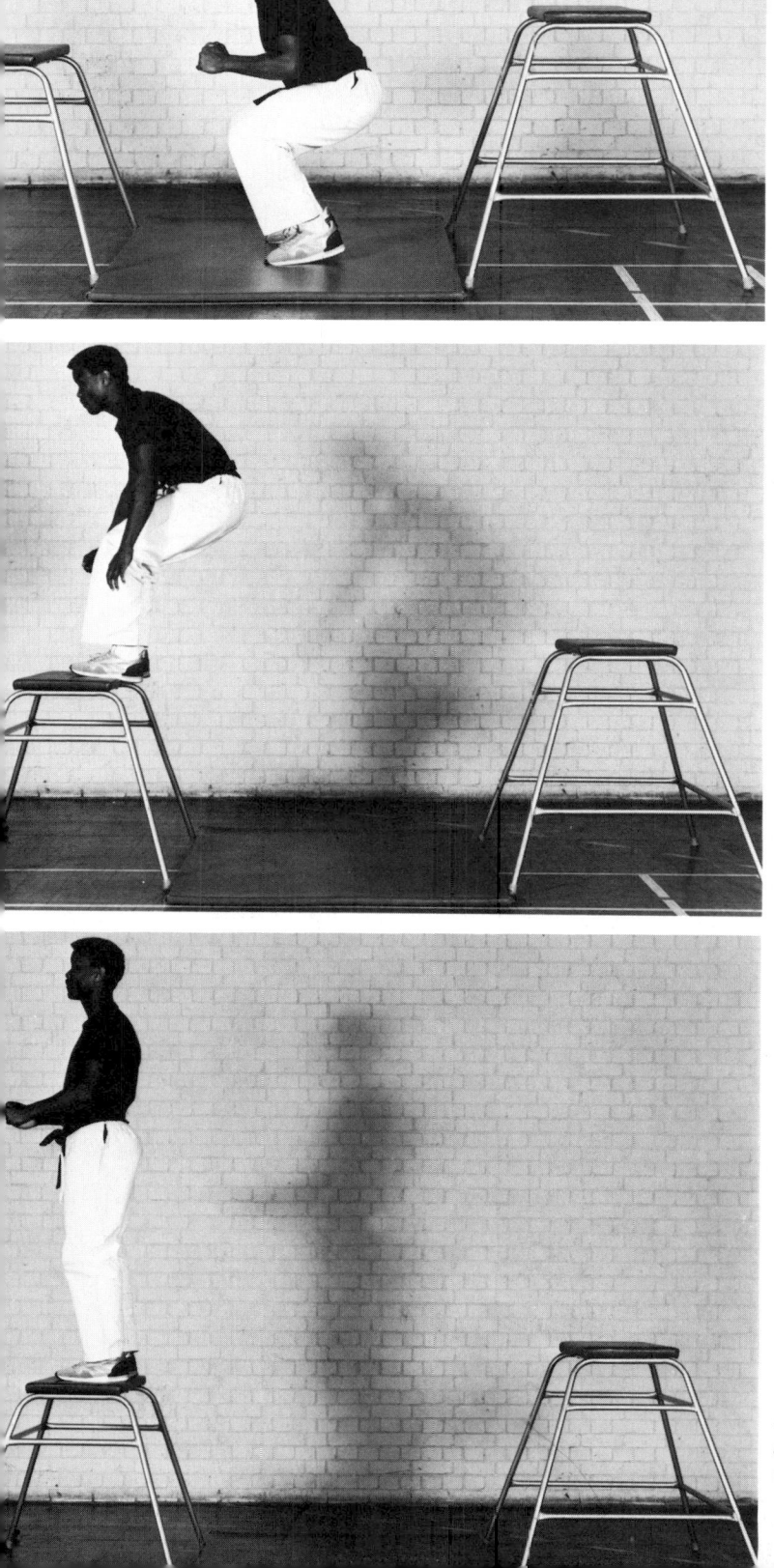

Plyometrics load muscle with energy

You can illustrate this theory by reference to the standing jump. Go into a half squat and jump straight up from it. Then make a quick bob down from the half squat before you spring. Which one gives the higher jump? The bob stretches the muscles on the front of the leg so they can contract more powerfully. Compare this with the front kick where the kicking leg bends as the knee rises, also stretching the muscles on the front of the leg. By applying the principles of plyometrics to the martial arts, it may well be possible to produce a faster kick or punch.

Plyometrics training needs good general strength in the muscles, otherwise it may result in frequent trips to the local physiotherapist! Before you start training, make sure your legs and joints are strong enough to cope with the loading. To reduce risk of injury, combine plyometrics training with other training forms.

Begin training by either jumping/hopping over obstacles, or by jumping down from a height and immediately jumping back up and onto a platform of equal or greater height. Jumping over obstacles is a good starting point but make those obstacles light and collapsible to avoid injuries to the fatigued martial artist. Rest a bamboo across a pair of chairs, or get members of the class to hold either end of a belt.

The equipment for jumping down and up again is more difficult to organise. The platforms must be light yet rigid – a gym box is excellent though you can use piles of mats at a pinch. If you use tables, make sure they are really strong or you may find them collapsing under you. The platforms must be no more than one metre in height, otherwise the knee joint can be over-stressed. Arrange the platforms in a straight line, sepa-rated by sufficient space for you to land and take off. If they are spaced too widely, then coordinating the take-off to gain enough horizontal distance becomes too important a factor.

The number of obstacles/platforms is arbitrary, though four to six with a walk recovery is ideal. Make your landing onto a sprung floor since solid floors are never suitable for martial arts practice. Start with four or five sets of four repetitions over four plat-forms, with a walk back recovery between repetitions and a one or two minute break between sets.

If you want to up-rate training, increase height of the platforms, increase the repetitions, or carry weights.

Use plyometrics for training the upper body too. Go from a deep press-up position, springing up to place your hands on a bench. Improve your endurance by imposing a time limit, or by shortening the rest period between plyometric sets. A lot of explosive energy is needed to lift the body up to a platform.

As a variant, exercises using side-to-side horizontal leaps between two lines might well be useful for prepar-ing the martial artist to deal with sudden changes of angle. For this application, it is important not to leap high.

Combining Exercises Into Schedules

Whichever form(s) of training you eventually settle for, you must be pre-pared to assess all new developments as and when they arise, for their suit-ability to your programme.

At this time, a good all-round option is a set of free weights coupled with a basic knowledge of how the body works, an understanding of how your martial art techniques work and an ability to evaluate the effectiveness of exercises you design to match the techniques you are trying to strengthen.

That's all!

Whilst creating all these new world-shattering exercises, do not neglect the humble all-round exercises, or the need for a properly balanced schedule. When training for the strong punch for example, don't neglect the need for a strong pull-back and exercise for that too.

Develop both your general and specific muscle fitness. Obviously what you work into your programme will depend upon the availability of training facilities but with a bit of ingenuity, you will be able to train the same muscles with whatever is available to you.

Whichever you go for, always work in the correct form, since this is more important than weight shifted. Correct form ensures that the right muscle groups are exercised optimally and the risk of injury reduced. Work explosively on the effort phase and in

Front squats will exercise your legs

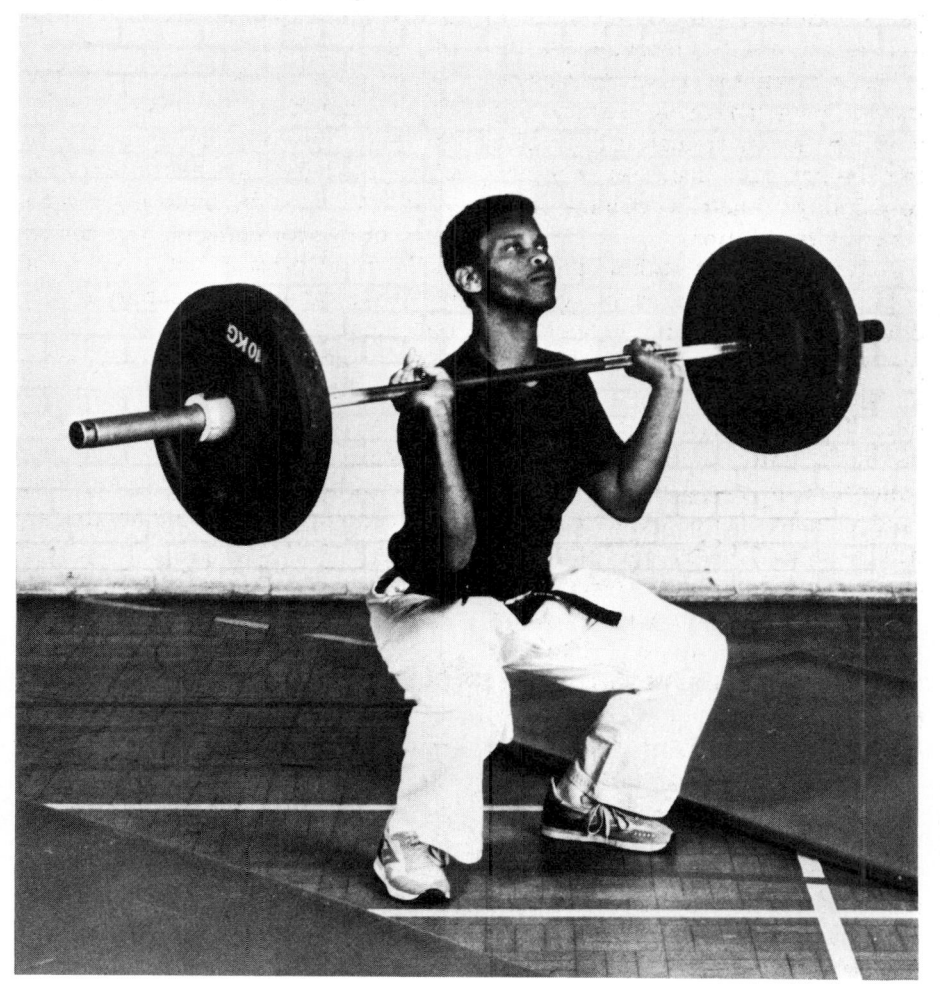

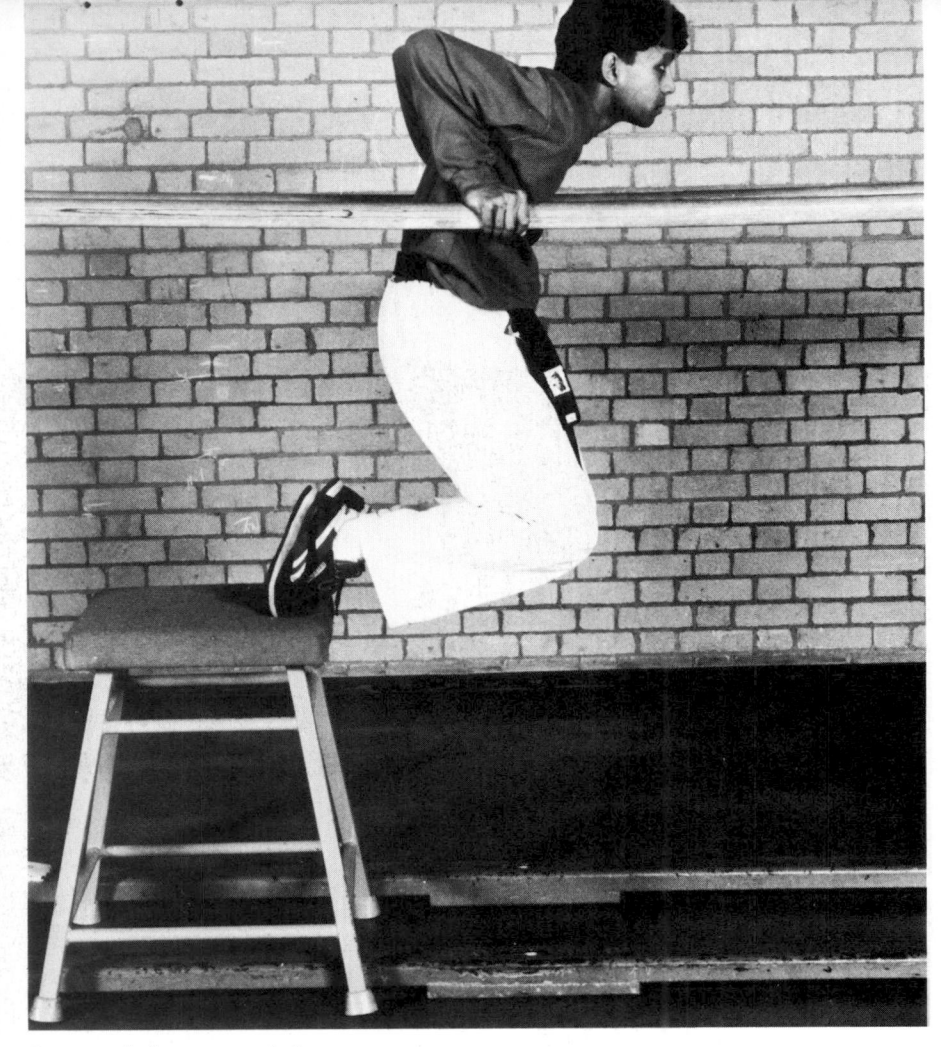

Dips work the arms and chest

a controlled manner on the negative phase. Don't bounce down after the active phase because not only does this increase injury risk but it also reduces load and hence exercise value. It is much harder to work explosively from a static position.

Begin by warming up properly so you are actually sweating. This practice reduces risk of injury. Warming down after rigorous training involves light stretching and gentle movements to reduce the onset of stiffness. This is particularly important with novice martial artists and more advanced students working out in later sessions.

Set yourself a target to aim for and keep a record of your performance. When you have achieved the goal three times in consecutive sessions, increase the loading. Do resistance training two or three times a week, with a day's recovery between each session. Top performers may want to work on a split-schedule in which different body parts are worked on consecutive days.

The following weight training schedule is suitable for novice martial artists.

Using free weights, do four sets of ten repetitions of the power clean.

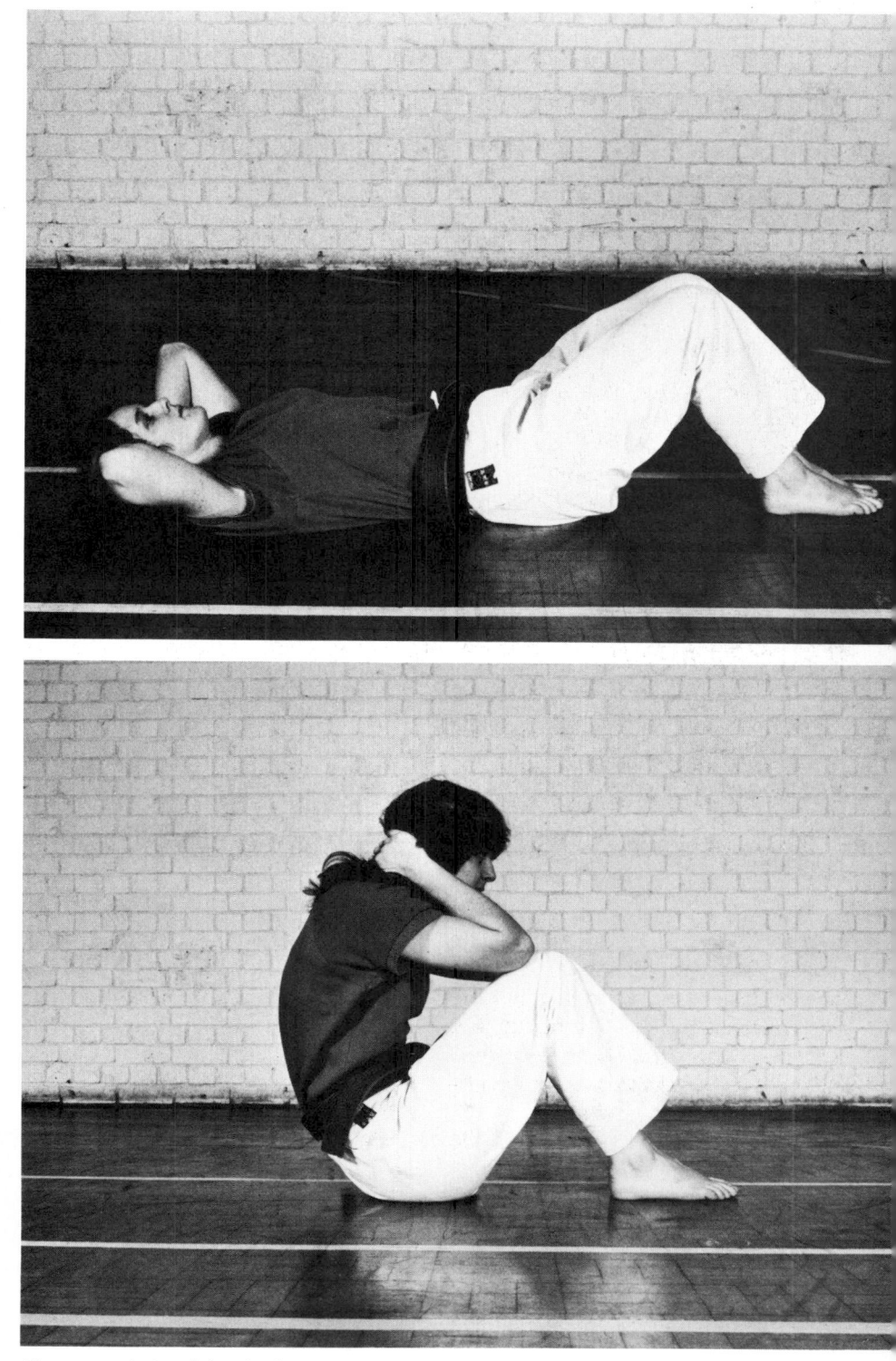

Sit-ups work the abdominals

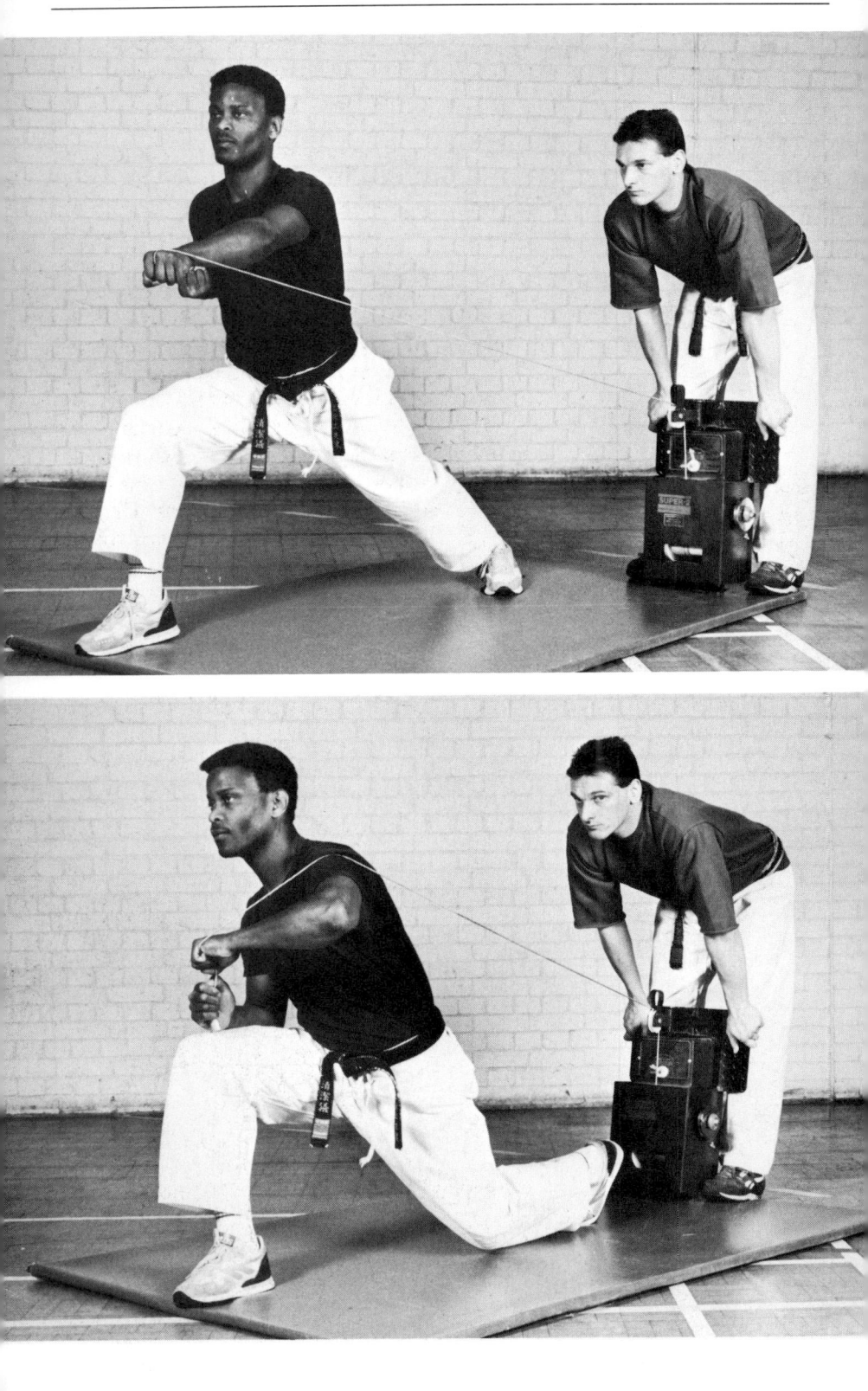

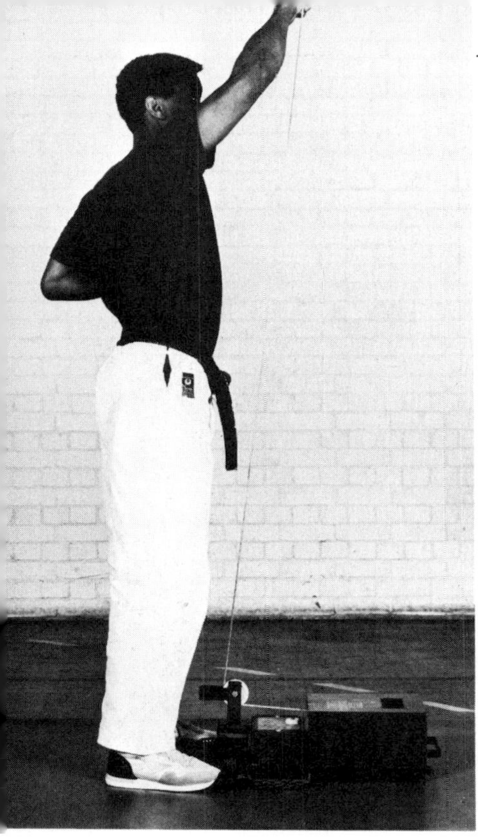

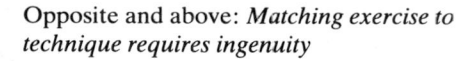

This will exercise all of your body. Do four sets of ten repetitions of the bench press to exercise your chest and arms. Four times ten repetitions of front squats will exercise your legs and back whilst four by ten 'good mornings'/dead lift will work the back. Four by ten explosive step-ups whilst carrying weights will exercise the legs. Dips work the arms and chest, so do four sets, each of ten or twelve repetitions. Three sets of twenty sit-ups and three by ten repetitions of leg lifts will exercise the abdominals.

If you use machines, do four by ten jump squats to work virtually the whole of your body. Four sets of ten repetitions of bench press will exercise the chest and arms, as will four by ten or twelve dips. Four times ten repetitions of leg press will suffice for the legs and you can also do four sets of eight repetitions using a single leg

Opposite and above: *Matching exercise to technique requires ingenuity*

Below: *Press-ups exercise your chest and arms*

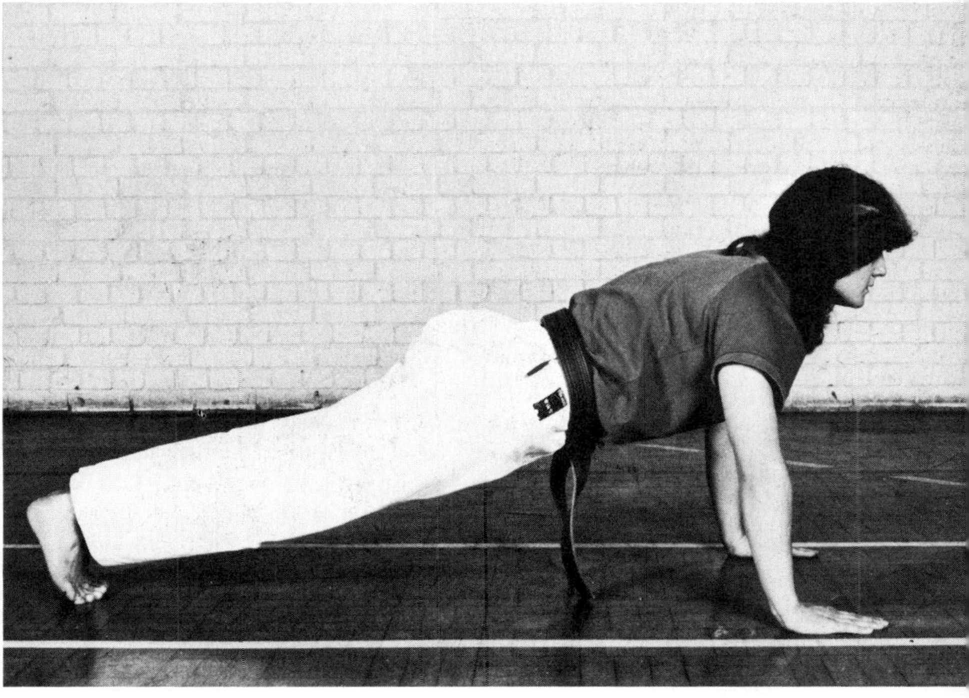

STRENGTH TRAINING

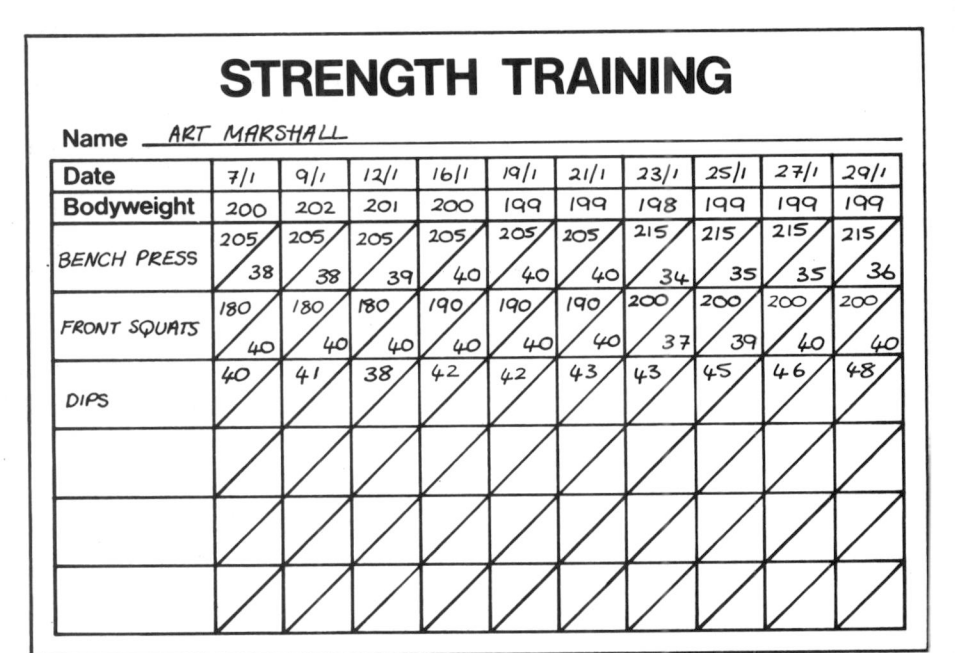

Name ART MARSHALL

Date	7/1	9/1	12/1	16/1	19/1	21/1	23/1	25/1	27/1	29/1
Bodyweight	200	202	201	200	199	199	198	199	199	199
BENCH PRESS	205 / 38	205 / 38	205 / 39	205 / 40	205 / 40	205 / 40	215 / 34	215 / 35	215 / 35	215 / 36
FRONT SQUATS	180 / 40	180 / 40	180 / 40	190 / 40	190 / 40	190 / 40	200 / 37	200 / 39	200 / 40	200 / 40
DIPS	40	41	38	42	42	43	43	45	46	48

Keep a record of your performance

push on the leg press station. Four by ten dead lifts utilising the bench press station will exercise the back. Work the abdominals with three sets of ten or twenty sit-ups.

If you go for body weight exercises, then do four sets of ten repetitions of height jumps/jump squats to exercise your whole body. Press-ups where you rest your feet on a chair will work the muscles of your chest and arms so do four sets, each of fifteen to twenty repetitions. You can also do four sets of twelve or sixteen reverse dips between chairs. Four by ten single leg squats will work your leg muscles but maintain balance by holding onto a bar, or a partner's arm. A second leg exercise uses five sets of eight step-ups on each leg. Four times fifteen round back hyperextensions will work the back and three sets of ten or twenty of the ubiquitous sit-ups will exercise the abdominals.

When matching exercises to technique, consider the speed of movement, the range of movement, the resistance to be used, the number of exercise repetitions, the number of sets of those repetitions and any other ancillary exercises that need to be practised in combination. As an example, let's consider how we might develop strength training exercises using free weights for improving front kick.

Front kick uses the muscles on the front and back of the upper leg, plus the calves and abdominals. The best overall exercise using weights is the squat. A word of warning at this point. Some medical opinion considers that this exercise can overload the knee joint so make sure you are fit enough to cope with this sort of training before starting. If in doubt, use a half-squat.

Adopt front squat, holding the barbell in front of the head for safety and best body position. Use light weights only. The front squat allows you to get rid of the bar easily and also prevents over-usage of the back muscles to counter leg fatigue and poor flexibility. Keep your body erect, otherwise the bar falls off.

Keep your knees and feet pointing the same way and you will avoid ankle and knee injury. Do the exercise correctly and don't compromise. Keep your feet flat on the floor throughout and don't let your heels rise during the squat. Even if your heels do have a tendency to lift through poor ankle flexibility, don't use heel blocks.

Other exercises for front kick include lunges, calf raises and any sort of twisting sit-up, especially those which involve leg movement.

As should now be clear, you must make a large number of decisions before beginning your course of training. This is no bad thing because a careful consideration of all the facts and alternatives may well produce a greater level of commitment than would result from the imposition of schedules by an outside authority, however authoritative.

Fast Reactions

Muscle conditioning is absolutely useless unless harnessed to the right technique and delivered at the right time. How you respond to a situation is governed by a number of important factors, the first of which is **perception**.

Although we take in a large amount of data at any one time, we process (ie pay attention to) only a small amount. If you find this difficult to understand, try reading this book whilst fending off your pet dog and tapping your feet in rhythm, all at the same time. This would be difficult for most people but the martial artist must take in a lot of data and selectively process only the most crucial facts which will give a clue to the opponent's intentions.

Perception training involves getting you to recognise and act correctly upon certain cues. Pressure can be applied either by making the cues less obvious, introducing a number of false cues, or 'feints', cutting down the amount of time you have to spot the cue and distraction through such other pressures as exhaustion.

An on-the-ball coach will have analysed the performances of any opponents you are likely to encounter and will be able to brief you on cues to look out for. In the longer term, you must learn to do this analysis for yourself.

Better perception allows you to see attacks at the planning rather than at the execution stage.

The second factor to consider is **decision making**. In certain martial arts, conscious decisions on how to deal with a potential or actual attack are almost eliminated by the development of automatic counters. This obviously makes them faster.

More experienced martial artists

Fast reactions

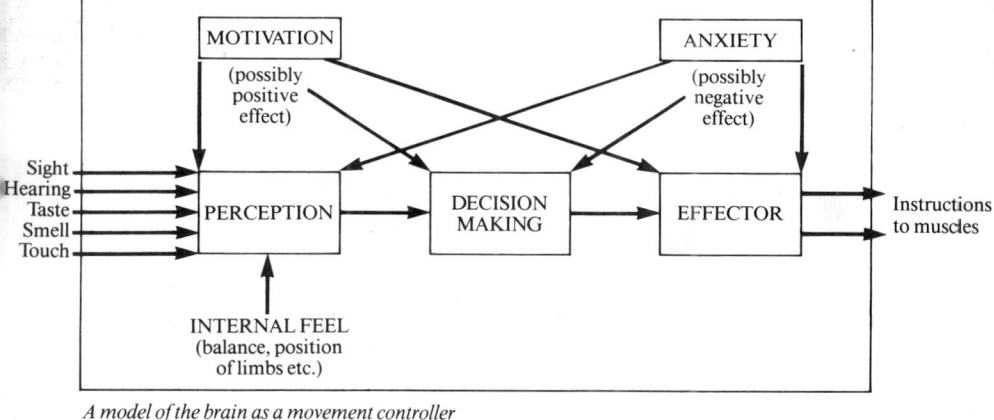

A model of the brain as a movement controller

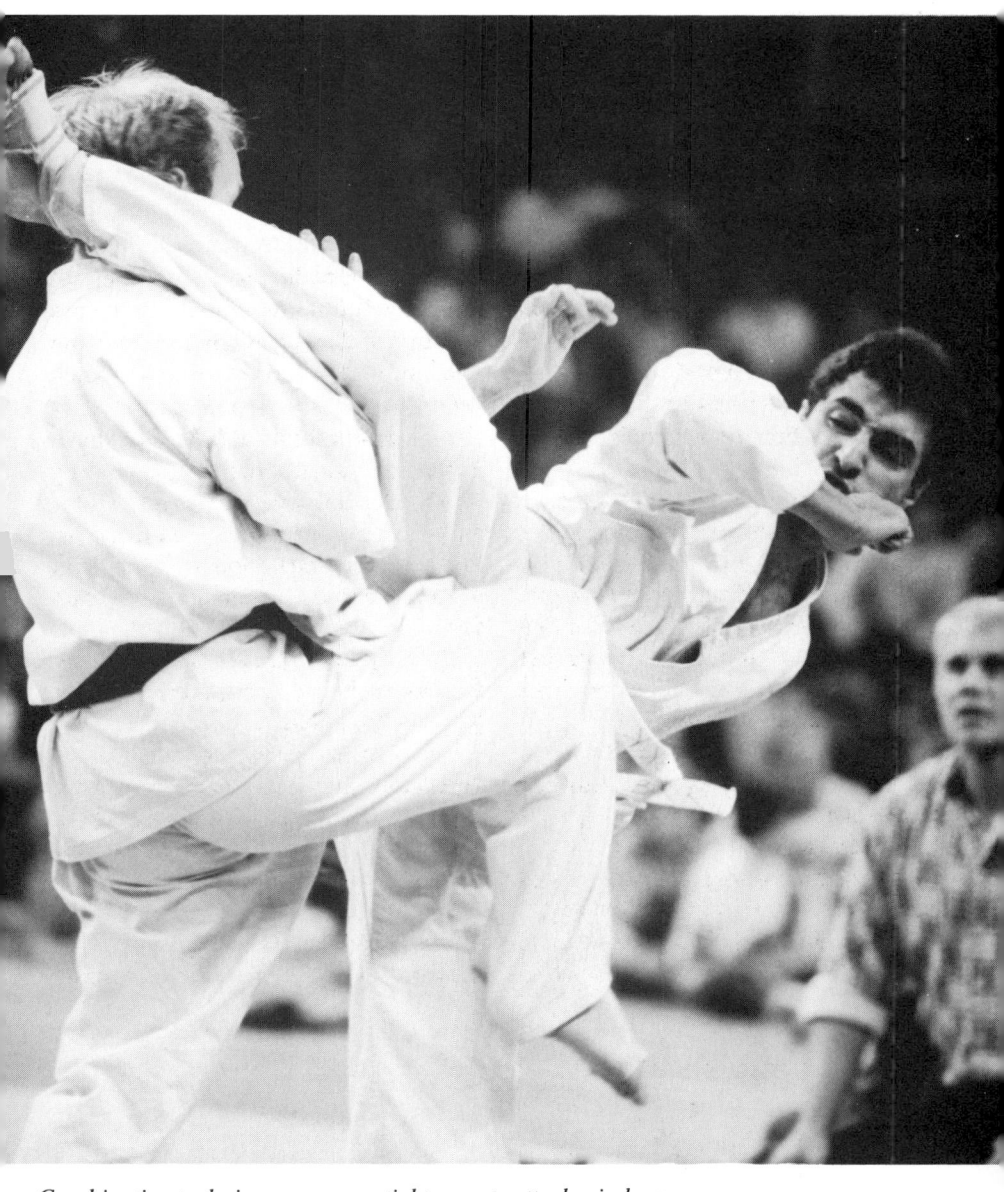

Combination techniques are essential to create attack windows

will have several options to select from and will minimise decision making by advance planning either before sparring, or prior to attacks. A good coach will be able to plan the appropriate responses in advance and direct the competitor appropriately.

The third factor is the **effector** mechanism where the brain sends instructions to the muscles to do a certain number of things in a specified way. When applying a hold or lock, the novice martial artist is slowed by the need to concentrate on getting the various bits of the specified action right. The more advanced student on the other hand, has practised the technique so many times that it can be performed much faster.

Individual techniques can be combined to form whole series of complicated, fast and consistent techniques. However to get the combination effective, training must be sharp, with no sloppiness or cheating.

It is essential to monitor this form of practice to stop serious mistakes from developing and repeating. Personal idiosyncrasies may be permissible, but dropping guard during a particular move may have catastrophic results. These mistakes do tend to occur after long practice when the martial artist is becoming tired. Every effort must be made to weed them out before they become incorporated into the programme.

The key to performing techniques effectively, with speed and maximum power lies in repetition practice termed 'overtraining'.

At the time of your grading or competition do remember that the optimum conditions for the development of speed and power occur when the neuromuscular system is properly rested.

Training for Flexibility

Flexibility is a component of fitness defined as the range of movement at a joint, or number of joints. Flexibility is essential for performing smooth movements and for generating larger forces produced when muscles contract over greater distances. This leads to the fast limb movements essential to martial art practice.

Flexibility is limited by a number of factors. The skeleton itself imposes limitations on such as the elbow joint. Most peoples' elbows will open out to around one hundred and eighty degrees only and further movement at the joint is limited by a bony protrusion from the bone of the upper arm (*humerus*). This 'door stop' is called the *olecranon process* and it is one of the body parts which suffers badly from incorrect techniques.

The knee joint has a similar door stop to prevent it extending more than 180°, for without some sort of skeletal limitation, these hinge joints would suffer injury. Other joints place less limitations of movement, particularly the ball-and-socket arrangements found in the hip and shoulder. A strong force applied to the shoulder joint can separate the ball from the socket, producing a dislocation. Therefore it is necessary to increase the strength of those muscles which provide stability.

Fortunately, in those areas where most flexibility is required, the skeleton is rarely the limiting factor. Most resistance is caused by ligaments, tendons and muscles. Ligaments hold joints together and are the bits that suffer, for example, when you turn over on your ankle. Tendons attach muscle to bones and the best known perhaps, is the *Achilles tendon* which runs downwards to the heel. Muscle consists of many tiny fibres, all bound together with an elastic connective tissue covering that prevents the muscle from being over-stretched.

Limitations to flexibility are the muscle length, the connective tissue and muscle contraction during stretching. Muscle size, fat and skin may also impose limits. Large muscles and fat get in the way but the skin will stretch as far as need be, though you may collect stretch marks (as body builders and pregnant women do). Still other factors affecting flexibility are age and sex. Age does reduce flexibility in older sedentary people and even without any training at all, women are generally more supple than men.

It is possible to train for flexibility by increasing the length of the tissues which are limiting movement and by encouraging relaxation of the muscles being stretched.

Some physical activities with limited skeletal involvement such as jogging, actually lead to a reduction in flexibility whereas others such as swimming, increase shoulder and

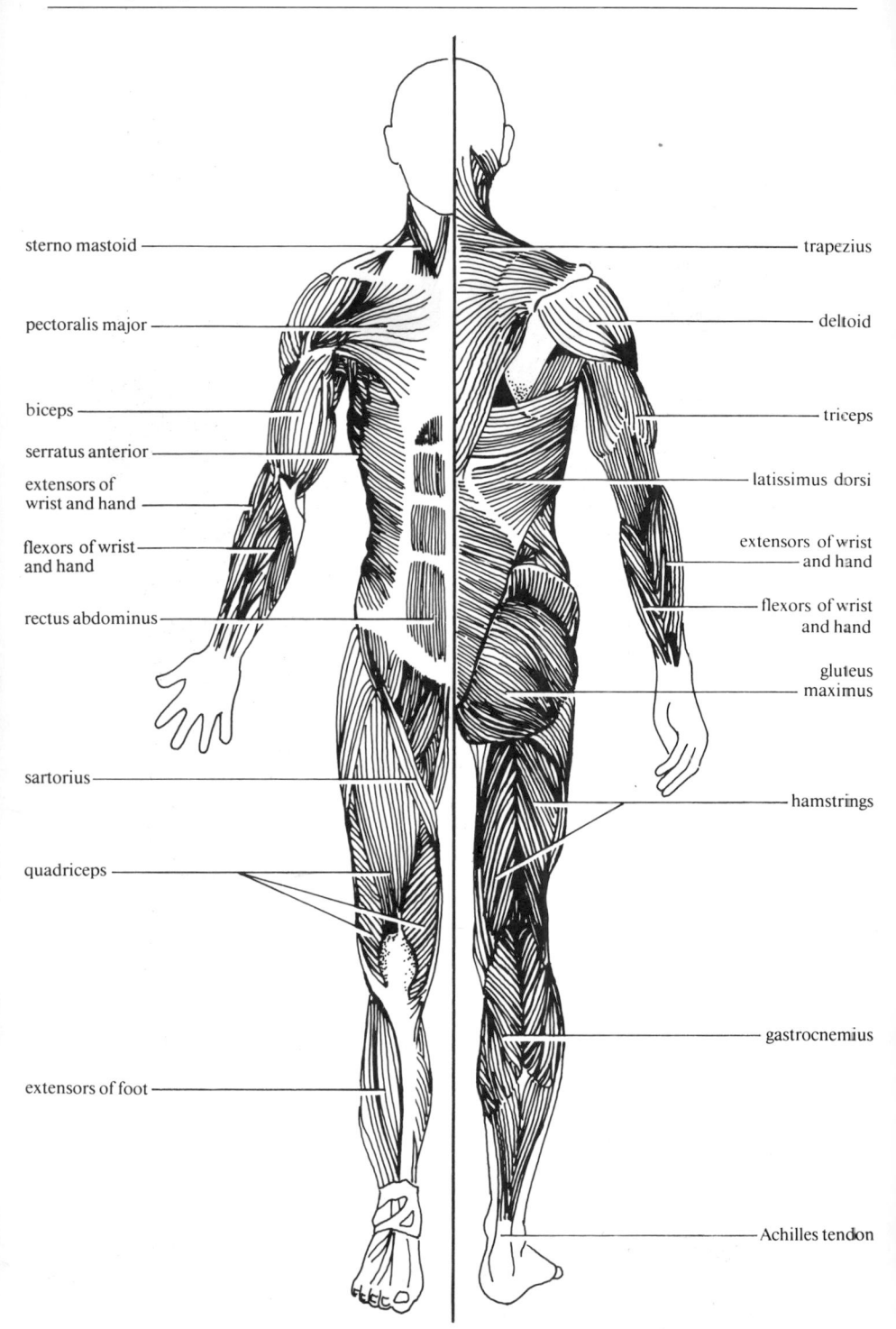

sterno mastoid

pectoralis major

biceps

serratus anterior

extensors of
wrist and hand

flexors of wrist
and hand

rectus abdominus

sartorius

quadriceps

extensors of foot

trapezius

deltoid

triceps

latissimus dorsi

extensors of wrist
and hand

flexors of wrist
and hand

gluteus
maximus

hamstrings

gastrocnemius

Achilles tendon

Flexibility is a function of joints and the muscles that hold them together

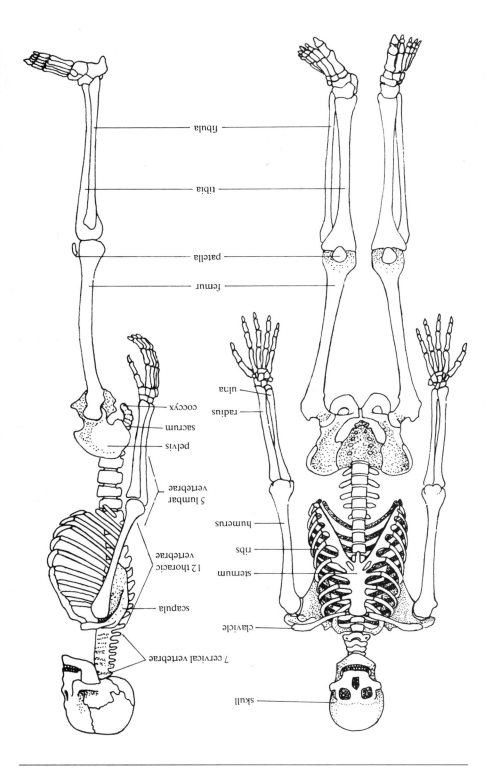

fibula

tibia

patella

femur

ulna

radius

coccyx

sacrum

pelvis

5 lumbar
vertebrae

12 thoracic
vertebrae

scapula

7 cervical vertebrae

humerus

ribs

sternum

clavicle

skull

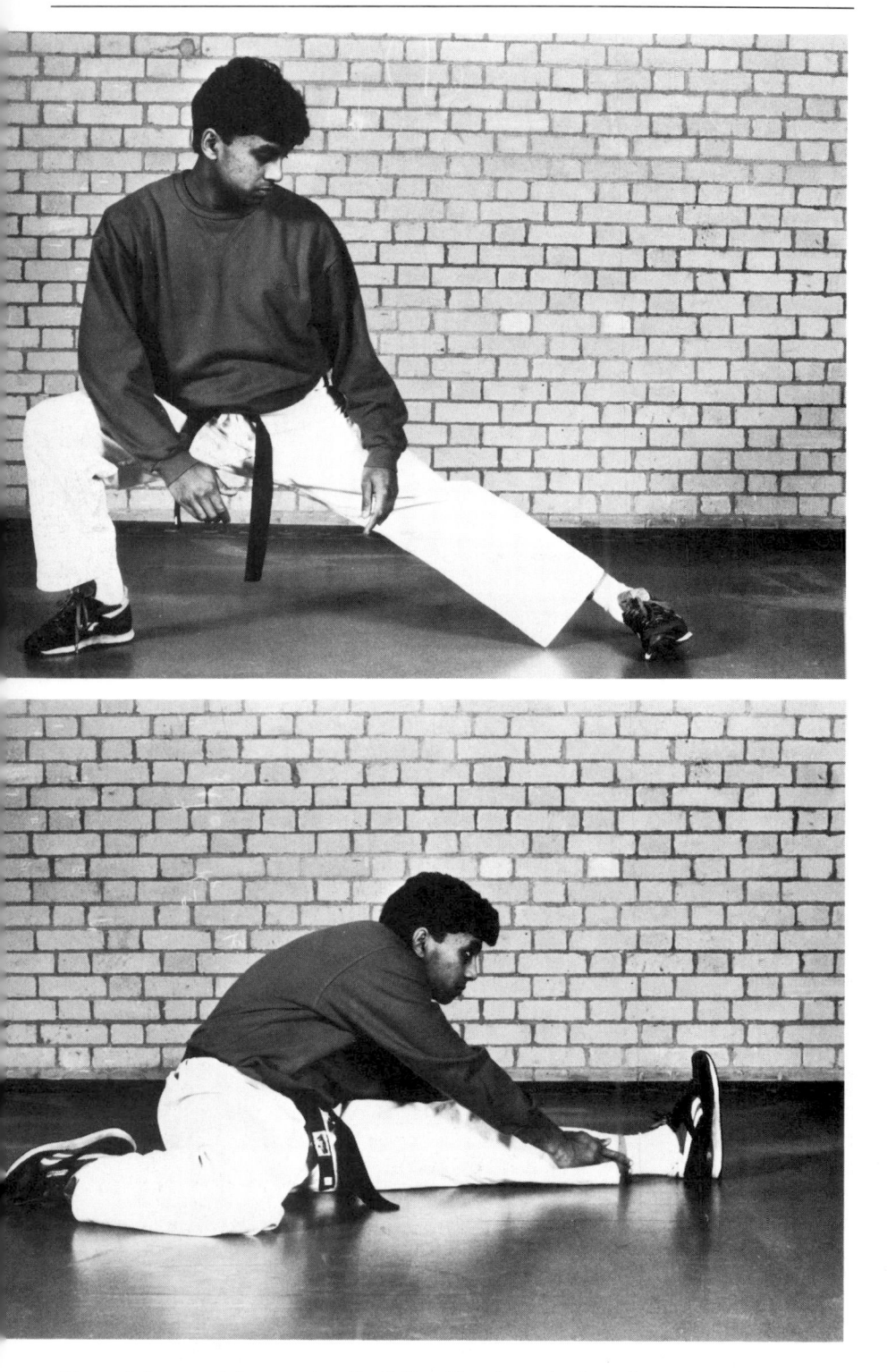

All martial arts training requires flexibility. Here is a selection of exercises you can use.

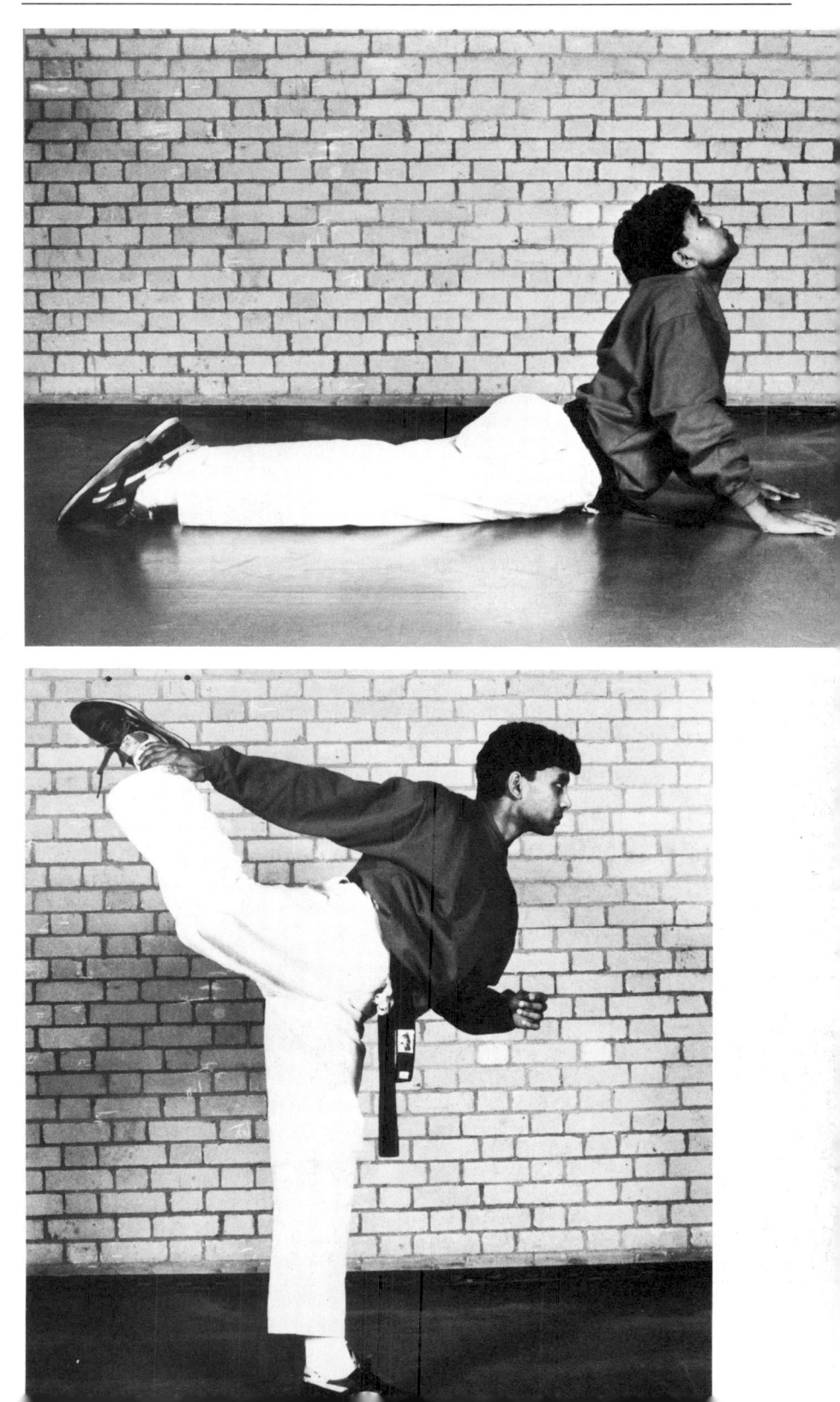

ankle flexibility. The martial arts use many explosive movements and if you are insufficiently flexible, you run a risk of injury. It is not a good idea to rely on continued practice of a technique to improve the flexibility you need to do that very technique. Use suitable exercises instead.

Joint mobility can be developed in three ways, the first being the 'ballistic stretching' so beloved of some martial arts. It used to be widely used in different sporting disciplines but it is not so popular today. To stretch a joint ballistically, you use a bobbing or bouncing action such as when you sit down, extend your legs out in front of you and lunge at your toes. This causes a sudden muscle stretch and the length sensors imbedded within the muscle immediately send a message to the spinal cord, the result of which is a contraction in the muscle being stretched. This is a simple, self defence reaction to stop muscle damage.

This muscle contraction is counterproductive because that same muscle is supposed to relax in order to produce the required degree of joint movement. Of course, you can apply such a sudden high loading to your muscles that they are not able to protect themselves with a contraction and injury results. Even when you don't go that far, you will discover that ballistic stretching is associated with muscle stiffness. Never practise any form of ballistic stretching with a partner because this is extremely risky.

The second method of flexibility training is called the 'passive stretch'. This involves gradually taking joints close to their limits of movement, so some discomfort is felt. This position is held for between ten and thirty seconds. The gentle application of stretch reduces the chance of reflex contraction. This type of training is easy to fit into a daily routine and if you get bored, do it at home in front of the TV. You can static stretch with a partner but since the partner can't feel the discomfort inflicted, he/she must be very careful indeed.

Static stretches are used during the cooling down phase following training because they have been found to reduce muscular stiffness. Compare this with ballistic stretching which actually causes stiffness.

The third form of flexibility training is useful to those martial artists requiring even greater flexibility and is known by the imposing title *Proprioceptive Neuromuscular Facilitation*, or 'PNF'. PNF is based upon the way a muscle responds after a strong contraction and exercises using it require the assistance of a reliable partner.

Go into a static stretch position and relax all the muscles in the area being stretched. Your partner assists you by following your stretch with correct pressure. Isometrically contract those muscles which would limit the stretch and hold the contraction for three seconds. Your partner must resist the movement. Then contract those opposing muscles which would make your stretch actually wider and finally relax all muscles and continue with an assisted static stretch.

The first isometric contraction of the muscle to be stretched, followed by contraction of the opposing muscle helps prepare the former for the final passive stretch and the previous limit is exceeded.

The following is an example of PNF stretching intended to improve hip flexibility.

Lie on the floor and lift one leg. Keep your leg straight and muscles relaxed. Allow your partner to take it

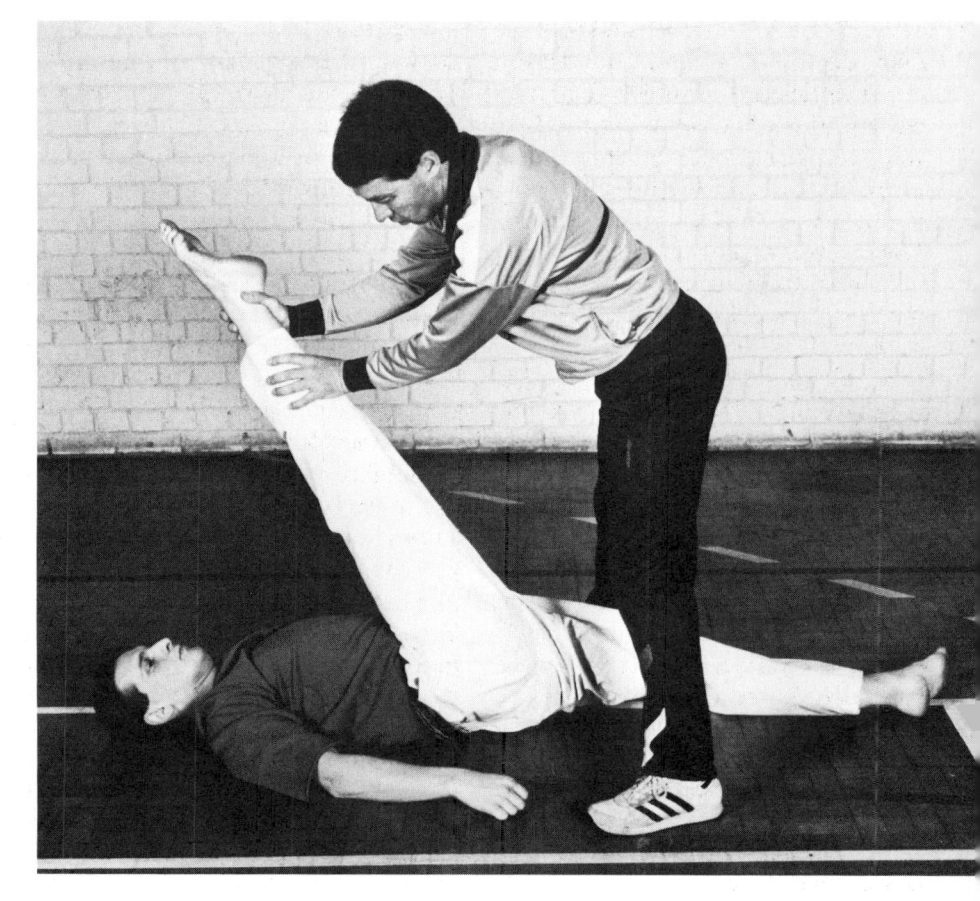

Perform PNF stretching with great care

to the limit and hold it there for a few seconds. Contract the muscles in the back of your leg whilst your partner prevents your leg from moving (ie isometric contraction). Then contract the muscles on the front of your thighs for a few seconds. Relax all leg muscles and allow your partner to increase the stretch, holding the new position for a few seconds.

Perform PNF stretching with great care and only after a thorough warm-up. It is not recommended for novice martial artists and suffers from the disadvantage of needing a partner. Nevertheless, research indicates that it is better at increasing joint mobility than static stretching alone.

Remember that the greater the range of movement at a joint, the greater the potential power that can be generated.

The experienced martial artist or coach are the only ones who can identify those parts of the body which need to be made more flexible for the particular discipline. You may be aware of your own limitations in performing a technique and this may indicate areas where improvement is needed. Novice martial artists will require an overall general flexibility programme whilst more advanced students perhaps go for increased flexibility in specific areas.

Psychologists report that static

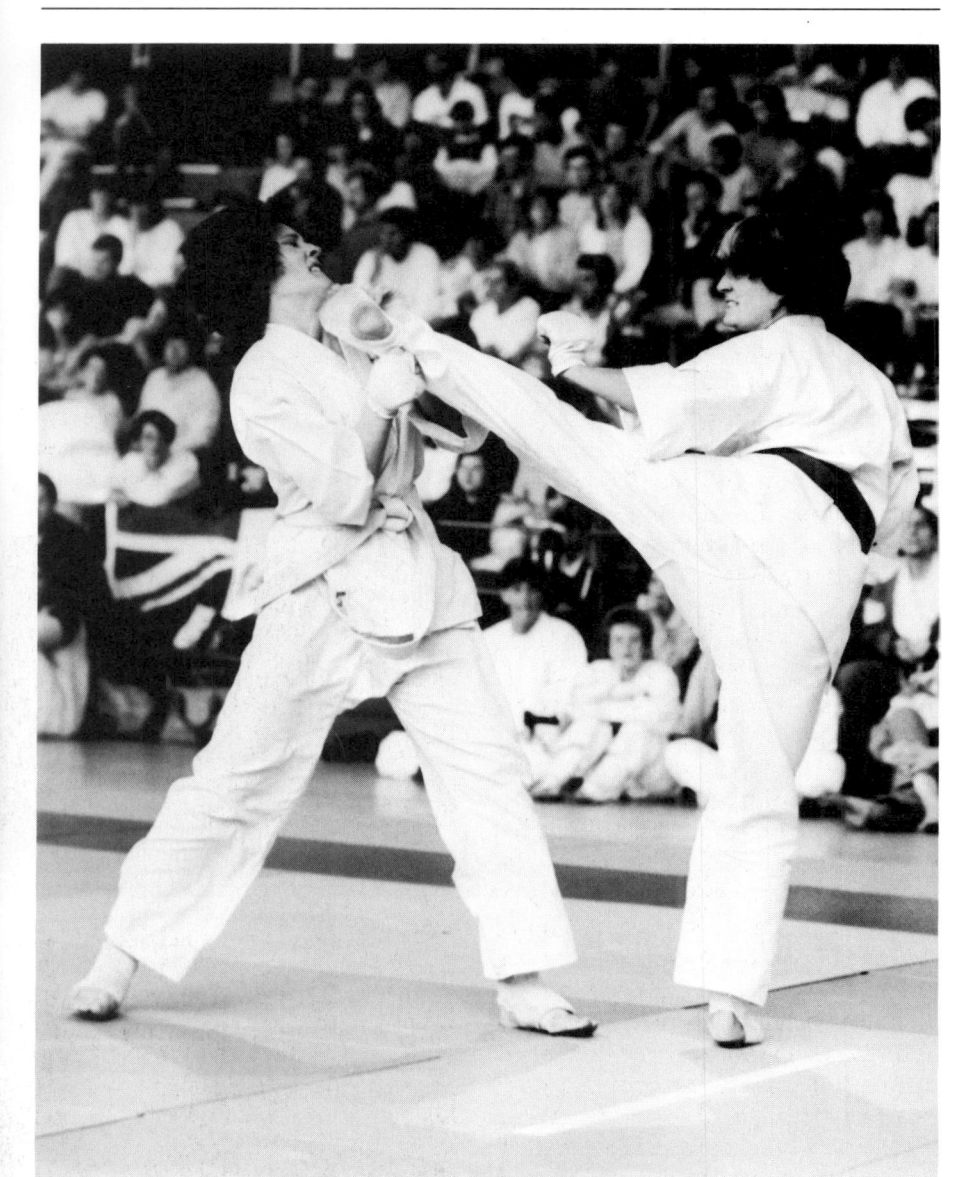

Body flexibility means being able to use all your techniques to best effect

stretching performed before an event may be useful in relaxing excessively nervous participants. It will also reduce the risk of injury if your martial art involves explosive movements. After the event, additional flexibility work will form part of the cool down necessary to prevent muscle stiffness. Include flexibility training into your daily programme too if you are serious about improving.

Do develop muscular strength along with joint mobility. If you don't, you may well develop great flexibility but you will also suffer from joint injuries because the muscles aren't strong enough to hold all the bits and pieces together.

Training for Stamina

What is stamina? Stamina is a vague term used to describe elements of both cardiovascular and local muscle endurance. Without a basic level of local muscular endurance you wouldn't even make it through the warm-up, much less the ensuing training session. Cardiovascular endurance is a prerequisite of more advanced training. It is the aerobic base upon which fitness rests and it is especially important for health. Both types of endurance must receive attention during a training session and in the preparation for grading or competition – especially during the early stages of training.

To have a cardiovascular effect, an activity must raise pulse rate to a higher than normal level and keep it there for a reasonable time. Moreover, this activity must take place often enough so the body is forced to adapt to the extra demand. Opinions on how far you should raise your heart rate and for how long vary but as a rough guide, work steadily at a pace which produces a heart rate of 130–160 beats per minute for a period of 15–20 minutes at least three times a week.

Your pulse is quite easy to find. Place two fingers just below the wrist on the inner thumb-side or on your neck near the side of the windpipe (but don't press too hard). Count the beats for 15 seconds and multiply by four. Try to keep moving as you take your pulse – a bit of practice will make this easier. Alternatively, invest in a pulse monitor which you wear on your wrist.

Don't go at it too hard. Exercising for the full period at regular intervals is more beneficial than hammering yourself once a fortnight. As you become more fit, your sessions will

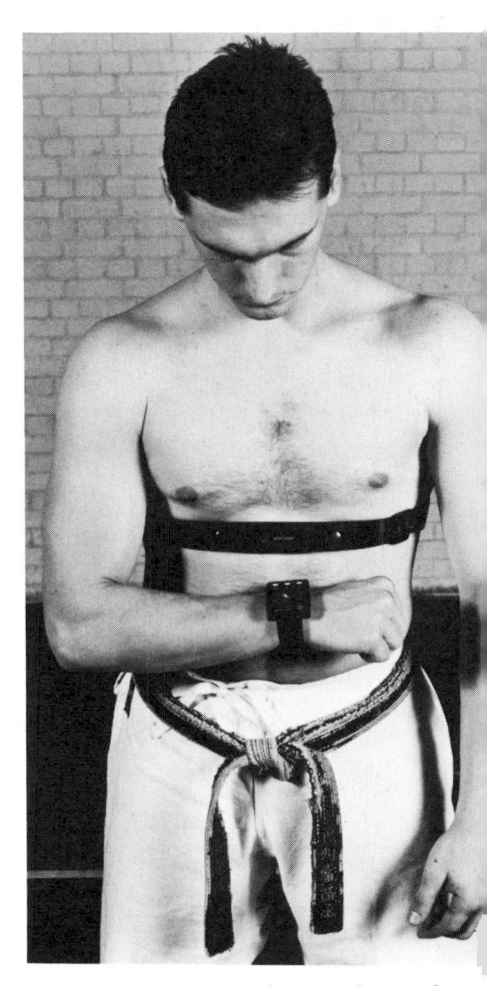

A pulse monitor is a sophisticated way of measuring your heart rate

become harder as you reach towards your new limits. Even top martial artists hurt during training. They just have to work harder to get tired.

'Work steadily' is an important guideline for this type of training. Research has shown that steady rhythmic activity is more effective in improving endurance at the basic level than bursts of activity. Any activity which can be done continuously for 20 minutes and works the body hard enough can be used. Running, dancing and swimming are popular alternatives. If you choose running, reduce the risk of stress injuries with a thorough warm-up and good shoes. Roadwork is hard on the legs – especially so for the heavier person. Cross-country is more interesting and usually less risky.

Whether you are a top martial artist or an enthusiastic novice, it is important to make training time effective. Long slow distance running was widely held to be the best way to build endurance but recent research seems to indicate that shorter, harder sessions are more effective. If you want to go for a high-level course of training, aim towards a target of three miles in 18/21 minutes. This will provide an aerobic base for later, higher quality work.

You do appreciate of course that this target is a rough guestimate based upon average values. Factors such as body size must be taken into consideration when planning targets but most martial artists should be able to manage seven minute miles.

You must develop local muscular endurance both generally and in those muscle groups used extensively in your martial art practice. This can be done in two ways. Firstly you can work out which muscles are involved in the techniques you use and then design exercises to work them. Use the correct range of movement at the correct speed and avoid the risk of injuries arising out of bad body positioning and 'bouncing'. Secondly you can use the techniques themselves, using a punching pad or bag. Take care not to lose technique in the desire simply to hit hard.

If you practise 'unloaded' techniques against the air, watch out for joint injuries caused by over-extension. This type of training can also lead to anomalous techniques and the wrong muscle conditioning. Nevertheless it is a common form of martial art training and is actually useful for group learning of techniques, but be sure to balance it with other methods.

Martial art skills need to be practised under pressure by martial artists at all levels. Fatigue produces pressure but it also leads to cheating – the technique is modified to make it easier and bad habits picked up this way can be difficult to shed. Avoid this by training with partners capable of analysing what you are supposed to be doing and getting them to point out deficiencies.

Errors or omissions can be pointed out with something like a bamboo practise sword (*shinai*) such as is used in many classical Japanese martial art clubs. It only takes a couple of gentle raps with the shinai against your head to encourage you to keep an adequate guard whilst kicking. If you don't possess a shinai, use a padded pole.

Exercise to a count but make that count random. Better still, key movement to a visual signal such as a nod of the head. This is more in keeping with a martial arts format.

The following types of endurance training can be used:

Continuous work

Select an activity which you can both actually maintain for the target time and monitor your performance in from session to session.

Fartlek

In loose terms fartlek ('speed play') training consists of steady effort mixed with bursts of activity. It provides a change from continuous work, is excellent for improving your recovery rate and forms a useful link between continuous and interval training. The bursts of activity can occur at regular or random intervals. You can't anticipate it when your partner calls out at random intervals and the burst always seems to come at the wrong time.

Fartlek is good for group training, with everyone running along at the speed of the slowest member. Then for 100 metres or for 30 seconds, everyone switches to sprint and tries to stay together. After the sprint, the group closes up again. By timing it right, the senior can exercise the group very hard indeed and rivalry will contribute to the high work loads.

A mixed-ability group can be exercised by what is called a 'collecting run'. Everyone runs together until one breaks into a burst which lasts for perhaps one minute. When the minute is up, the leader about-turns and runs back, collecting up the stragglers. When all are collected, they turn back and continue the run. This works everyone with the fittest people running furthest.

Individuals can intersperse running with sprints, hillwork, or similar. The problem lies in ensuring a high work load because individuals tend to be too kind to themselves.

Intervals

This category is the one most used by top martial artists. The basic idea is that you reach your limit in stages, each one separated by a partial recovery rather than through one continuous push. The timing of rest periods to allow only a partial recovery means that the body must learn to tolerate an oxygen debt (ie work *anaerobically*). This is essential for martial arts practice since the activity bursts involve maximum efforts at high speed and in quick succession.

Take a percentage of your single best effort and repeat it with rests in between. Use this system with martial art techniques, running, or with weights. For example, if you can do 40 roundhouse kicks in a minute, interval training will require you to do four sets of 30 kicks per minute with 30 second rests between sets.

A second method mixes tasks that load you almost to your limit with an easier activity that provides an active recovery. A third method could use a punch, kick or throwing movement performed to a count. You stay with it for as long as you can, then take a 20 seconds rest before resuming. Work for perhaps five minutes total and try to minimise the number of rests you need to take. As soon as you can manage without rests for the whole period, increase the work rate.

A fourth alternative uses intervals of very hard exercising broken up by short rests. Exercise sets are grouped together into larger sets each of which are separated by longer rests. This is known as *plametric* work. As an example you might do four sets, each of three depth jumps followed by a walk recovery, then take one minute's rest before repeating the four sets. Otherwise do four sets of four 60 metre

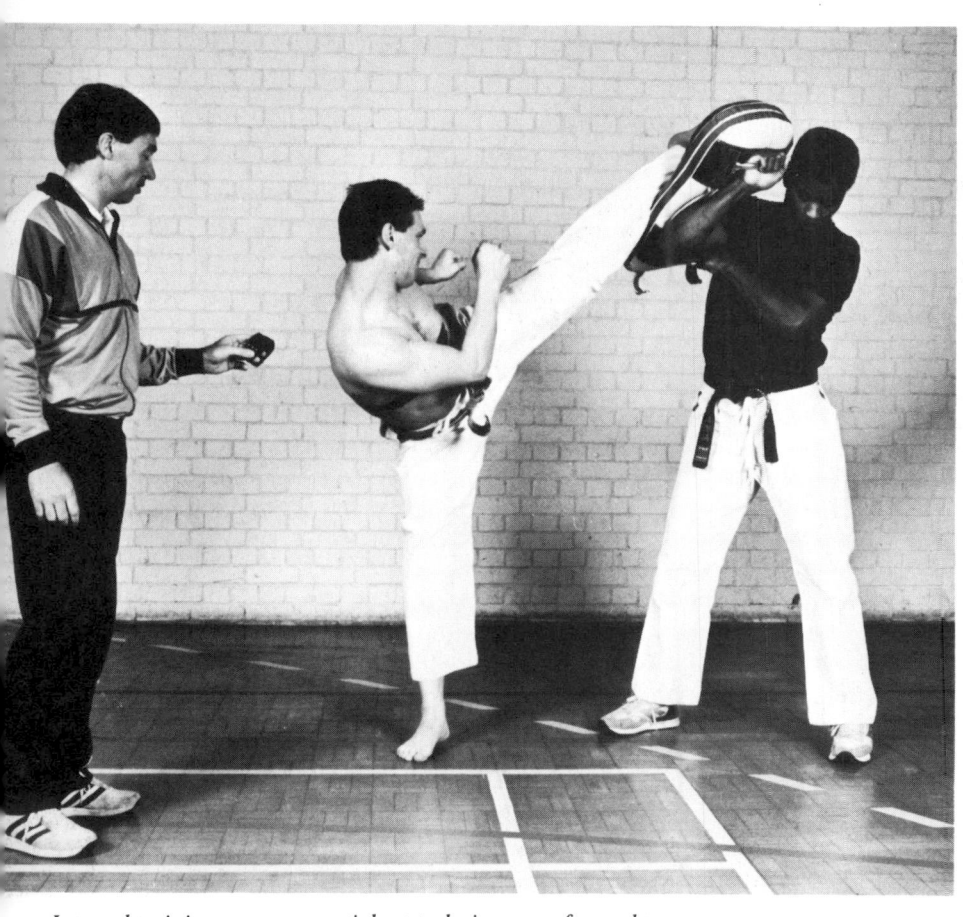

Interval training can use martial art techniques performed to a count

sprints with 15 seconds rest separating each sprint and one minute separating each set.

A fifth regime requires you to work as hard as you can for as long as you can, then rest until your pulse rate drops back to a pre-determined figure. The only difficulty arises from determining what that pulse rate will be.

If the exercises you are doing are very severe, then good form can be encouraged by what is termed the 'pyramid' system. You might choose to do a double kick into the punch bag, so work flat out for 20 seconds, rest for ten seconds, then work for fifteen seconds. Rest again for ten seconds, then do ten seconds work, rest, then five seconds and finish.

Deciding the durations of the work and rest phases is an art more than a science. You must know how severe the exercise is and key the timings in with the work demand generated by your choice. Three minute rounds are a good basis for martial artists to work to since they are related to bout lengths in competition. Consider also how many bursts of activity you will work into the work phases and how long each will be. The more strenuous the exercise you have selected, the shorter the work phase with longer rest periods.

Research seems to indicate that a

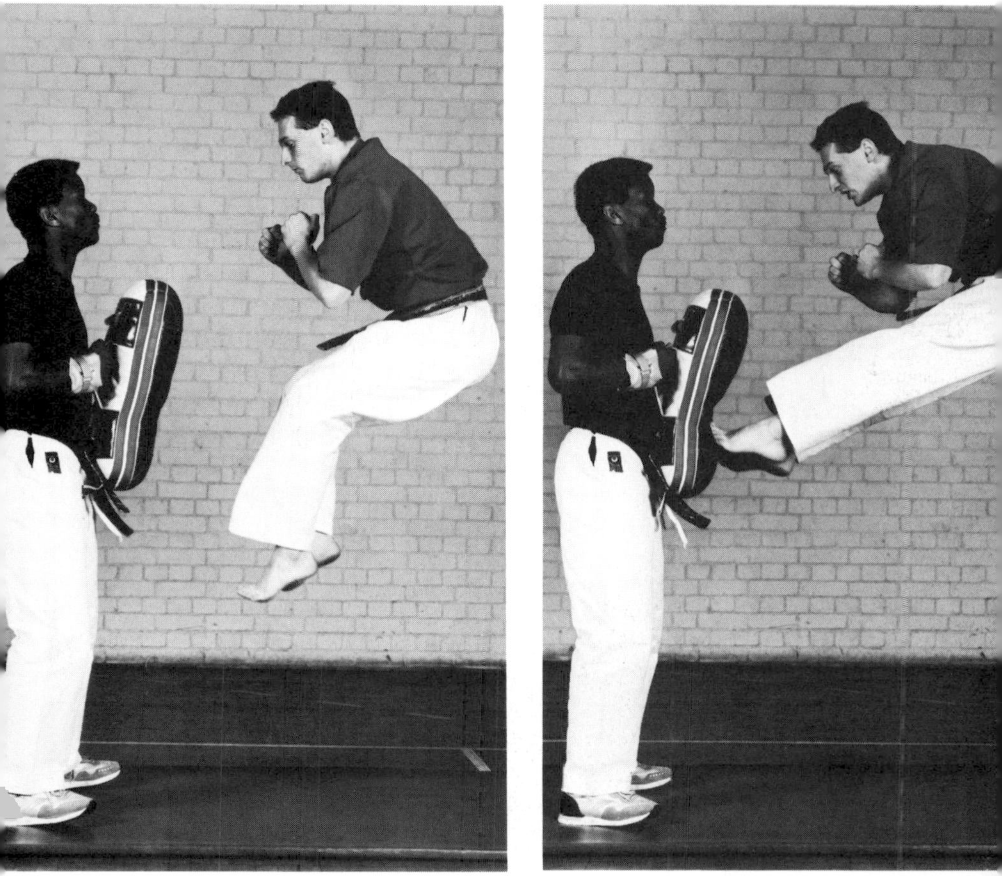

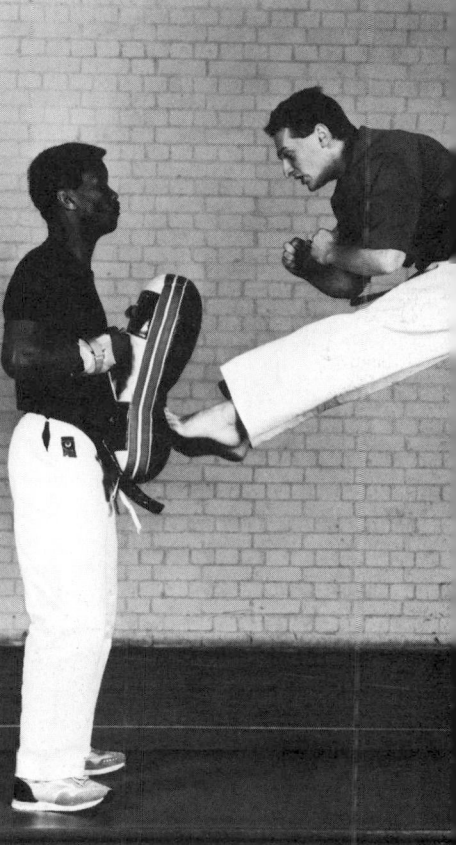

Increase your work rate to match your developing fitness

Calculating a worthwhile break

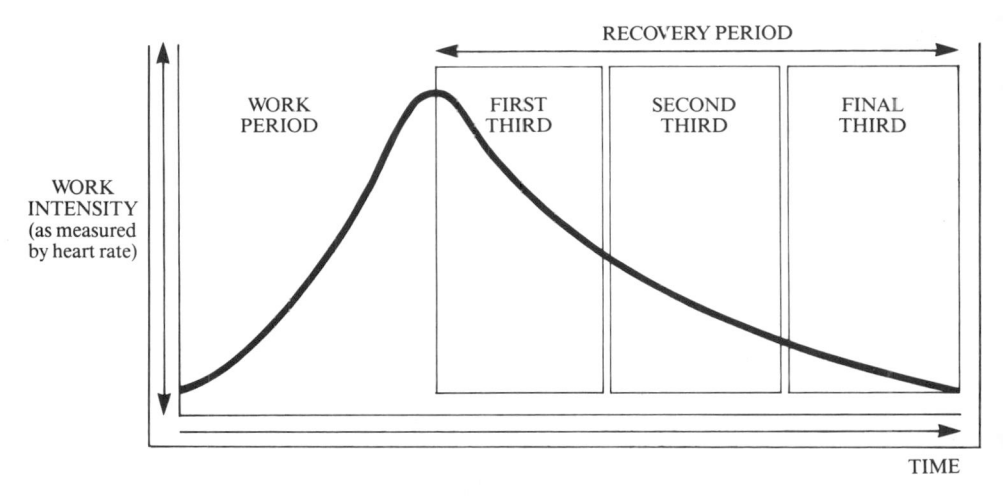

worthwhile break is required. This will last for about a third of the time needed for complete recovery. Shorter rests produce a greater oxygen debt and may tip over into an anaerobic training mode if the work is hard enough.

When designing your schedule, recognise your performance limits. Even a highly trained person can manage only 40 seconds in all-out sprint. Lower levels of fitness mean shorter periods of flat-out exercise. A schedule which demands maximum output and quality over six sets, each of 30 seconds is pushing it somewhat. In such a format, expect either to lose technique quality, or to have to resort to cheating.

Interval work is a good medium for exercises which build agility and coordination and it is the basis of over-training, ie putting skills under pressure.

Traditional Training Methods

The need for supplementary fitness training to benefit martial art practice has long been known. If legend is to be believed, then there is one particular instance where the supplementary exercise came before a martial art and that is in the case of *Shaolin Temple boxing*. This mainline development of Chinese martial arts is said to have come about from two exercises taught to the monks of Shaolin Monastery by the Indian monk Boddidharma. Although the exercises are now widely regarded as martial art practice forms, they are not. They were intended as a means of making the monks of Shaolin fitter to endure the rigours of their austere religious training. In time, these two exercises came to be used in conjunction with martial arts training proper.

The Shaolin Temple is significant in early martial art development and the first clear supplementary training regimens derive from there. The six foot staff was a traditional weapon of Shaolin and practised extensively by those monks with a martial arts interest. The staff was made from dense, heavy timber and possessed both inertia (resistance to movement) and momentum (the tendency of a moving object to continue moving). It was used both as a weapon and as a means of strengthening the arms, shoulders and upper body and various training patterns of linked techniques were devised for this purpose.

The staff would be swung in wide arcs, the body twisting with it. It would also be used in short, jerky thrusts or cuts. In the latter training method, movement was always arrested with a sudden jerk as the muscles of the upper body were tensed. This was found to greatly benefit the unarmed combat systems because the short, fast movements and muscle tensing generated power in punches and strikes. The staff is still used for this purpose in many forms of modern-day kung fu.

The 'wooden man' was another training aid used by the Shaolin monks to develop strikes and punches. It consisted of a balk of timber sunk deep into the ground and wedged upright with stones. Short spars representing crude arms and legs jutted from the trunk at different angles. The practitioner would stand close to and move around the wooden man, gripping the spars and striking the trunk. This training was performed in conjunction with a special skin dressing and made the forearms and hands less sensitive to impact damage.

The wooden man is still used by traditional schools of kung fu. Modern variants are supported on two springy rails resilient to impact.

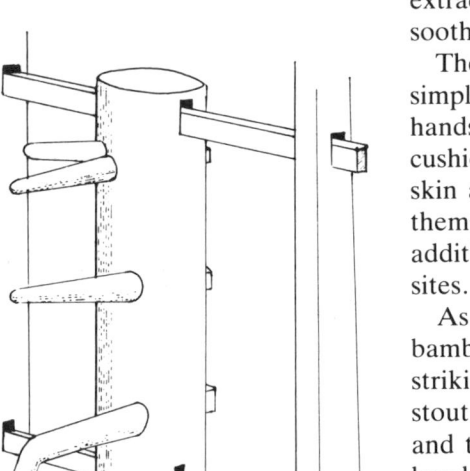

The kung fu wooden man

A heavy iron bar was held in the crook of the elbows and flung into the air by simultaneous straightening of the arms. As it fell, it was caught just behind the wrists and rolled back to the elbows, from whence the cycle was repeated. This training also toughened the forearms.

The hand and fist were trained using cloth bags containing earth hung against a wall. These were repeatedly punched and struck with palm heel, knife hand etc. When the hand became used to this level of training, a gradually increasing quantity of sand was added to the bags until the pure sand stage was reached. To develop claw- and spear hand, the fingers were driven first into earth, then into sand and finally into pebbles. In more severe schools, iron balls were heated in a metal bowl and the fingers driven into that.

All this type of training was associated with application of an extract of herbs which appeared to soothe bruises and cover lacerations.

The purpose of such training is simply to transform the arms and hands into more effective weapons by cushioning the bones with thickened skin and by strengthening the bones themselves through deposition of additional bone material on impact sites.

As has been previously mentioned, bamboos were used to train for faster striking techniques. The ends of tall, stout canes were lashed to the wrist and the arm drawn back against the bamboo's natural springiness.

Traditional Okinawan karate training methods resemble those of earlier mainland China. The six foot staff, for example, was extensively used both as a weapon and a training aid for unarmed combat. Short thrusting moves and cuts were assembled into training routines called *kata*.

Many movements from the staff kata were reproduced with bare hands and can still be identified in present day katas. With the phasing out of staff work in karate practice, the original meanings of these techniques have been lost and they are now submerged in a welter of incorrect speculation.

The old Okinawan karate masters were renowned for the speed and force of their techniques and some authorities have claimed this came about through supplementary training with the staff. When karate was introduced to the Japanese mainland, use of the staff was no longer taught and perhaps modern karate has suffered as a result.

The Chinese punching pad was replaced by the Okinawans with the *makiwara*. This is a springy post, the lower half of which is sunk into the ground and the upper half is faced

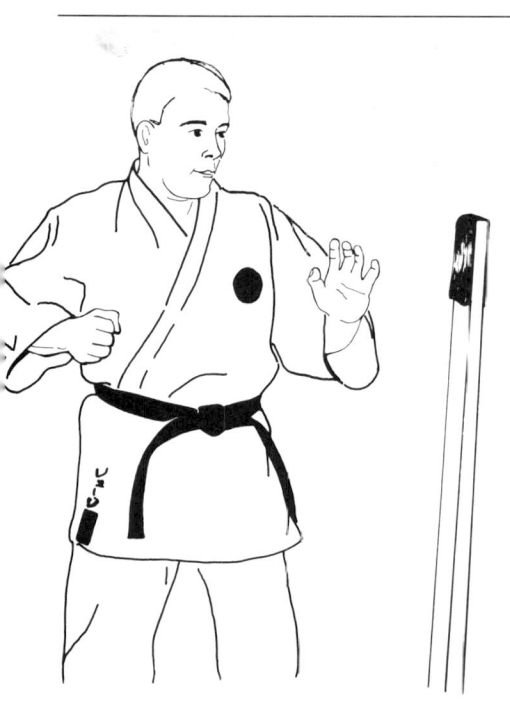

Stand with your left side inclined towards the punching pad

Strike the pad with the fist

with a rice straw pad. The pad is repeatedly struck with the hand or arm, beginning gently and gradually building as the limbs get used to training. The makiwara is very good for developing a correctly-shaped fist and in the illustrations, the teacher is standing with his left side inclined towards the punching pad. Note that the pad in this case is made of hard rubber. This is more hygienic and easier to obtain than rice straw.

The teacher turns his hips into the pad and punches it, with knuckles turned palm-downwards. Unlike the typical karate punch, there is no forearm rotation on impact. The drill is the same for other hand techniques.

The *chi'ishi* are lollipops with stone heads and a wooden haft by which they are gripped. These are used in a way vaguely reminiscent of the old Indian clubs and are intended to strengthen blocking techniques. Typi-

cally the practitioner squats down into a low horse-riding stance and lifts up the chi'ishi with one hand. It is then rotated through 180° until it is upright and held out from the body. As the arm tires, so the chi'ishi is returned to the floor once more. Both inside and outside grips can be used, each producing a different training effect. The exercise is repeated and as the body becomes accustomed to training, a heavier chi'ishi is used.

A second exercise is performed from a feet-apart standing stance. The practitioner reaches forwards and lifts the chi'ishi, taking it around and behind his back before squatting into horse-riding stance and simultaneously bringing the chi'ishi slowly over his head and down into the arm-extended position.

A third exercise uses the chi'ishi in a thrusting motion, driving it out quickly to the side of the body. A

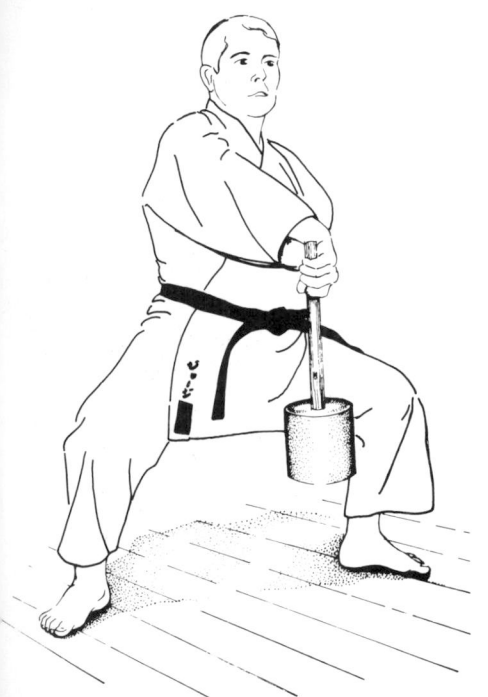

Lift the chi'ishi with one hand...

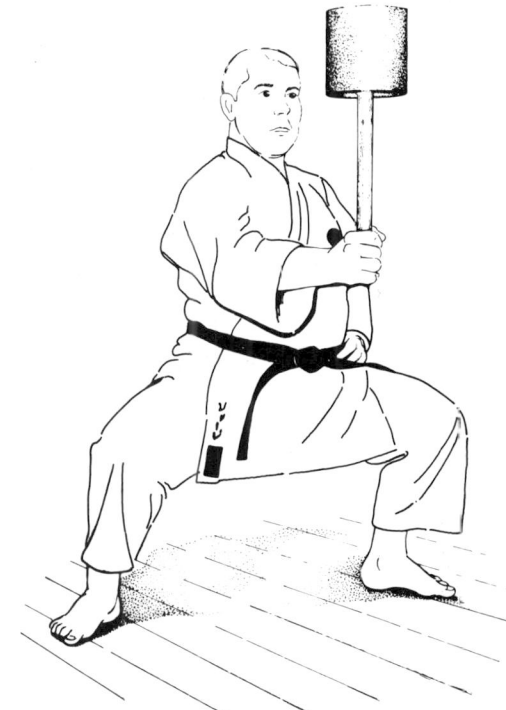

and twist it upright

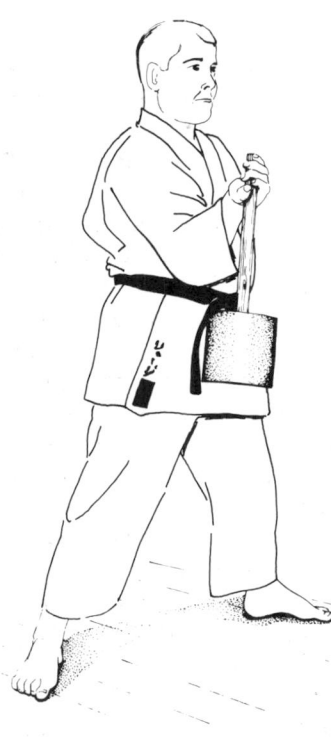

Lift the chi'ishi

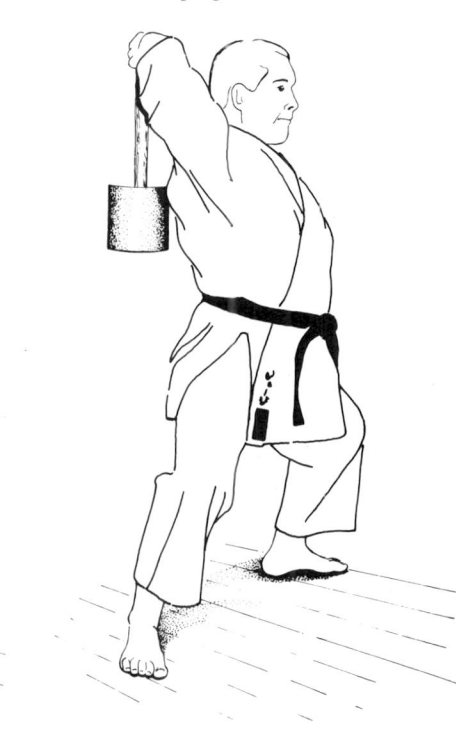

Swing it behind your back...

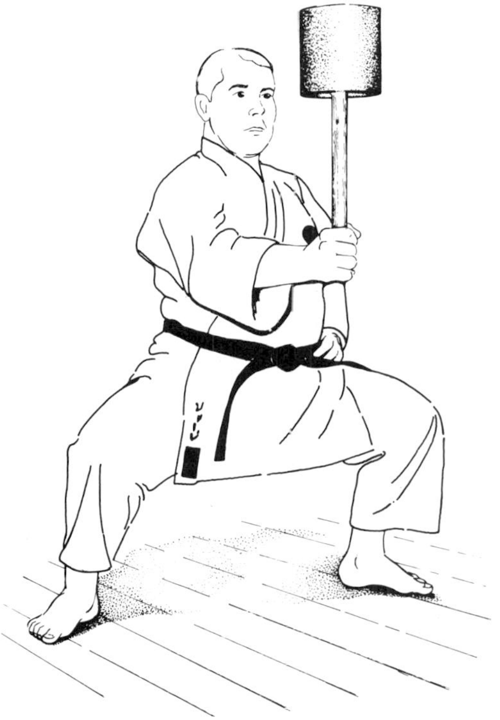

and bring it down in front of your chest

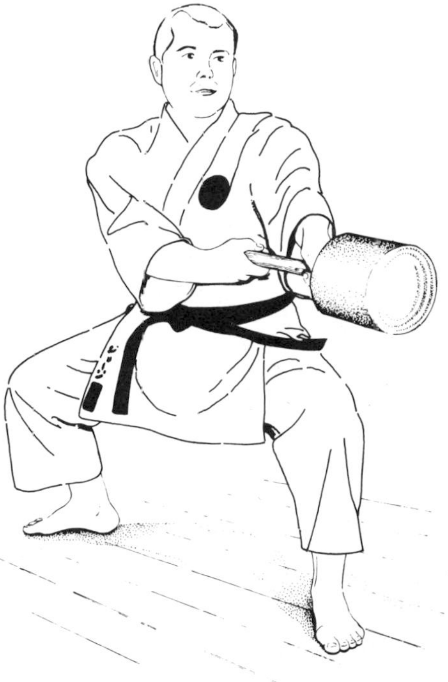

Thrust the chi'ishi to the side of the body

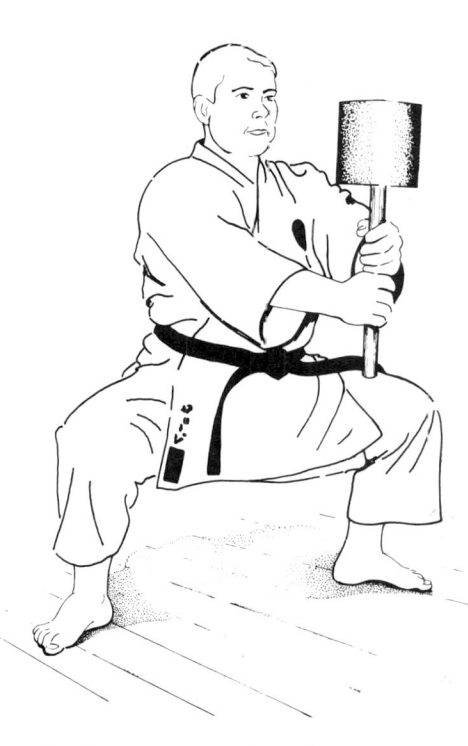

Apply a contra-rotating grip

fourth exercise applies a contra-rotating grip to the handle of the chi'ishi which is held out from the body by both arms. A fifth exercise rolls the chi'ishi handle along the forearm. This latter routine conditions the forearm and makes it less susceptible to bruising.

In the modern training hall, the chi'ishi is made by pouring concrete into a paint pot from which projects a wooden handle. A couple of nails stick out from the submerged portion of the handle, to anchor it firmly into the concrete.

The *ishi-sashi* are flat bottomed iron weights with an integral carrying handle. They are used in a normal weight-training manner and also for strengthening the kicking action. For this latter purpose, a weight is lifted by the instep and upper surface of the toes.

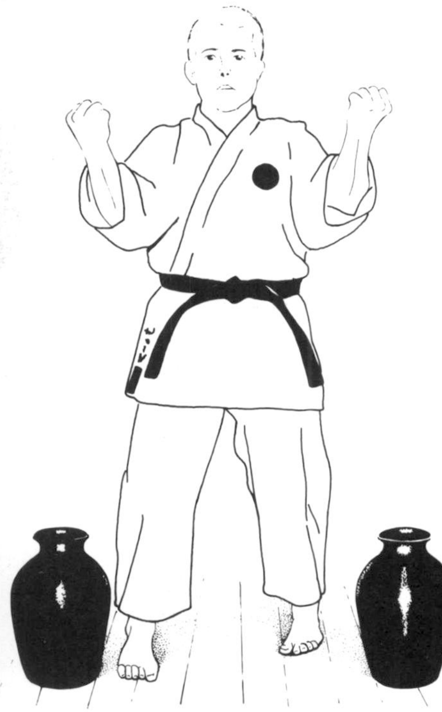

The nigiri *are earthenware jars*

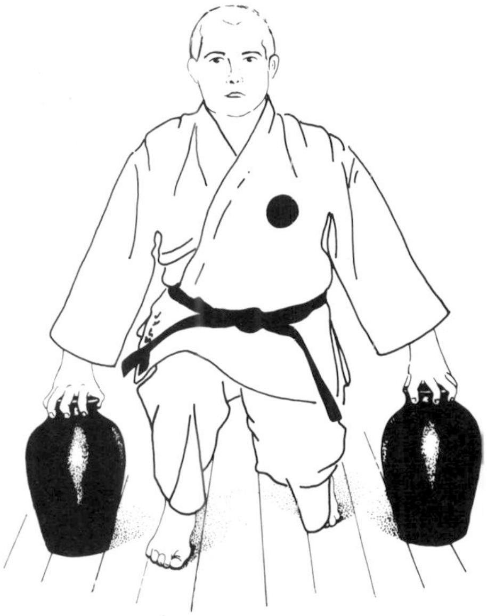

Squat down to pick them up

The Japanese used a variant of these weights known as the 'iron sandals'. These were flat iron weights strapped to the feet and used to increase the force of a kick. They are sometimes used for ballistic stretching of the legs, a practice which we would not recommend.

The *nigiri* are earthenware jars with a neck diameter sufficient to allow the thumb and finger ends to grasp. The practitioner squats down to pick them up and carries them whilst advancing up and down the training hall. Sometimes they are swung well out in front of the body, other times they are held out to the sides. The legs may also be worked by carrying nigiri whilst holding a low stance. When these exercises can be performed easily, weight is gradually added by filling each jar with stones or sand.

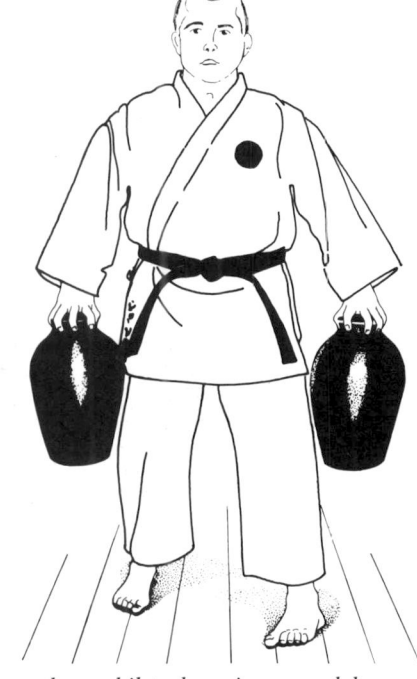

Carry them whilst advancing up and down the training hall

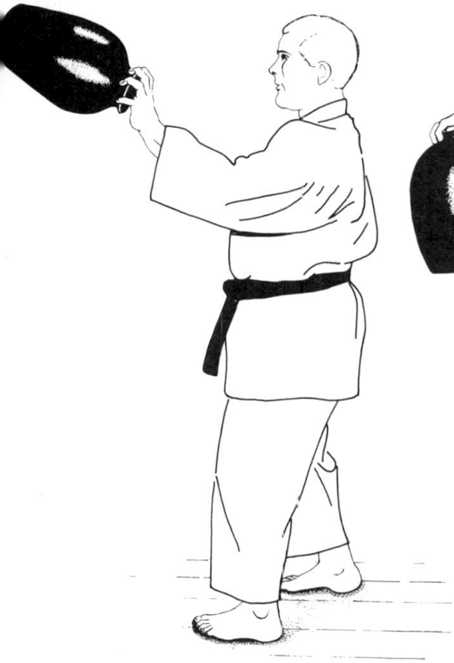

Swing them to the front… 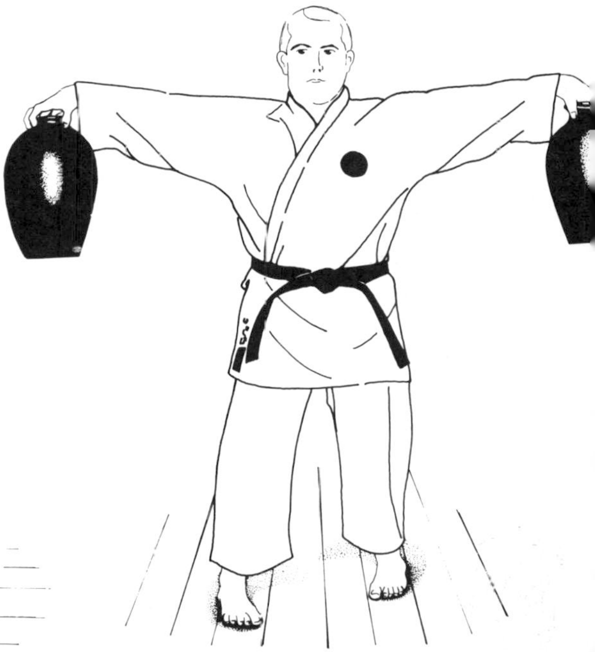   *or to the sides*

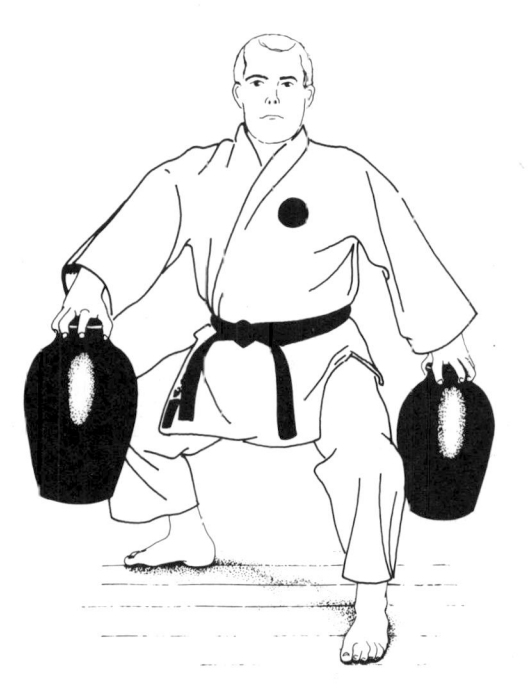

Using them whilst in a low stance works the legs

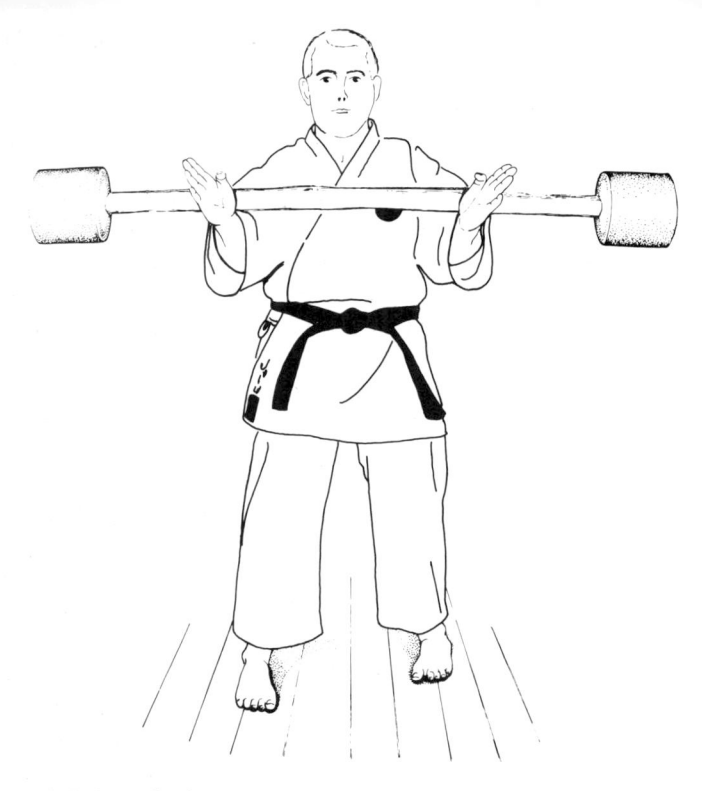

The tan *is rolled along the forearms*

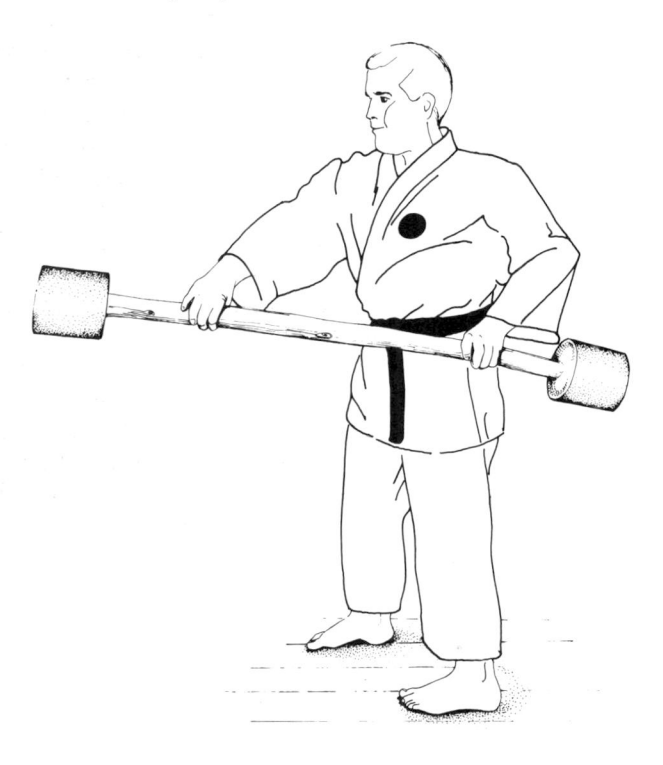

It can also be swung from side to side...

The *tan* is a primitive weight training device made from two heavy stones pierced by a long wooden shaft. It was used as one would utilise any such modern training weight and in addition it was rolled along the forearms, to condition them in much the same way as the practitioners of kung fu used the iron bar. It is also used in a broad swinging action that twists the spine, or with vertical rotation that turns it through 180°.

The *kongoken* is an iron oblong weighing at least 45 kilos. It is used with a whole series of specialised weight training exercises, one example of which is a form of leg squats. The kongoken is rested with one end on the floor in front of the practitioner and the other on the back of the neck

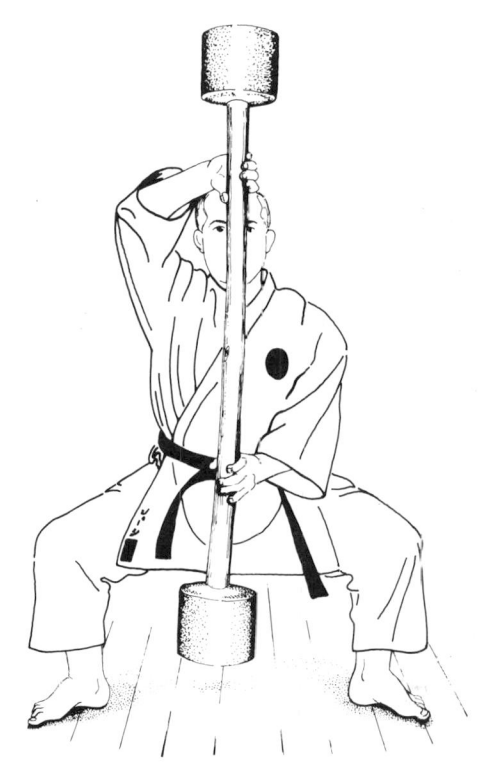

or turned through 180°

and shoulders. The practitioner drops into a low horse-riding stance and then straightens to an erect, feet-apart stance. To make press-ups more arduous, the kongoken can be rested on the back of the neck.

Earlier forms of Korean martial art used a punching post similar to the makiwara to train the hands. The Koreans still train to break wooden boards as part of their examination syllabus.

Jiu jitsu and aikido practice still involve staff and stick training as a means of strengthening the grip and making the shoulders more flexible.

Not all supplementary training used equipment. Many years before Charles Atlas developed his system called 'Dynamic Tension', the Okinawans had produced a training pattern called *sanchin* which pitted opposing muscles against each other. This is a later development of even earlier mainland Chinese forms. The whole body is tensed and the arms held out from the body and bent at the elbows. The hips are raised up and forwards and the knees driven outwards.

Movement between successive sanchin stances is in the form of fast semicircular steps.

This kata and its Chinese predecessors were believed to be the cornerstone of powerful karate and early practitioners often spent as long as three years doing nothing else! The kata was said to build great strength, stability and a body better able to withstand hard knocks.

Peaking Performance

Whilst there is a need for progressive training in the martial arts, you may wish to prepare yourself to do especially well in a particular grading or championships. Getting as prepared as you can be for a particular event is known as 'peaking'.

The more time you spend in preparation, the more effective it will be. Don't expect a bit of extra training the night before to do you a great deal of good. Set yourself a plan of preparation with realistic intermediate targets to work from and this will help you both to feel in control and to cover all training aspects in a logically connected manner. This is an important aid to motivation.

When you develop your programme, remember that:

1. The programme must develop all the components of fitness together with the technique work that you have decided is necessary.
2. All higher level or anaerobic training must be built on a sound aerobic base.
3. The training routines you are using must come to simulate what you will face at the event you are preparing for.
4. Setting intermediate targets along the way will maintain motivation and maximum training effectiveness.
5. As the event approaches, shorten your training session and aim for highest standards.

Do realise that the martial artist who can work at 100% intensity on every factor required is either a world champion, or will be, given time. Unfortunately not all of us can manage this.

Peaking in the martial arts will usually fall into one of three categories:

1. Peaking for one particular date.
2. Peaking for a short period, say two or three weeks.
3. Peaking for a limited number of events spread over a 'season'.

As a general rule, a true peak can only be achieved for a short time, perhaps one or two weeks and to do this requires a preparation time of between eight and ten months. More and longer peaks can be catered for but the level of performance reached will be lower because the martial artist is not so well tuned for each one.

The organisation of a martial artist's time into sections, each with different aims is termed 'periodisation'. Consider the following:

Period 1 – Pre-Preparation

It is important to have a period in your training year when there are relatively fewer gradings or competitions. In many martial arts, this tends to occur between middle July and early

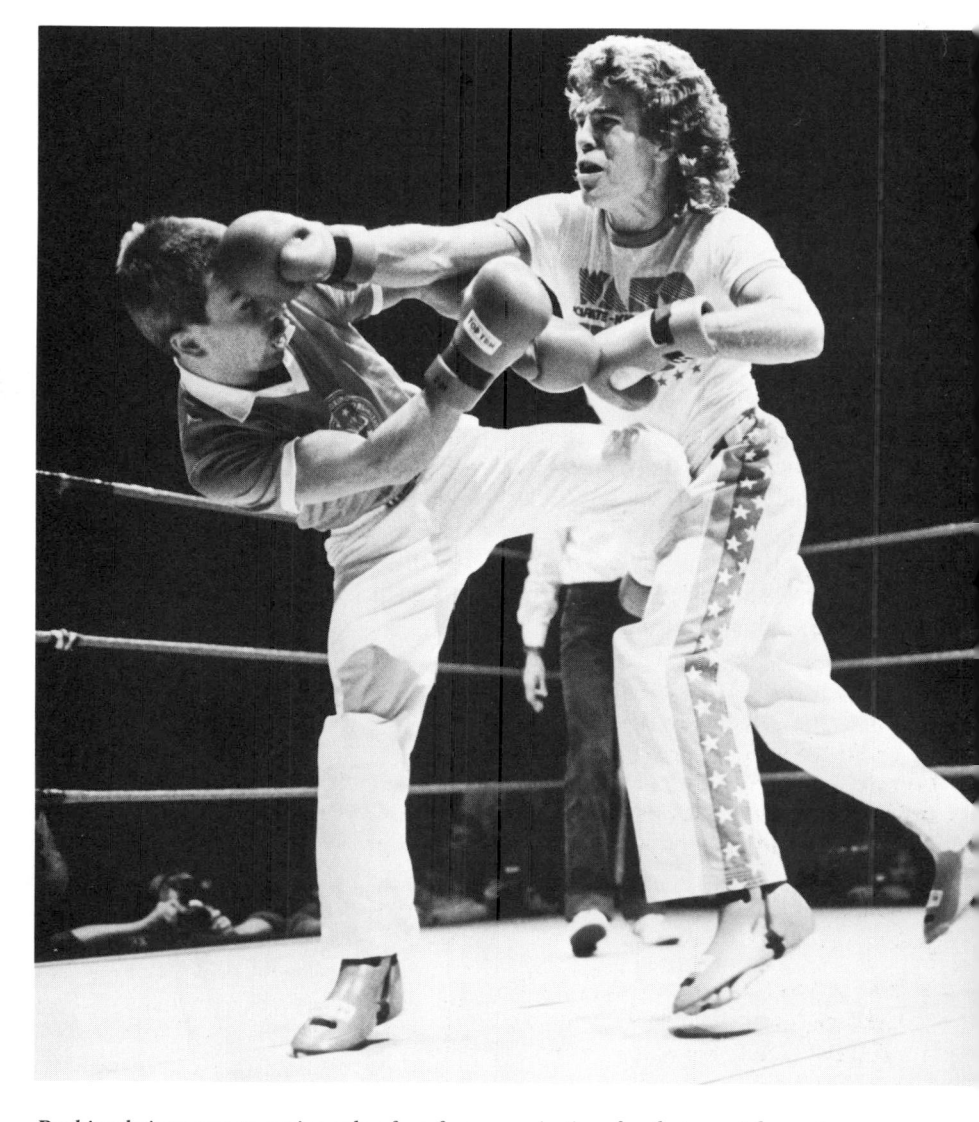

Peaking brings you to a pinnacle of performance in time for that crucial event

September. This is a valuable respite, providing a necessary rest from the high-intensity training associated with gradings and competitions, and helping to prevent the staleness that can occur when you never get a break.

It is not a complete rest however, because you can fill it with aerobic, flexibility and strength work. Improving your aerobic base at that time may help you support more strenuous training later in the programme. You can also use it to establish greater strength in the bits and pieces that are either recovering from injuries, or may be at risk of injury later on. You can fit more flexibility training in too, concentrating on areas of particular weakness. Work on those techniques and patterns you need to improve and set about learning new ones.

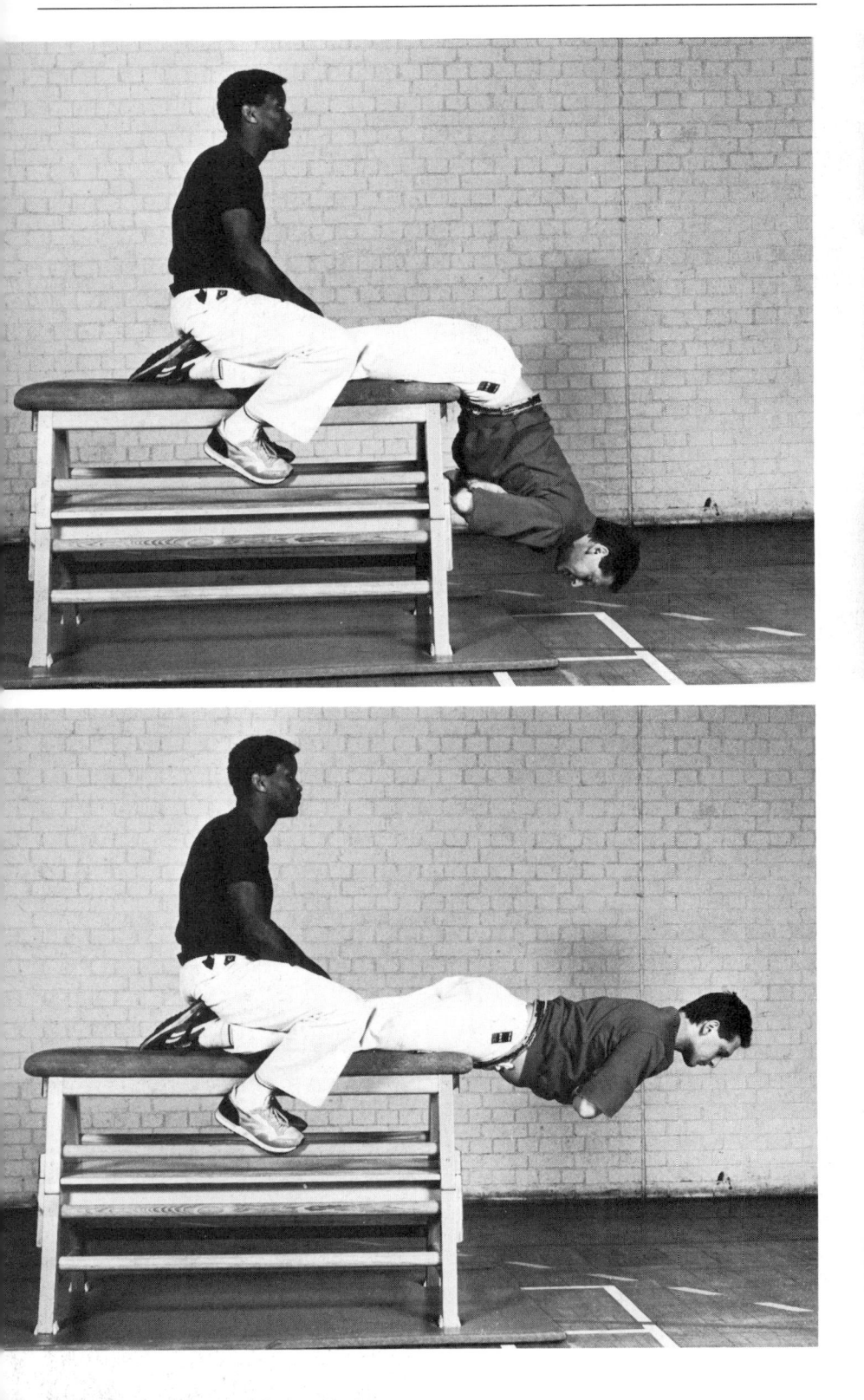

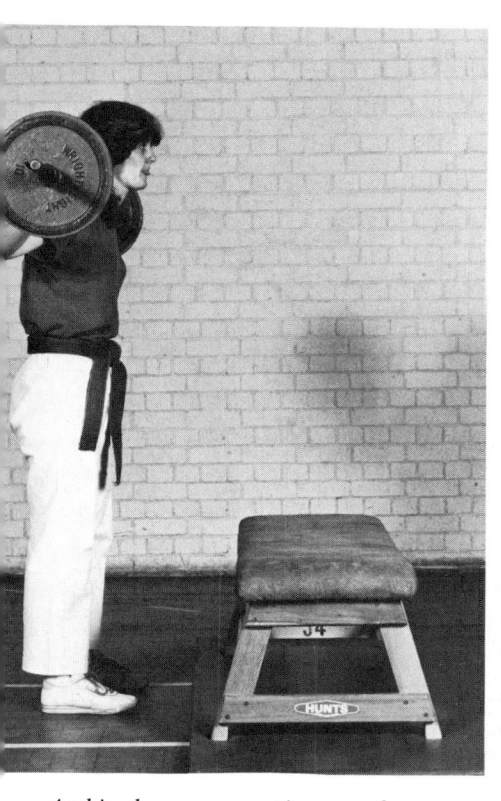

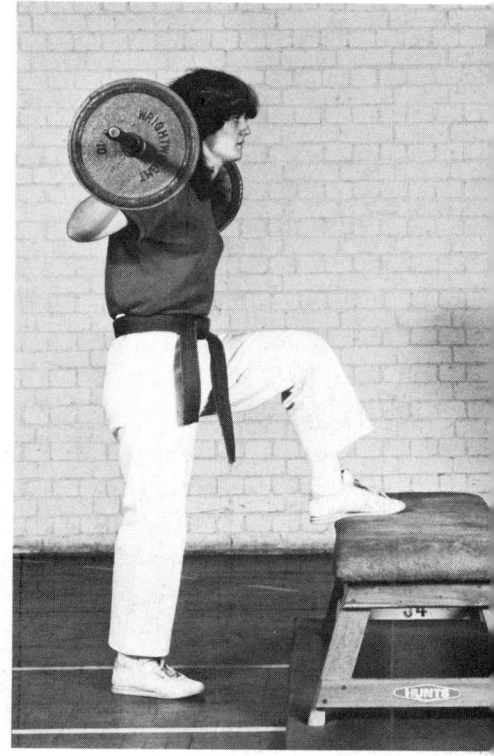

At this phase you must increase the intensity of your training with exercises. Use either body weight exercises (left) or weight training (above and right)

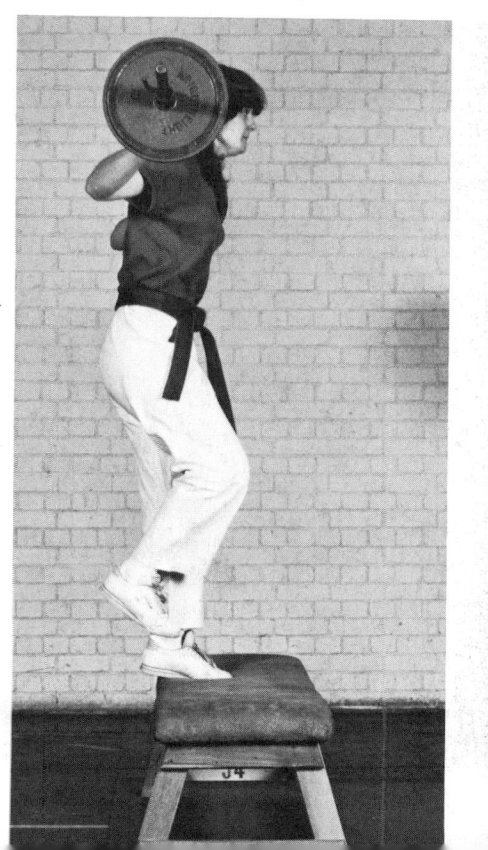

Period 2 – Preparation

As the event programme starts to gear up, increase the intensity of your training, covering aerobic, anaerobic, strength, power and flexibility. If you are fairly advanced, you can concentrate on the last four, otherwise cover them all. Match this acceleration with technique and skill training because now is the time to bring yourself progressively and reasonably quickly to peak performance, using the fitness-base you built up in Period 1.

Period 3 – Into Action

This is the period when most of your competitions and gradings will occur. Keep training though it may not now be possible to maintain the same consistency as in the earlier periods.

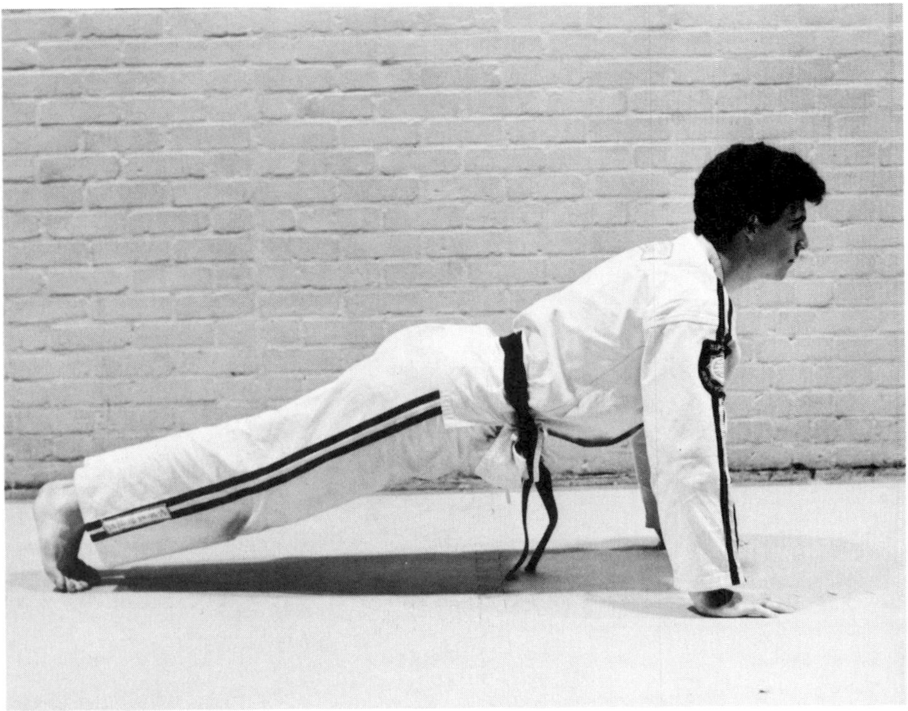

Make sure you gradually reduce the intensity and duration of training in the week before a scheduled event and in the final two days, go for low intensity activity (including skill work) to allow the body to recover from the fatigues of training. Mental

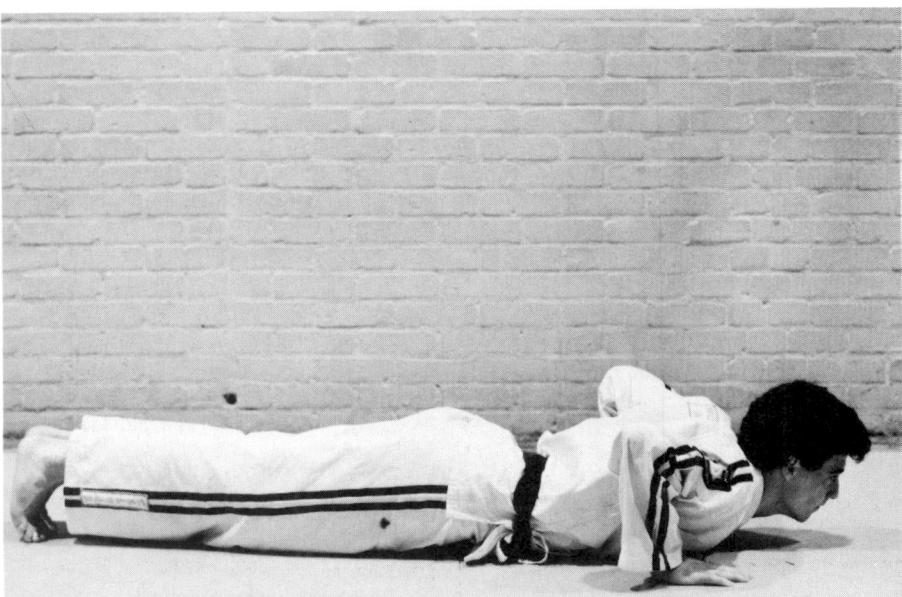

preparation is important during this time.

Return to training after the event, so you can begin preparing for the next. Stay at a high level of fitness by scheduling at least one intensive training session a week, covering such things as power and anaerobic endurance. Maintain your flexibility programme.

As your grading or competition approaches, go for lower intensity training Below left and right. *Alternative forms of press up*

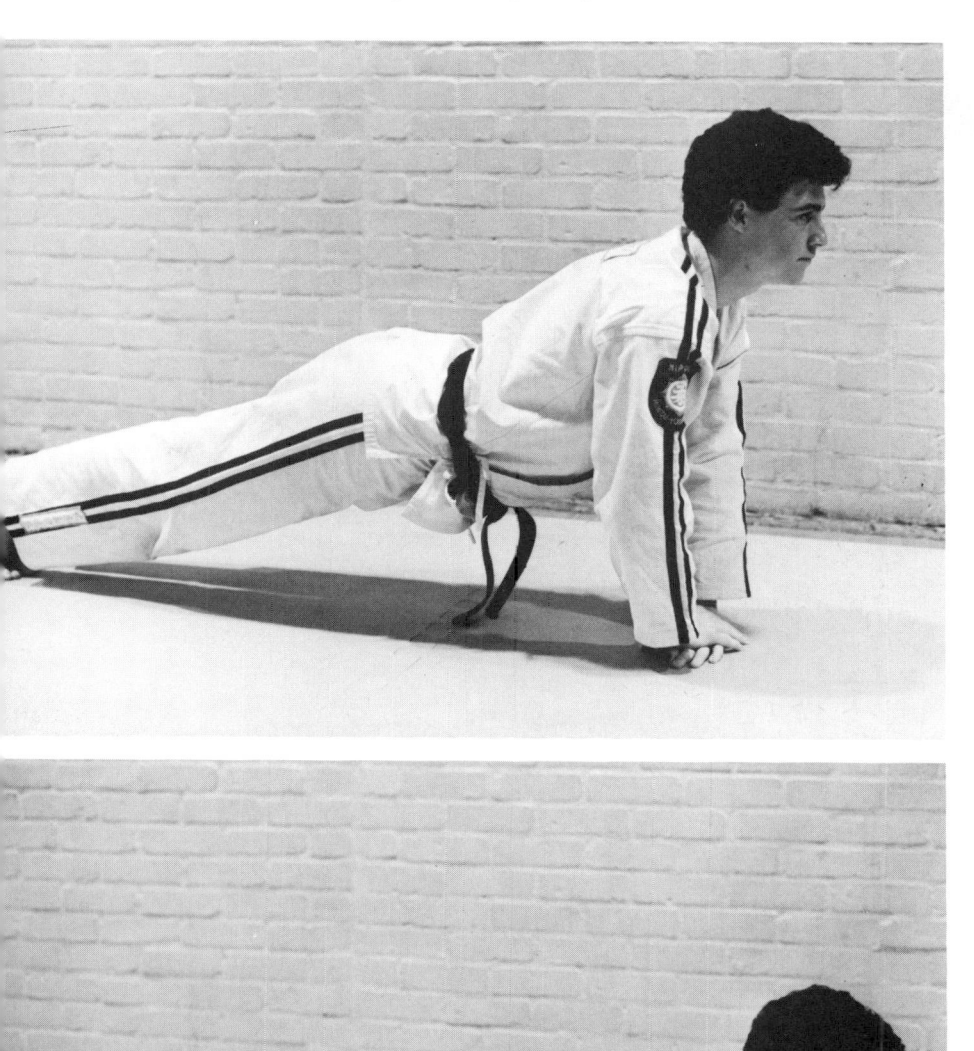

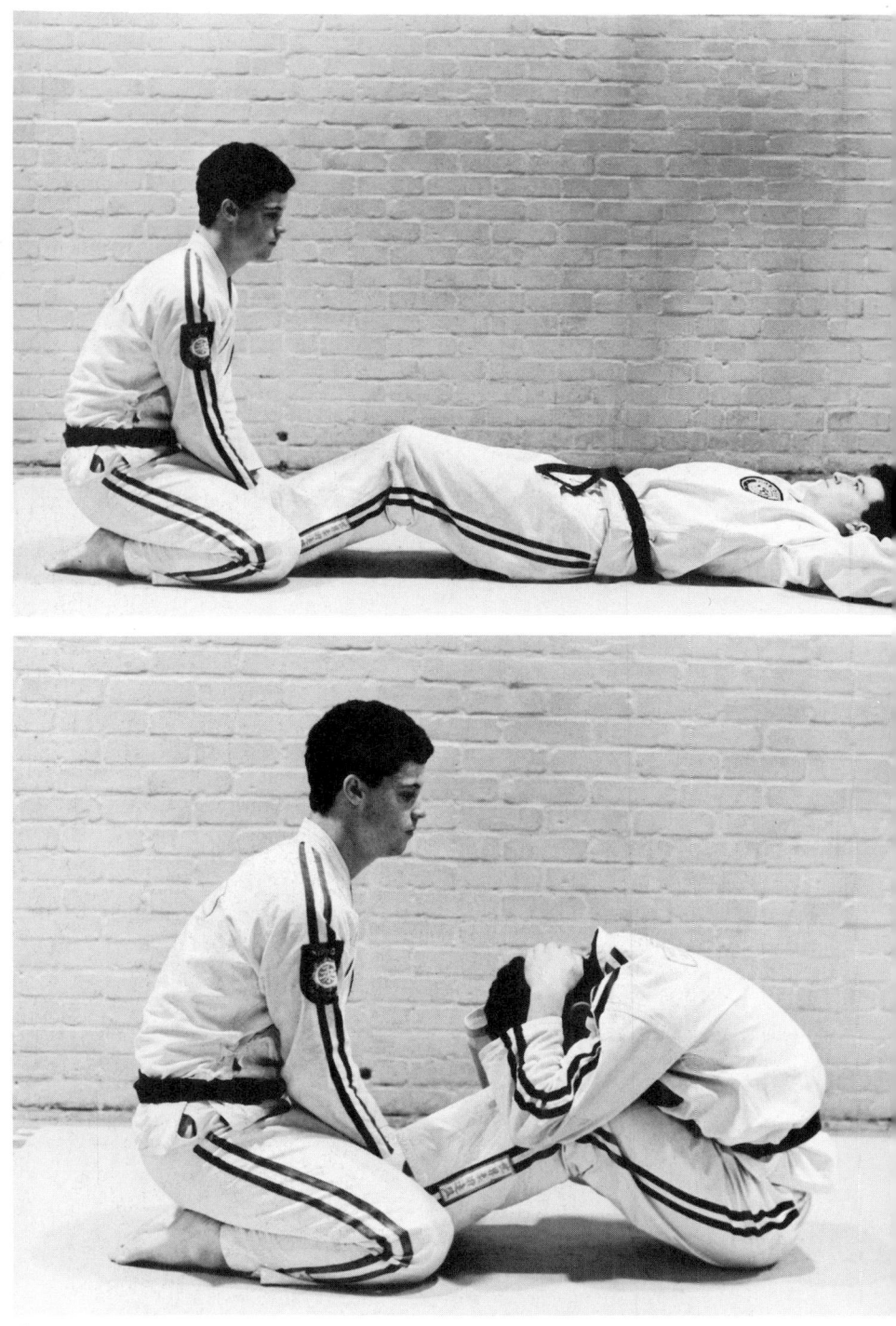

Sit-ups

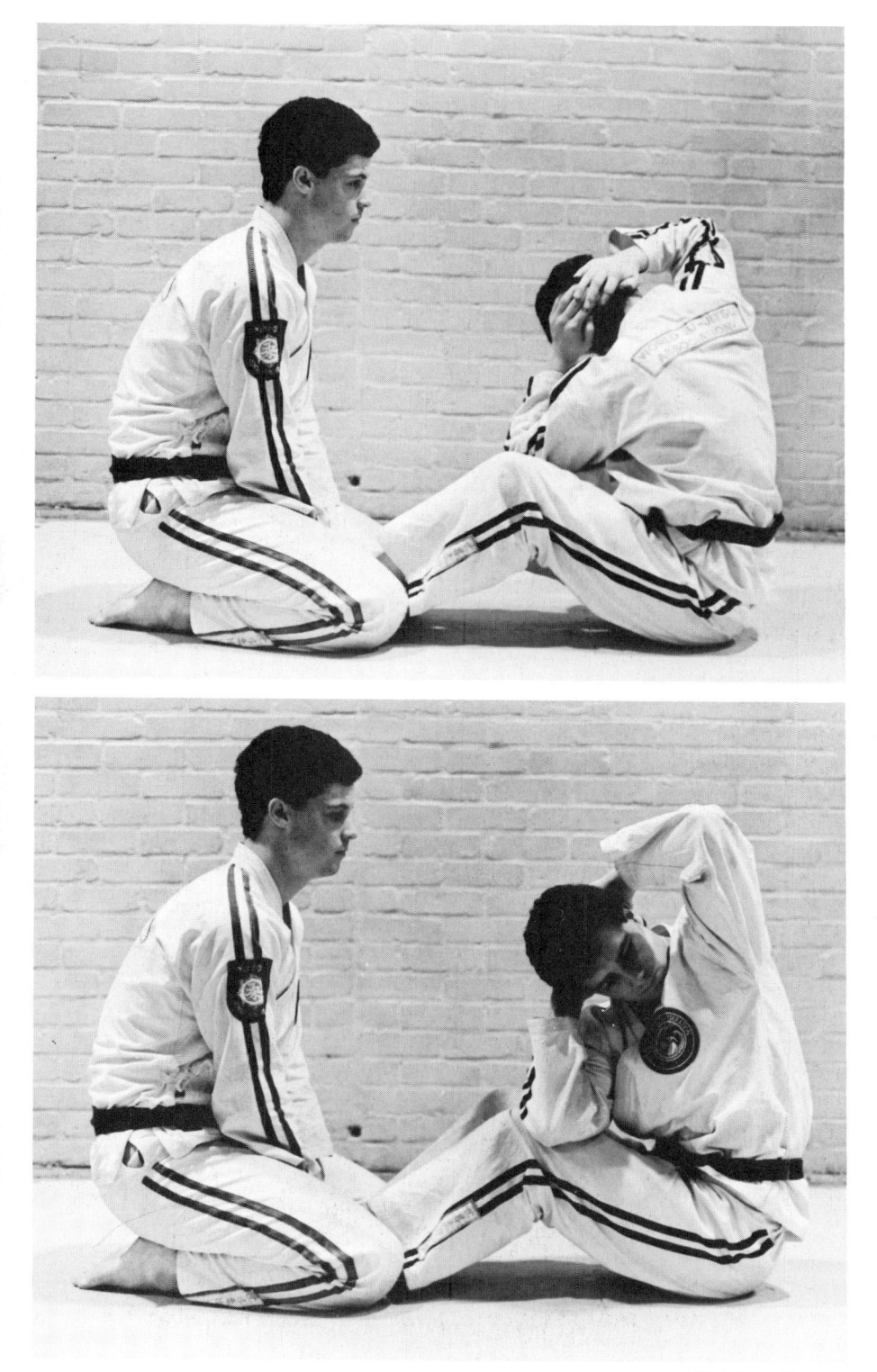

Twisting sit-ups

Period 4 – Transition

This is the time when you schedule your holidays and take a complete break from the martial arts. Go for swimming and gentle running to maintain a basic aerobic condition. In short, have a complete break from all the training and techniques of martial art so that when you come round once more to Period 1, you will be raring to go and fit to fight.

The overall training plan might well look something like this:

Lower intensity, lighter weight circuit training with short recovery intervals.

↓

Heavier weights in regimes, leading to momentary exhaustion and longer rests to allow partial recovery.

↓

High quality pyramid-style training regimes. Loading to near maximum but with rests suitable for virtually total recovery.

|

or

|

Long, steady-state work on basics plus running etc.

↓

Higher intensity work over shorter periods such as free practice or its equivalent over a 10/20 minute period.

↓

Training as near as possible to what you have to face in the event, over two – three minute periods with long recovery periods.

Hopefully you will get enough from this book to give you some ideas of what you should be working at. You and your coach are the proper people to make decisions on your training programme and these will take into account how committed you are, what factors you need to emphasize and what you are aiming for.

Think through the options available and weigh the pros and cons before settling on the programme of your choice. Keep an open mind and be prepared to consider additional information from any source.

Cooling Down

As previously mentioned, it is not at all unusual to feel stiff a day or so after a hard training session. Coordinated smooth movements become difficult and there is discomfort when the affected muscles contract. Some say this could have been avoided had you taken the session a little easier but this is easily said to a highly motivated martial artist who wants to win a competition or succeed in a grading. It seems that in certain circumstances, this stiffness is inevitable.

But is it? Would it be possible to train very hard and then adopt a procedure that would help alleviate discomfort over the next few days? The answer is almost certainly 'YES'. A physiologist named de Vries suggested a 'warm down' programme to follow training. This is now more commonly referred to as a 'cool down'.

The cool down has two stages. The first begins with about four minutes of gentle jogging, followed by a minute's walking. The second stage uses static stretches which concentrate on the muscles that were most used during the training session proper. During the first part of cool down, the heart and respiration rates are gradually returned to more normal levels. It may be that during the second stage, stretching assists in the removal of waste products from the muscles.

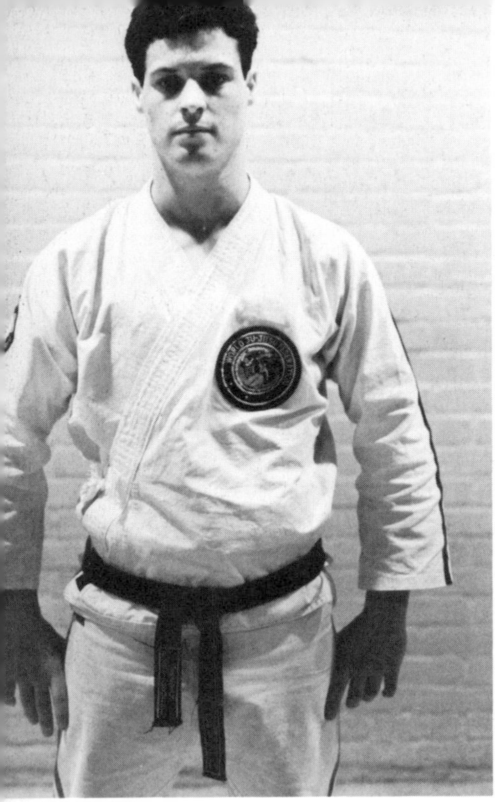

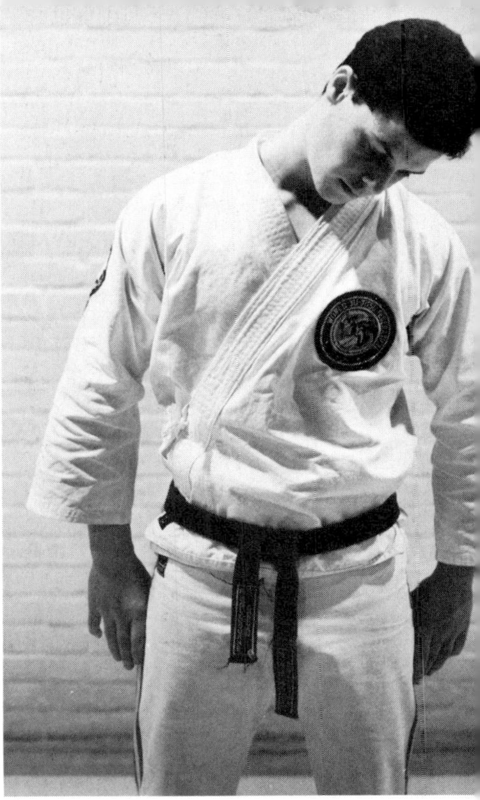

It is important to cool down properly after training. Begin with head circling

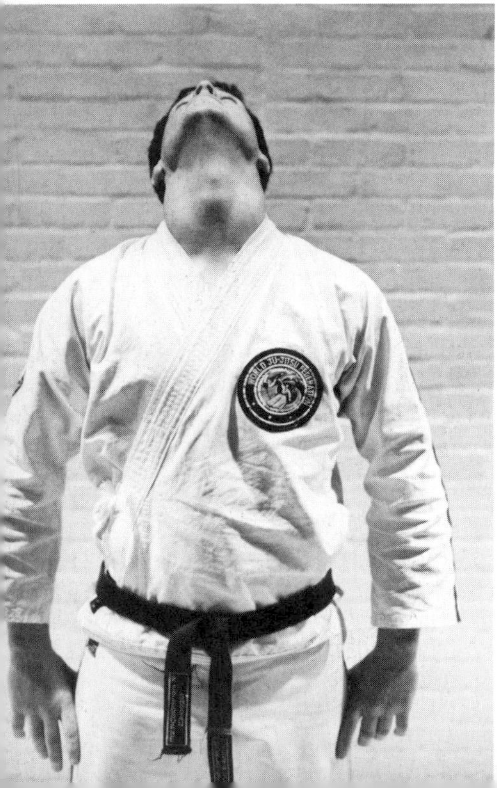

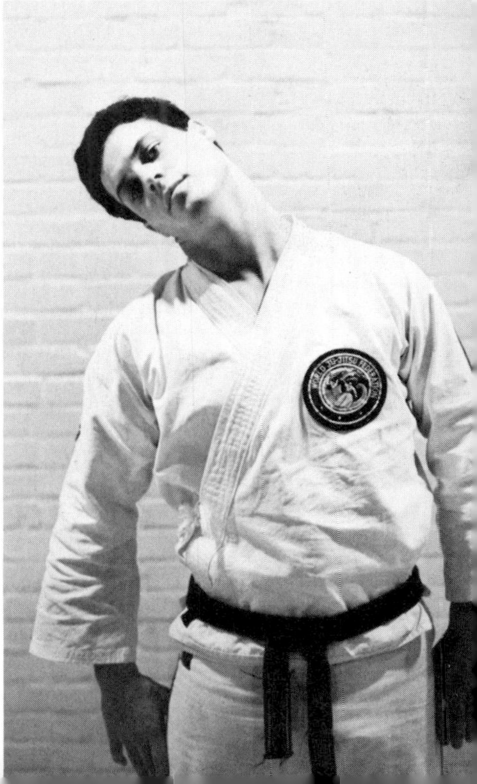

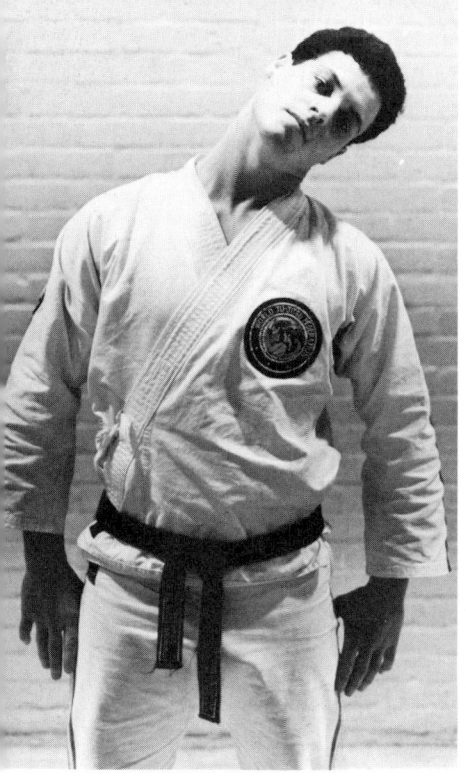
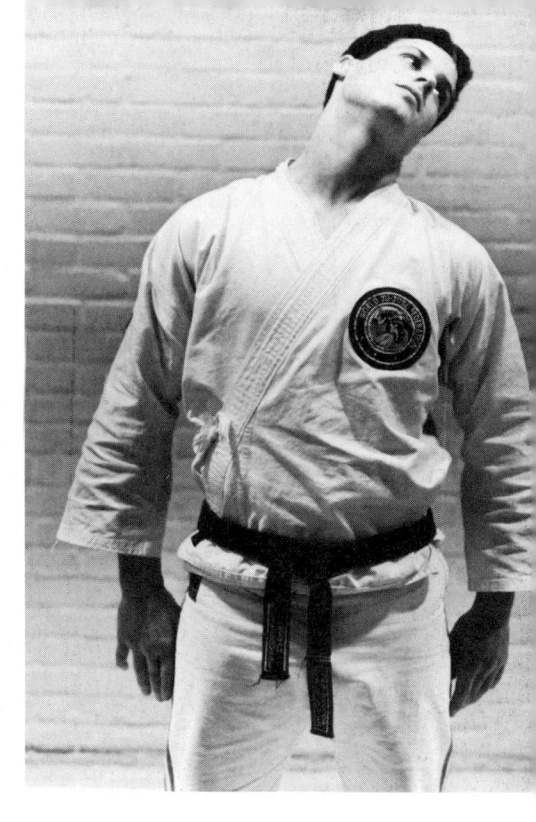
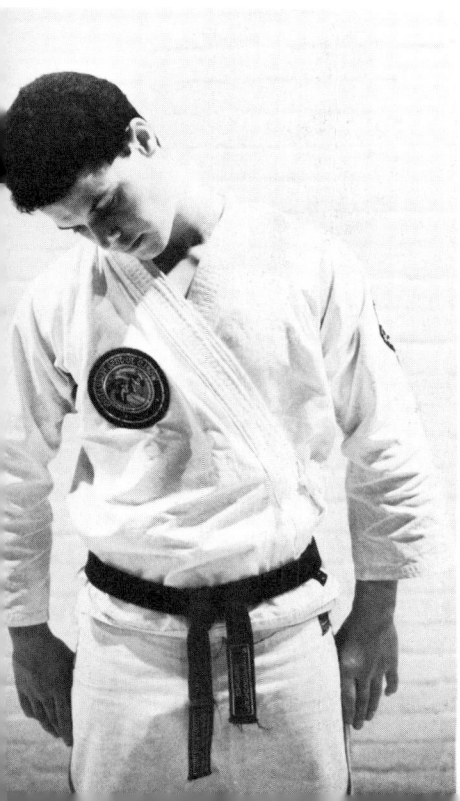
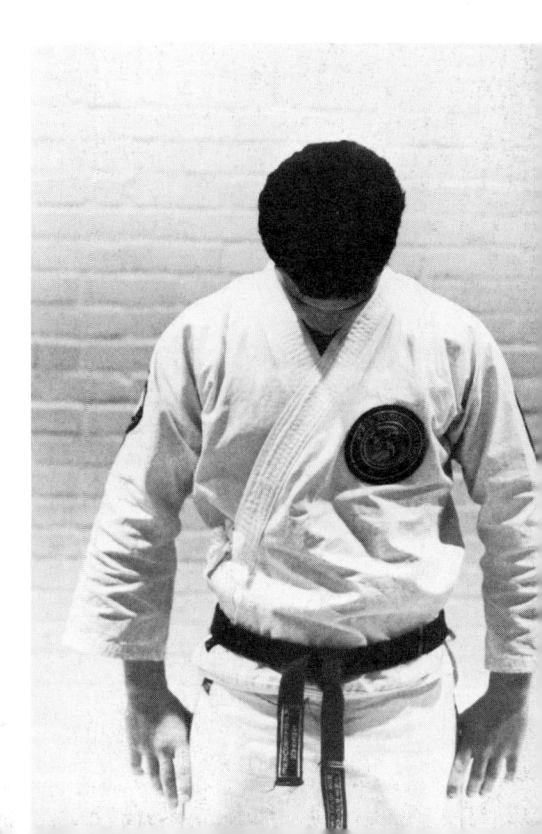

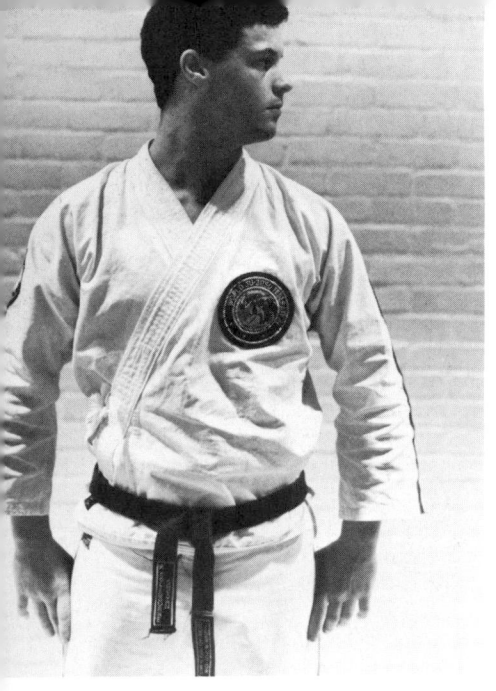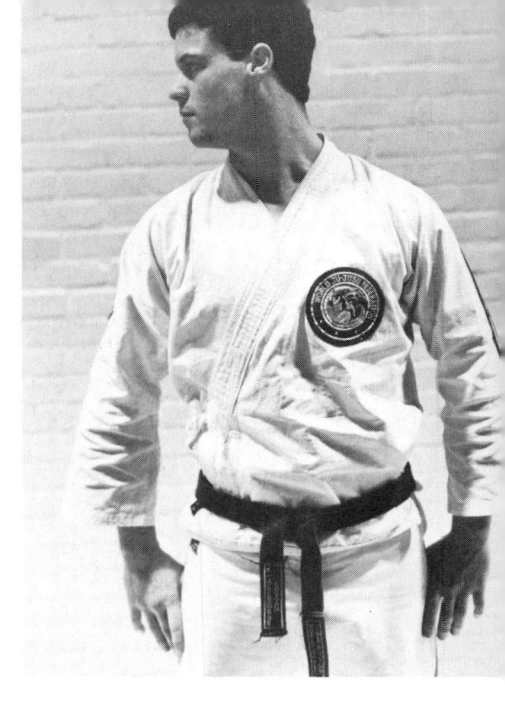

Turn your head from side to side

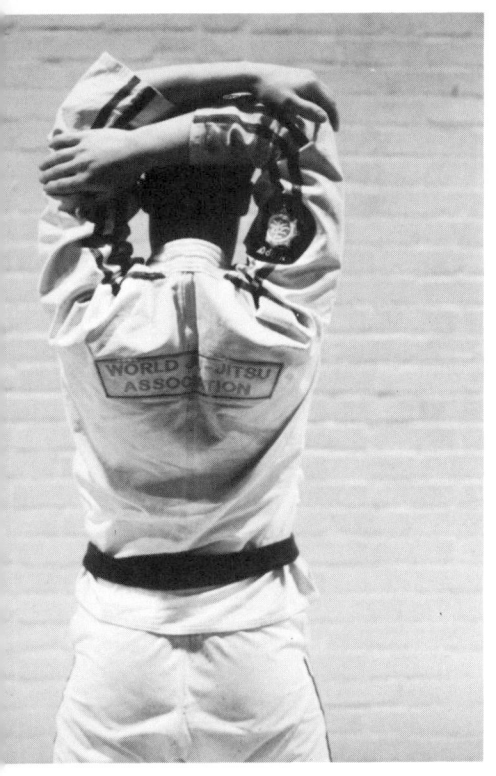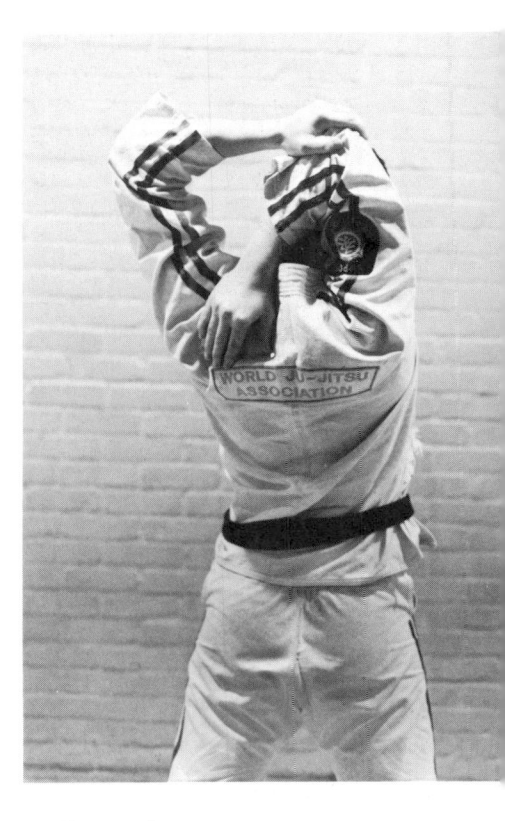

Link arms

Pull your elbow

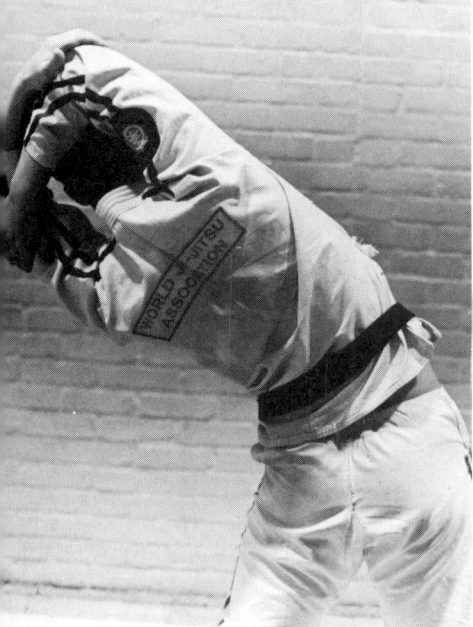

Lean to one side…

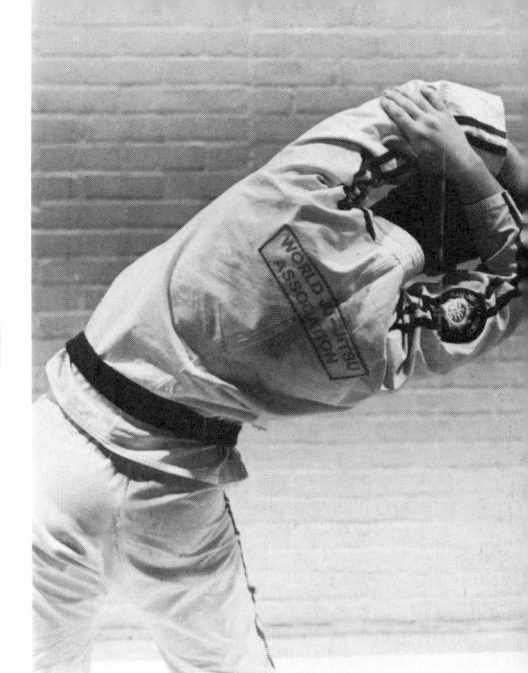

Then to the other

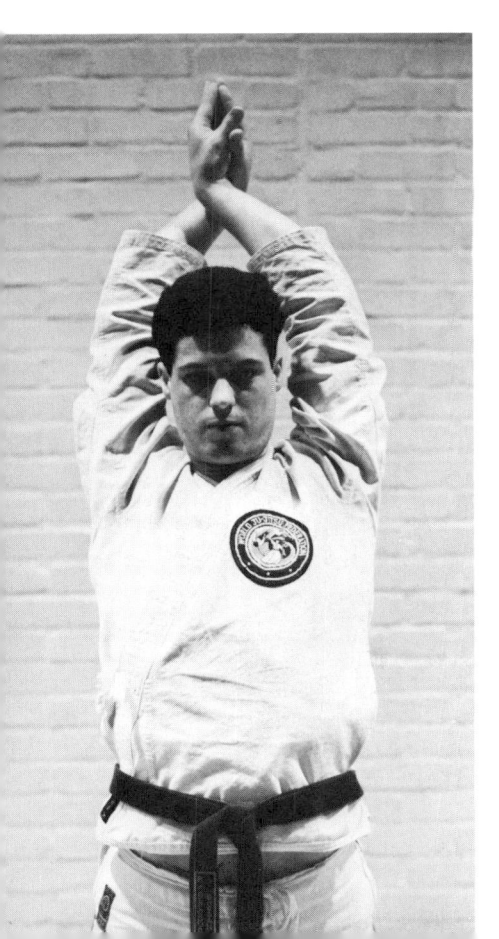

Thrust your arms above your head

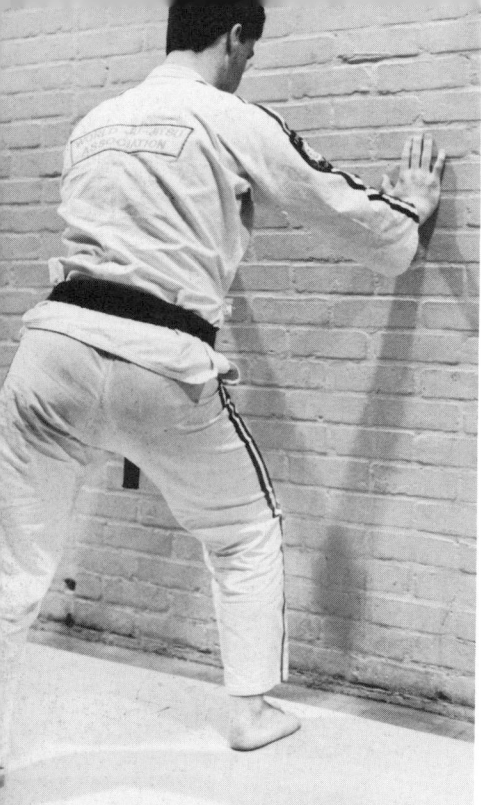 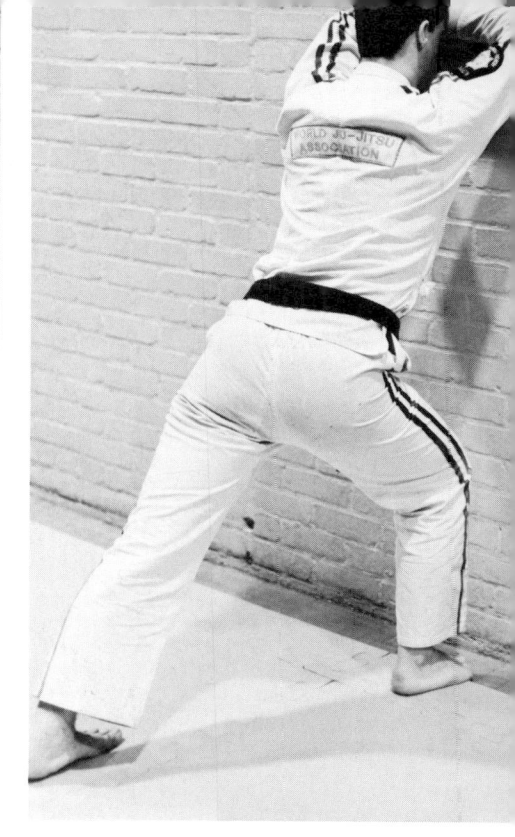

Stretch your Achilles tendon by pushing against a wall with your hands...   *or your elbows*

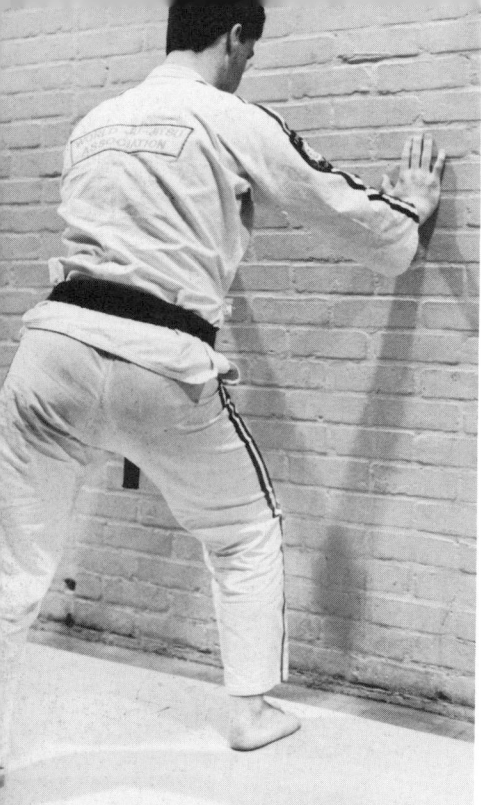

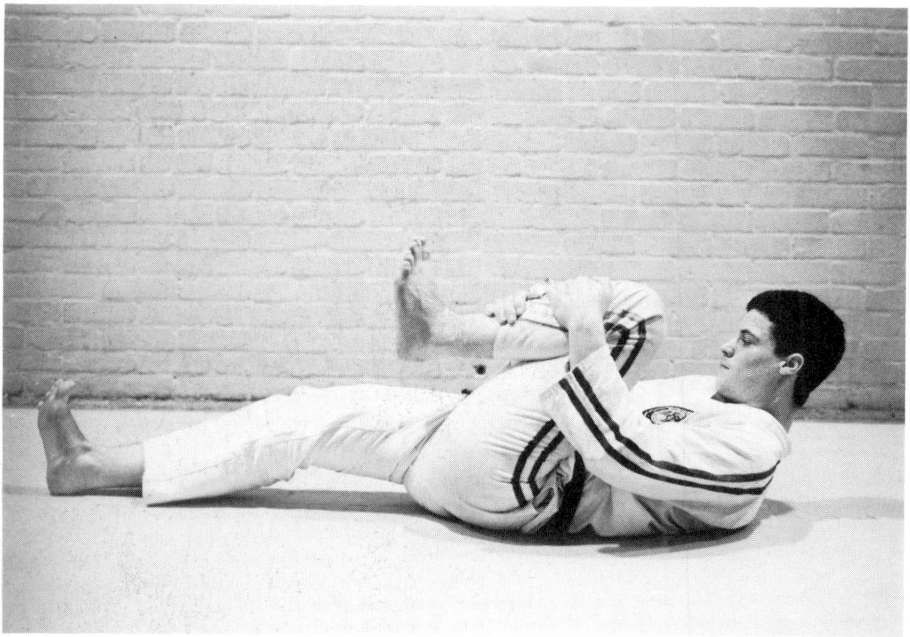

Draw your knee to your chest

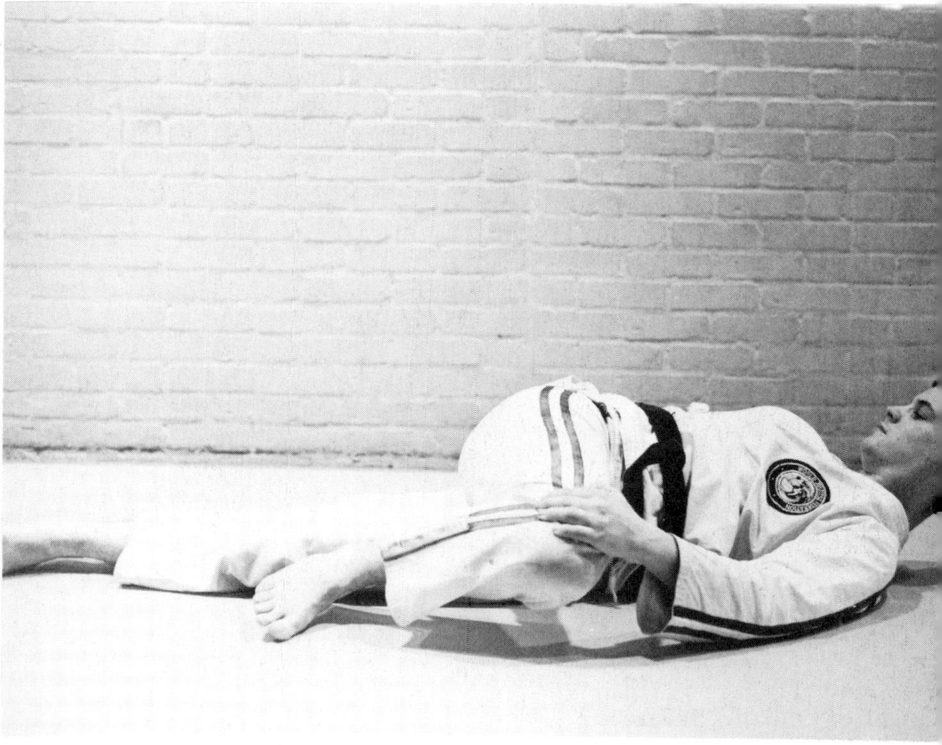

Pull your knee to one side

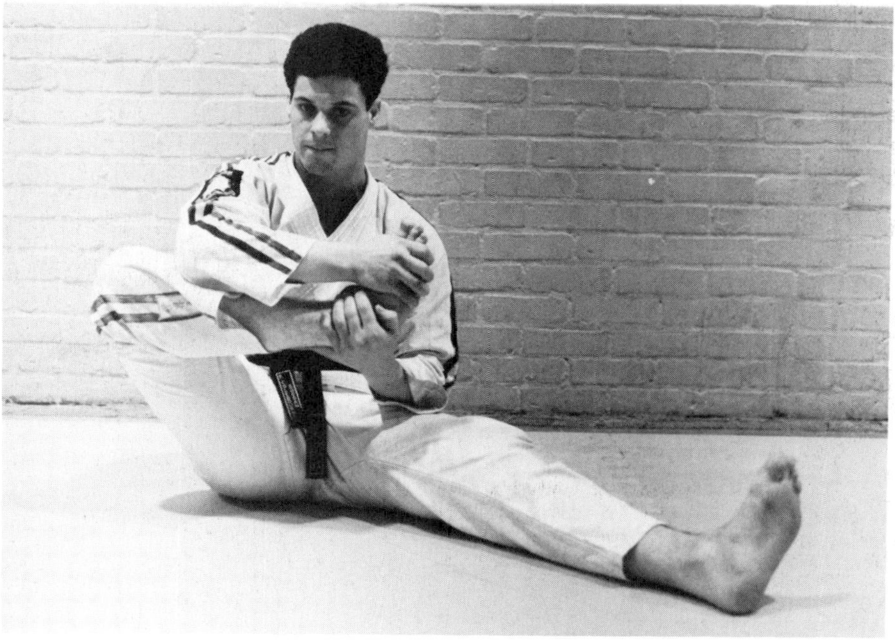

Pull your foot to your chest

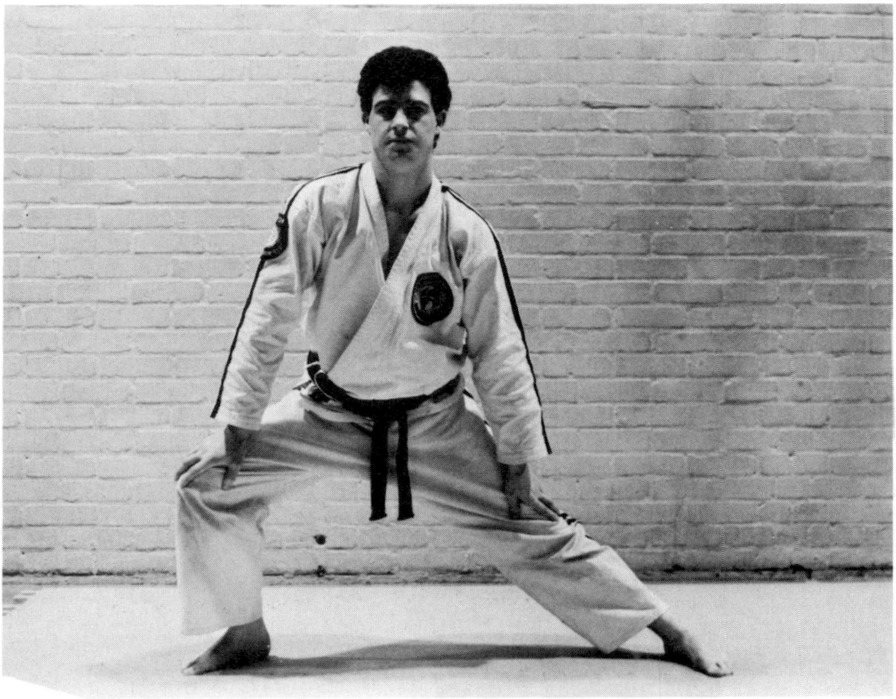

Lower weight first on one side...

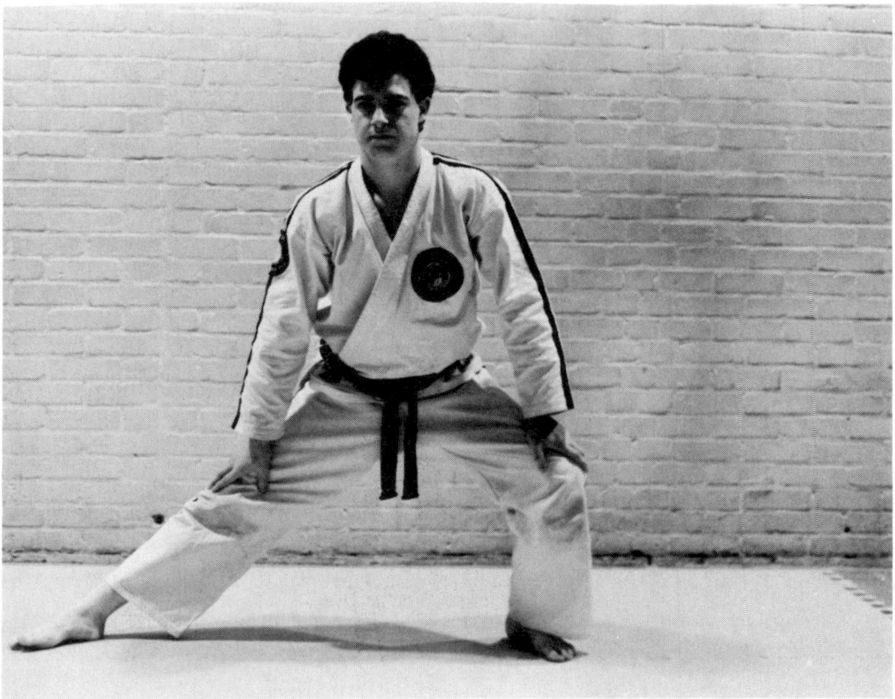

then the other

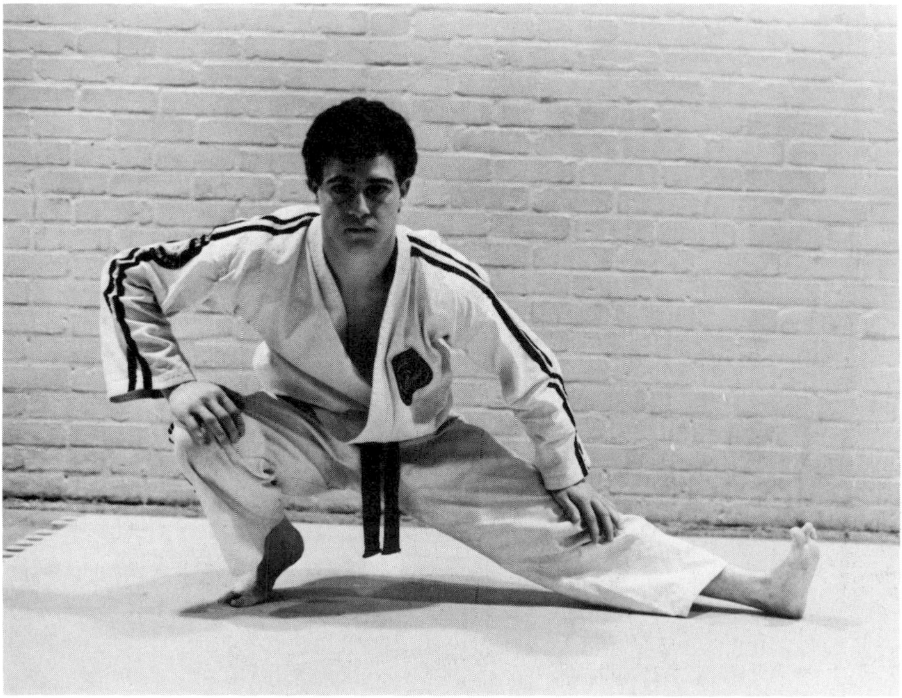

Sink down on one side...

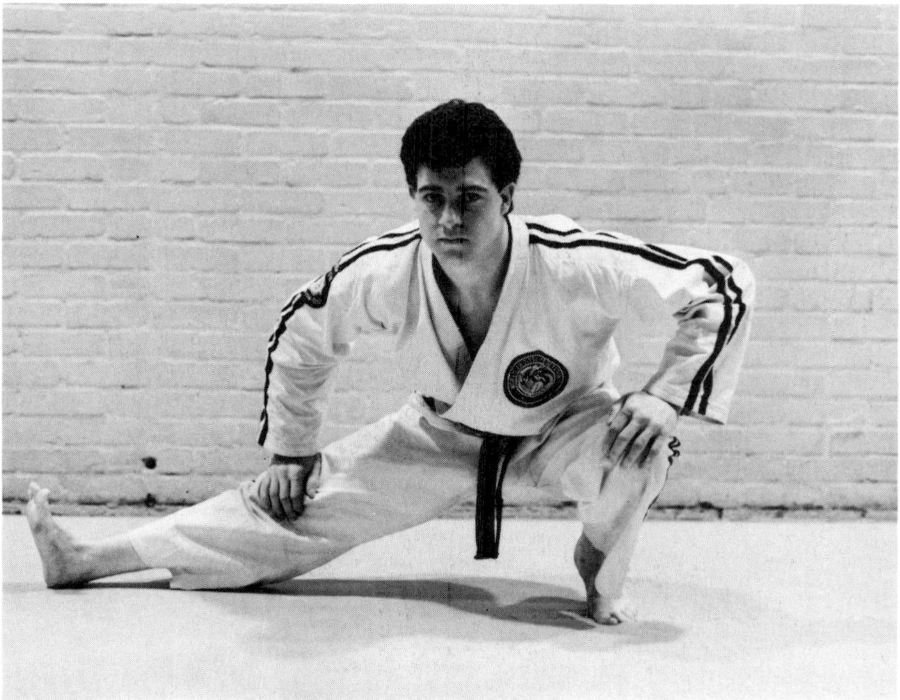

then the other

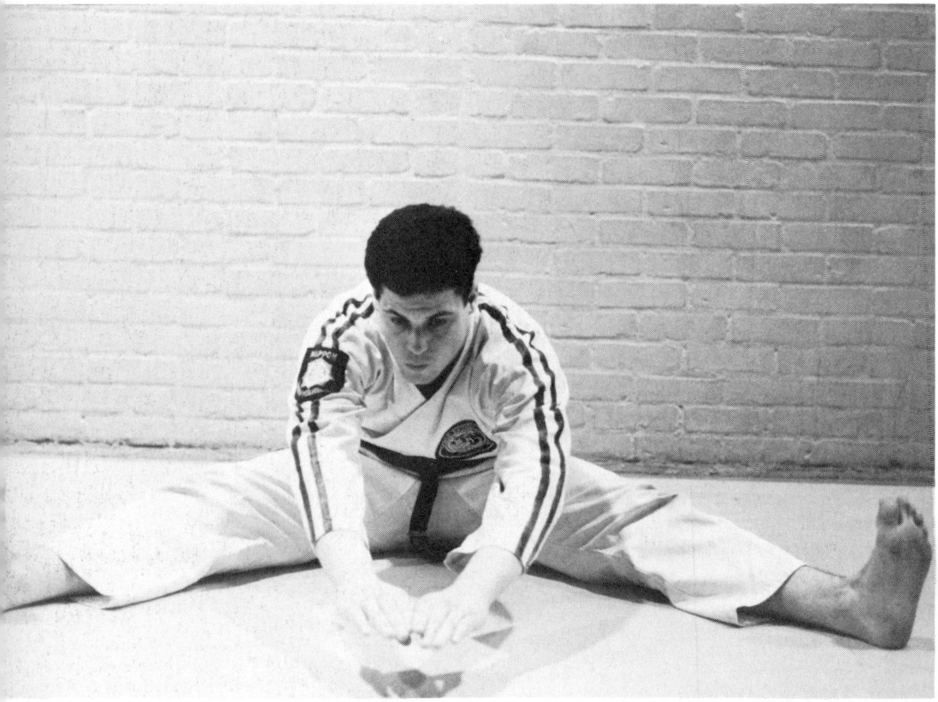

Reach between your splayed legs...

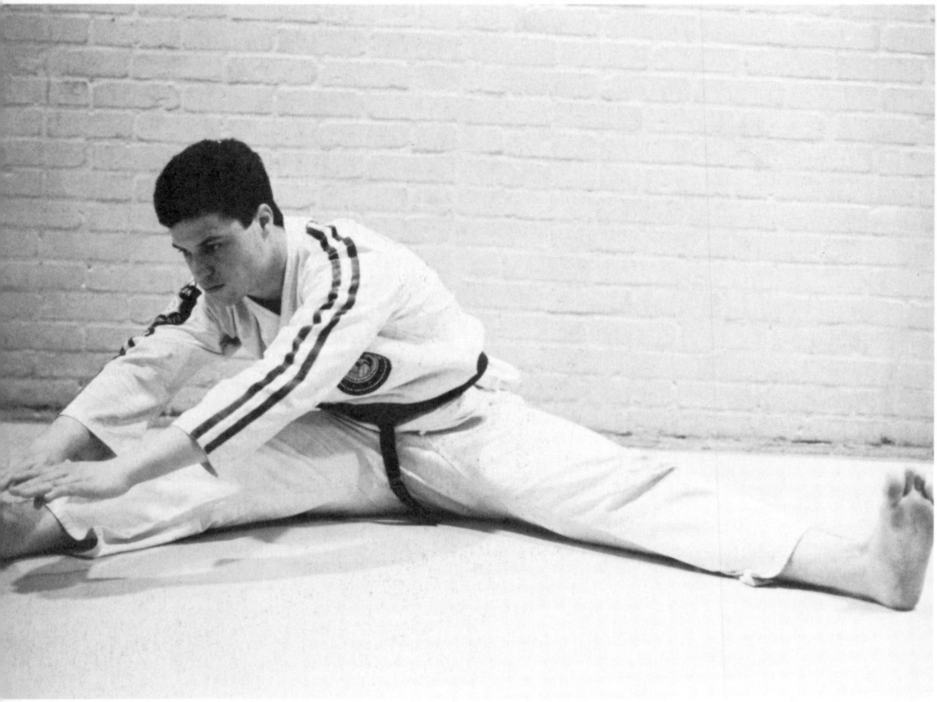

Swing your arms to one side...

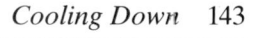

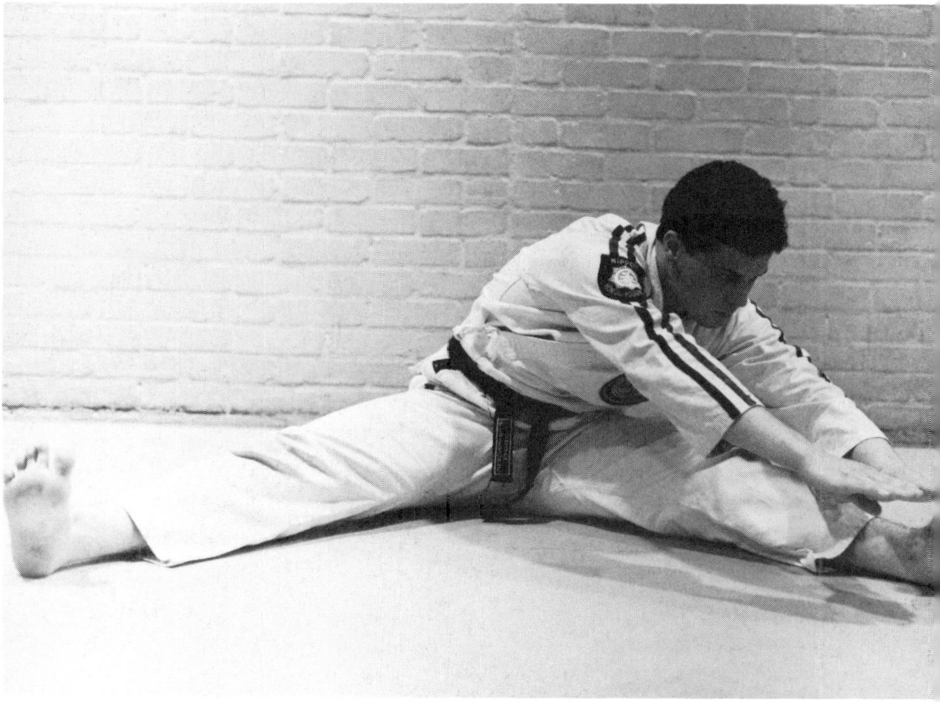

then the other

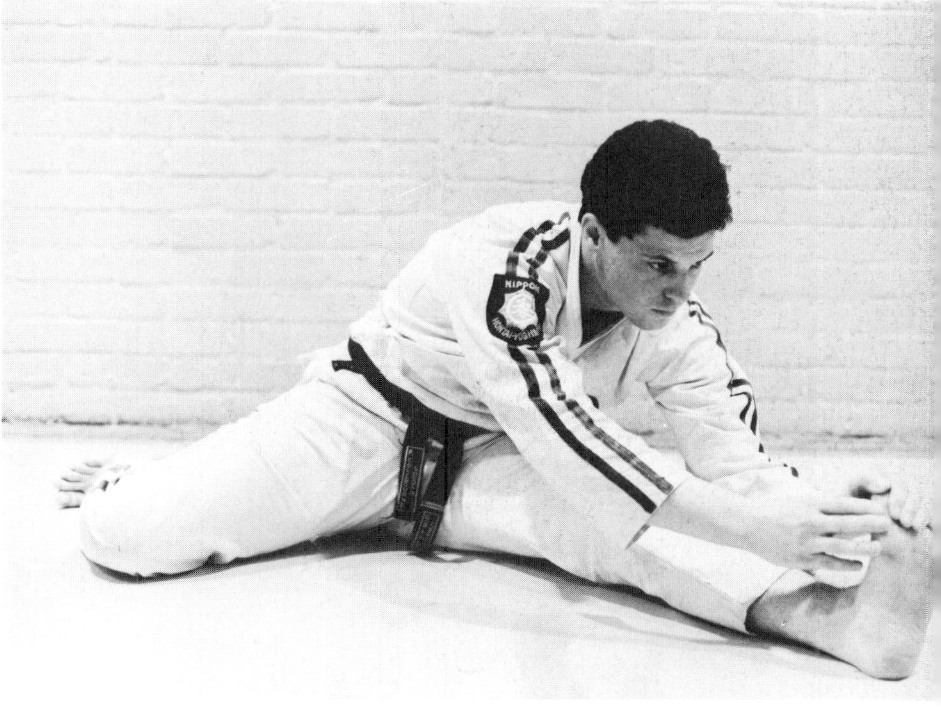

Pull your body forward

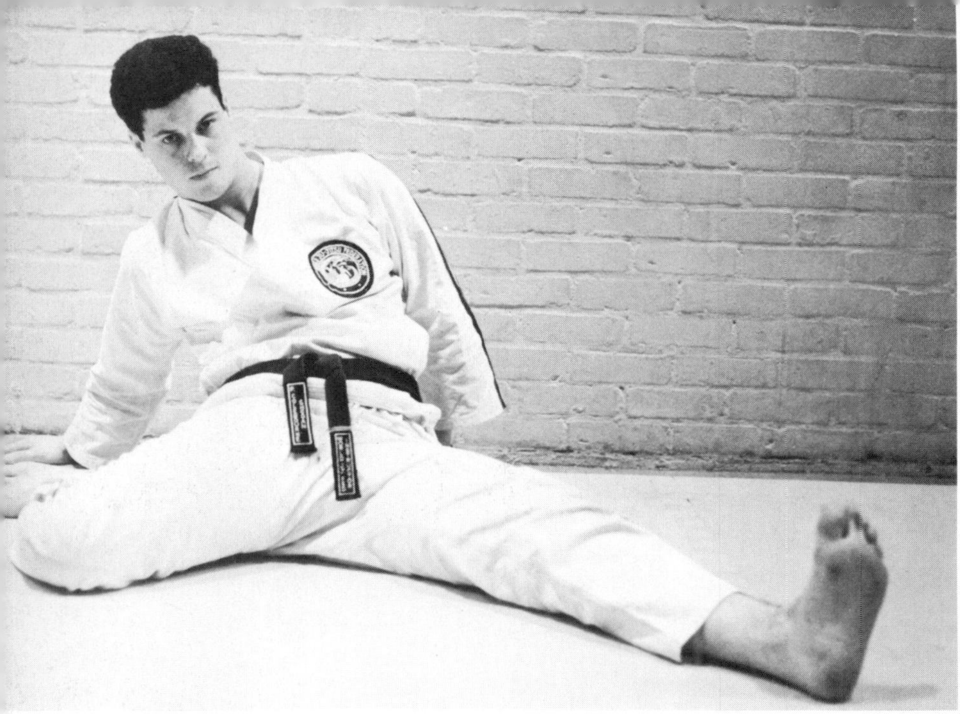

Lean right back

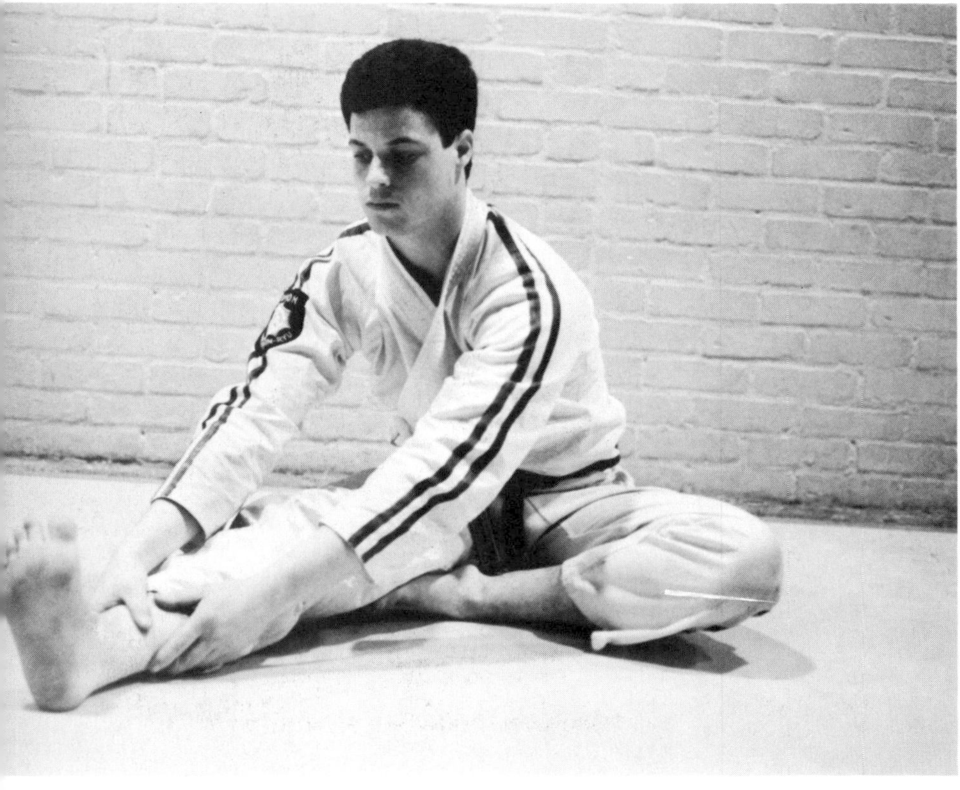

Keep your leg flat to the floor

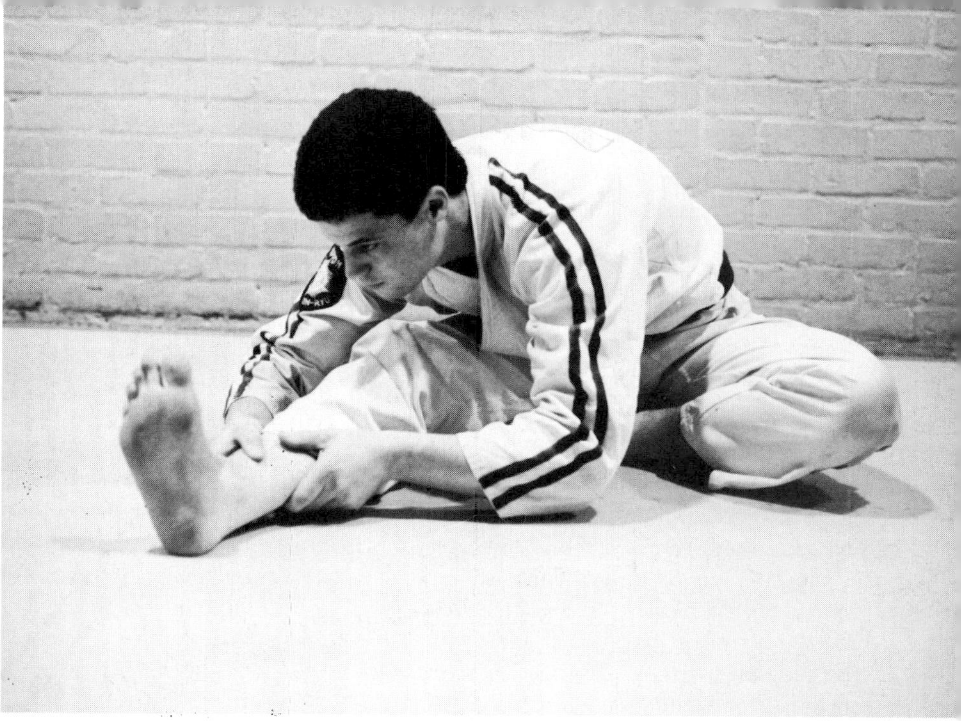

Pull yourself down

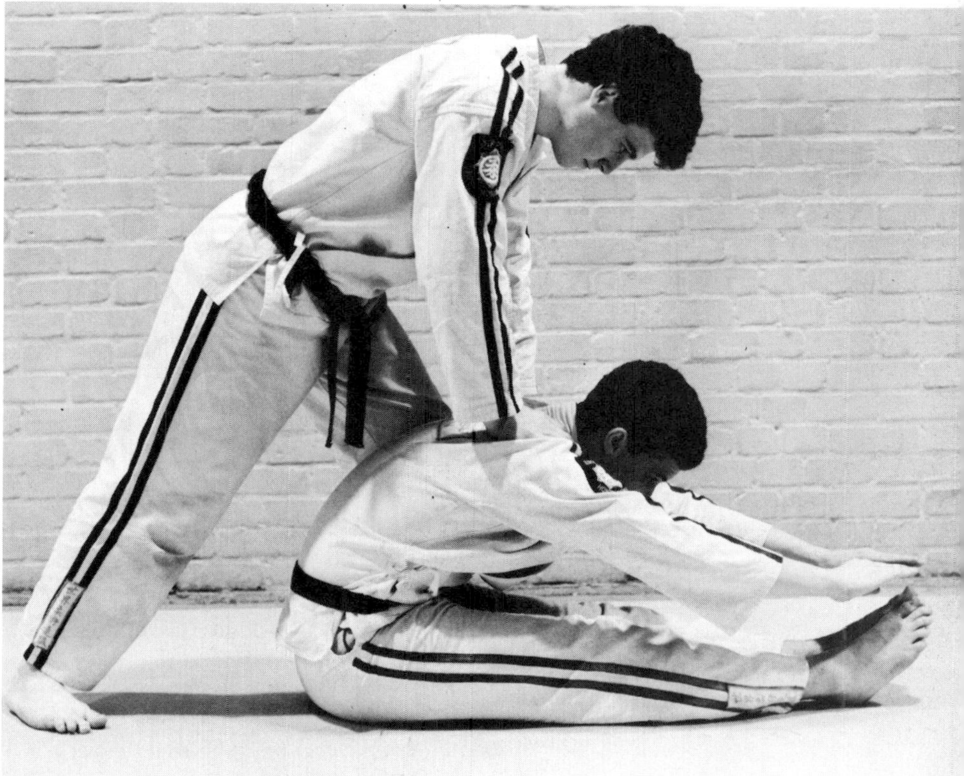

A trusted friend can be a great help

Martial Art Injuries and Management

The average family doctor may not be the best person to consult when you have suffered a training injury. Some overworked or uninterested members of the medical profession regard a martial arts injury in the same light as self-inflicted injuries. Picture if you will, the martial artist waiting for an hour in the surgery, next to wheezing old souls, screaming children and pregnant females. He limps in to see the doctor, who looks up briefly from writing up the last patient's medical card and says rather tersely, "What's wrong with you?"

"It's my knee – it hurts!" says the martial artist by way of explanation.

"When does it hurt?" asks the doctor.

"When I do this," replies the martial artist, gingerly demonstrating a side kick.

"Well don't do that, then," says the doctor. "Next please!"

You therefore have two options; one is to take the advice of the doctor and delete side kick from your repertoire of techniques. The other is to somehow rehabilitate your injured knee so that it becomes capable once again of doing side kick. A Sports Injury Clinic may be able to help.

Sports injury is not a speciality study, though doctors with interest in the subject have got together into groups such as 'B A T S' – the British Association of Trauma in Sport. These doctors are pooling their practical knowledge of sports injuries and the future at least looks hopeful.

We are going to offer you some practical advice on managing common martial arts injuries but the first thing we must say is that ultimately, the effectiveness of any treatment is affected by the patient's attitude to it. For example, if you have a bad headache caused by a thump or bad fall and you happen to believe that paracetamol works for you, then take it and good luck to you. If you have great confidence in the pills and potions of so-called 'natural medicine', then by all means do your own thing.

One martial artist used to bang his toes during front kick and discovered that alternating hot and cold soakings followed by a brisk walk during which the injured toe was made to flex, caused the pain and swelling to abate in record time.

Research by martial arts interested doctors is beginning to reveal some quite fascinating facts. It appears that the practice of certain martial arts can actually cause injury. Take for example those impact-based systems which advance up and down the training hall punching and kicking at the empty air.

"Snap it back!" calls the instructor, obviously unaware of the damage this is causing to each and every practitioner. The elbow is a hinge joint that has a natural limit of movement. When you slam your arm out unchecked, the elbow joints slam straight and the bits of bone, string and cardboard all grunch together in a nasty way.

Because the body is capable of withstanding abuse, the odd such happenstance can be tolerated but if you are spending four plus hours a week doing it, then after a couple of years (or even less), the chances are that the joint will seize up. Surgical intervention is then necessary to remove all the bits and bobs which are now floating around the joint capsule and getting in the way.

The knee joint is similarly limited in its movement and repeated damage caused by snapping the lower leg out hard damages the ligaments and nips bits off the cartilage. Repeated abuse can damage the cartilage so badly that it interferes with normal action and recourse to surgery is then required to have it removed. Unfortunately the cartilage is there for a purpose and taking it out is rather like going to a garage with a car mis-firing on one of its four cylinders whereupon the mechanic identifies the failing spark plug, unscrews it and throws it away. It doesn't mis-fire any more but you now have a three cylinder motorcar!

Staying with kicks for a moment, Doctor Jim Canney of MediMAC has discovered that if a roundhouse kick is repeatedly done incorrectly, it places a tremendous twisting stress on the barely moveable joint where the bottom of the spine joins the pelvis. This stress leads to inflammation of the *sacroiliac* and curiously this produces identical symptoms to ham-

A doctor is essential at all tournaments

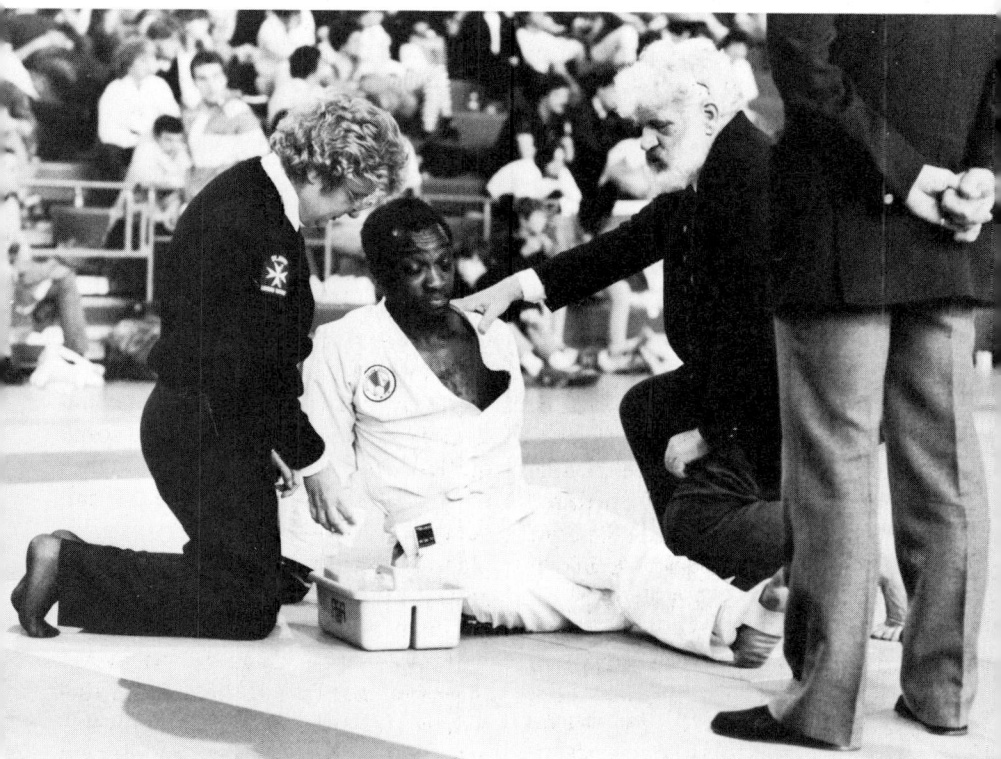

string injury. So even if you leave off leg-stretching exercises the strain won't get any better and you will continue to suffer unnecessarily for months afterwards.

Rule One for punches is:- DON'T fully straighten your elbow.

Rule Two for kicks:- DON'T snap your lower leg out straight.

Rule Three for backs:- DO twist fully on your supporting leg when doing side kick and roundhouse kick.

The grappling-based martial arts tend to be less damaging on the body. Having said that, do make sure you release your partner when he/she taps up. Don't be tempted to put that little bit of extra pressure on momentarily before releasing because if you do, you could end up causing a fracture. Be careful when applying chokes which cut off the supply of blood to the brain. When the person lapses into unconsciousness it is because you have succeeded in killing off a couple of thousand brain cells that are never going to be replaced.

Jiu jitsu practitioners can suffer with knee injuries brought about by applying a throw incorrectly. You lever your partner up and over your shoulder and twist your hips only to find your knee collapsing under the load. When your knee is bent, it is carrying ten times body weight and with someone on your shoulders, any weaknesses make themselves quickly apparent.

Now let's consider the various types of injuries you'll come across and how to manage them. You can damage the skin, the muscles, the bones and the joints, or any combination of these. You can also damage the nerves and we include in this the brain.

Starting with the skin, the most commonly encountered condition is the blister. Prevention is better than cure, so when parts of your foot begin to feel sore, stop and tape them up with a cushion plaster. What you don't want is to have the blisters burst and then grind dirt from the floor into the raw flesh. Sticking plaster on its own won't withstand training and even if you clean the skin first, it soon comes loose. If you put a sock over the plaster, you may be alright whilst practising on mats but on a sprung wood floor, you'll end up skating all over the place. Carry a pair of kung fu slippers with you and slip these on.

Medical opinion appears to vary on what you should do for a blister. Some say just cover it with a plaster. Others tell you to burst it with a sterile needle. To sterilise the needle, dip it into a strong antiseptic solution and use one of your own needles – not someone else's! Generally the blister bursts soon after it forms. As long as you keep it clean, you should get no problems and healing is rapid.

If the lacerated skin is not likely to be further damaged, then don't bother with a dressing. If it is bleeding, cover it with a light dressing which allows a free access to the air. Dressings often impede the rapid healing of a laceration so if you can leave it uncovered, do so.

If there is dirt in the laceration, try and wash it out. Don't use regular applications of antiseptic unless you believe the wound stands a chance of becoming infected. Antiseptics can actually cause infection because they can alter the characteristics of the skin and kill off useful surface bacteria.

If you suffer a really bad laceration – such as a toenail tearing the eyelid during a high kick – get the person to hospital. Don't bother dressing the injury. Cuts can be allowed to bleed a little, if only to dislodge foreign bits and bobs. If an arm is cut, do a 'Heil

Hitler' and lift it up until bleeding stops. If your foot is cut, you can lie down and elevate that too. If your nose bleeds, pinch the nostrils together and keep them closed until bleeding stops. Press a towel into a bad gash from which blood is pumping. If you haven't got a towel, your fingers will do. Do not apply a tourniquet unless you have to carry the patient to a place where he or she can be picked up and taken to hospital.

Bruises are common in all the martial arts. Sometimes they are severe and a clot of blood forms under the skin. This is called a *haematoma* and it can become so bad that a surgical intervention will aid more rapid healing. Bones are well supplied by a web of bloodvessels which overlie the surface. When you bang a bone, you damage these bloodvessels and the familiar blue discoloration develops. As the body's repair crew gets working, the blood is broken down and removed, the process indicated by the change in colour.

There is no need to treat a bruise. If you have a bruised shin, then wear a shin pad and don't engage in any activity which is likely to damage it again. If you do, then all that will happen is that it will take longer for the discomfort to go away. If you are in the middle of a grading or competition, a freezing spray can give temporary relief but avoid over-spraying the affected part. If you bruise your knuckles, wear fist mitts to protect them from further injury.

If you bang your toes or knuckles, use ice to get the swelling down and when you get home, or perhaps the next day, try the contrast, hot and cold baths using two large bowls that you can fit the injured parts into. Fill one with cold water to which you have added ice cubes; fill the other with

water as hot as you can stand. Put the injured part in the one bowl and after three or four minutes there, transfer it to the other. If you like, just apply a cold-pack to your injury, wrapping ice cubes in a tea cloth or towel. Either treatment eases discomfort and you should go for mobility immediately after it. Don't give things a chance to seize up!

Severe impacts or bad landings can cause fractures. If someone is thrown awkwardly, for example, and tries to break their fall with an extended arm, a fracture may occur mid-way up the forearm. Break your falls with a bent arm, not a straight one. If someone breaks their arm or collar bone, they won't like you touching it very much, so don't! They will brace it with the uninjured hand in the position of maximum relative comfort and this will suffice until they reach hospital. Don't bother calling an ambulance if the patient can walk.

A broken leg is entirely different. Don't play about with splints, just call for an ambulance and leave the patient where he/she is until it arrives. Give nothing to eat or drink in case the hospital needs to operate.

The two most common fractures encountered in the martial arts need no treatment. Broken ribs make breathing difficult but there is little the hospital can do once it has examined them, except strap them up. This is not to be recommended because not only can the strapping cause pain through the constriction it causes but it can also give rise to allergic rashes. And when you come to peel it off a hairy torso... The other common fracture, that of the toes, requires only the strapping together of adjacent toes.

When recovering from injury, it is very important to keep joints mobile and muscles in shape. If limbs are immobilised through treatment, maintain flexibility of joints above and below the injury site. The most common complication arising from a broken wrist for example, is arthritis of the shoulder caused from not exercising it whilst the wrist is in plaster. When exercising non-fracture injuries, always move affected joints to their limits and even to the point of discomfort. It is not cissy to take painkillers because these permit more movement of the joint and a faster recovery.

Sprains, strains and dislocations all take their toll of martial arts training. Dislocated fingers are a frequent concomitant of impact-based martial arts. A fast-travelling kick makes unexpected contact with stiffened fingers and dislocation may result. If you don't know what you are doing, go to the hospital. By the time you get there, the digit will have swollen to twice its size and the anaesthesia of shock will have worn off. If you know exactly what you are doing, then and then only may you act quickly after the dislocation and simply tug on and bend the dislocated joint. The tugging pulls the bones back so they are end-to-end and the bending causes the joint to relocate.

After a reduced finger dislocation, the affected digit will swell up like a chipolata sausage. Use ice for your first aid treatment. Later on, contrast baths may speed recovery. Work the joint very gently and if you feel in need of cossetting, strap the injured finger to one of those next to it.

Twisted ankles occur where ill-fitting mats are employed, or when the foot doesn't turn freely during a throw. They can be extremely painful and if you don't look after them, symptoms can persist for ages. If the ankle feels very painful, visit the hospital for an X-ray to confirm that nothing is broken. Then get the swelling down using ice in the first instance and contrast baths later on. Allow the ankle a day's rest, keeping it elevated if you can. Crepe bandage can be put on to cushion the injured part and a properly applied bandage may help reduce swelling.

Wobble boards are good for working an injured ankle. They are circular boards attached to the flat surface of a hemisphere. Stand on the board and try to keep your balance.

When the acute swelling has gone down, begin walking around on the foot, putting weight gingerly onto the injured part. Repeated ice treatments or soaking in hot water will make it feel better after a session of working-out.

Don't overload it though and allow plenty of rest between sessions.

For those martial artists using lots of strikes and kicks, think seriously about buying a properly fitted gumshield. These not only save teeth but protect lips and gums too. They can even protect against concussion. At the other end of the body, a boxer-type groin guard is useful for protecting the testicles. Don't use the loose cups that slip inside a jockstrap because they move around like plastic pastrycutters.

Passing finally to nervous tissue injury, do think carefully before practising a martial art that allows full-power strikes to the head. Brain cells don't regenerate if they are knocked about and the full effect of brain damage appears gradually. The brain has the consistency of thick porridge and when the head is accelerated through impact with a foot or fist, the brain tissue moves at unequal speeds and thumps against the inside of the skull.

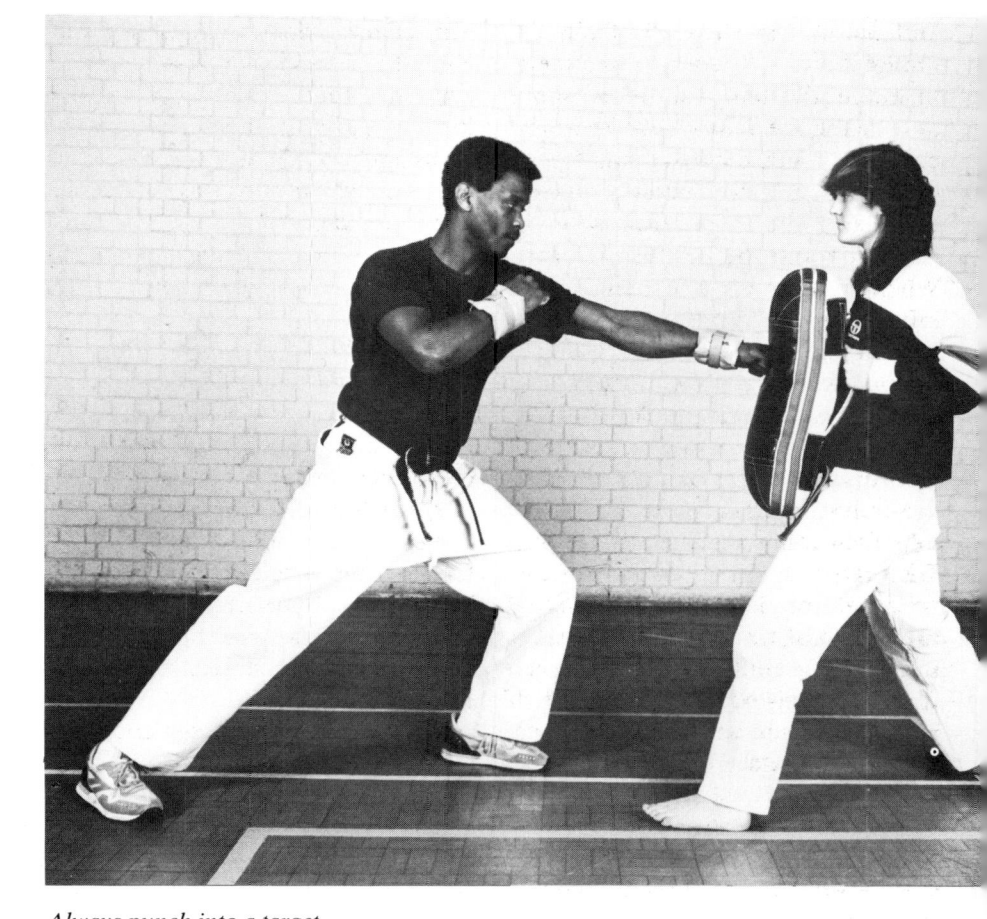

Always punch into a target

This both crushes the brain cells and shears off the connections that link cells together.

If you are knocked senseless, even if only for a couple of seconds, you must withdraw from further activity likely to cause a repeat of the injury. If you get another bang on the head a short time after the first, then the damage done will not be doubled, it will be made worse by a factor of several times. The effects of serious head injury can persist for up to a year after the accident and during this time, the martial artist may suffer from loss of concentration, headaches, disturbed vision and impaired hearing.

Brain damage is the one martial arts injury you don't hurry along. You simply ease up for a period of at least six weeks. You can train during this period but such training should not involve the risk of further head injury.

Now Read On

I hope you enjoyed reading this book and your appetite for further knowledge is well and truly whetted. There is no doubt that your enthusiasm to do better plus extra information will lead to an improvement in your training and I recommend you now contact the National Coaching Foundation.

The Foundation exists to promote more effective participation in all physical activities and it has arranged a programme of 13 four-hour courses covering a wide range of topics. Though these courses are not specifically aimed at the martial arts, the information they provide can be adapted to our needs. Since each course only costs £5, you can enrol for several without breaking the bank. The courses are not all theory and there may well be some practical work to do in the ones you select.

Get the Foundation's programme by writing to:

The National Coaching Foundation,
4 College Close
Beckett Park
Leeds LS6 3QH
Tel: Leeds (0532) 744802

Here are the courses you can choose from:

Structure of the Body
This explains how the muscles, bones and joints of the body work. Some exercises are looked at to see how they benefit training.

Prevention and Rehabilitation of Injury
This provides guidance for first aid practice and covers ways in which you can get back into full training after injury. The course explains how injuries arise and suggests ways of reducing risks.

Nutrition and Sports Performance
This course looks into the nutritional requirements of people in training, explaining about the different types of food available and their benefits.

Developing Endurance
Methods of increasing endurance are discussed and the way in which they work is looked at. Various ways of measuring changes in endurance are studied.

Development of Strength and Speed
This course explains the principles of strength training and how they can be applied. Speed drills are set out and the course looks into reaction time and mobilisation.

Developing Flexibility
This course links in well with the previous one. It covers methods by which flexibility can be measured and increased. Factors affecting flexibility are explained.

An Introduction to Sports Mechanics
This shows how far mechanical principles can be applied to body action and

ways in which this knowledge can help you with daily training.

Use of Video in Coaching
The course shows how a video can be best used to reveal how athletes are actually performing technique during training.

Understanding and Improving Skill
This course explains how skills are learned by people in training and suggests how training routines can be adapted to improve the rate of learning.

Mental Preparation for Performance
The course suggests ways in which someone in training can be helped to deal with the effects of stress accompanying gradings and competitions.

The Coach and Athlete: Working as a Team
For training to be beneficial, the coach and students must form a good working team. The course looks at ways in which this relationship can be developed and maintained.

How to Plan your Programme
This course shows how to set up reasonable training schedules for different targets and how to monitor progress towards those targets.

Effective Coaching
Different situations need different approaches. This course shows different methods of communicating information within the training programme.

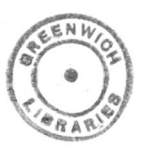

Glossary of Forbidden Drugs

Psychomotor Stimulants

Amphetamine
Benzphetamine
Chlorphentermine
Cocaine
Diethylpropion
Dimethylamphetamine
Ethylamphetamine
Fencamfamin
Meclofenoxate
Methylamphetamine
Methylphenidate
Norpseudoephedrine
Pemoline
Phendimetrazine
Phenmetrazine
Phentermine
Pipradol
Prolintane

Sympathomimetic Amines

Clorprenaline
Ephedrine
Etafedrine
Isoetharine
Isoprenaline
Methylephedrine
Methoxyphenamine

Miscellaneous CNS Stimulants

Amiphenazole
Bemegride
Doxapram
Ethamivan
Leptazol
Nikethamide
Picrotoxin
Strychnine

Narcotic Analgesics

Anileridine
Codeine
Dextromoramide
Dihydrocodeine
Dipipanone
Ethylmorphine
Heroin
Hydrocodone
Hydromorphone
Levorphanol
Methadone
Morphine
Oxocodone
Oxomorphone
Pentazocine
Pethidine
Phenazocine
Piminodine
Thebacon
Trimeperidine

Anabolic Steroids

Clostebol
Ethyloestranol
Fluoxymesterone
Methandienone
Methenolone
Methandriol
Methyltestosterone

Nandralone
Oxandrolone
Oxymetholone
Stanolone
Stanozolol

And other related compounds in all categories.

Recommended Reading

Fit to Exercise
BURKE E J AND HUMPHREYS J H L
Pelham Books, 1982

Measurement in Physical Education
MATHEWS D K
W B Saunders Company, 1978
Fifth Edition

Physical Fitness and Athletic Performance
WATSON A W S
Longman, 1983

Physiology and Performance
The National Coaching Foundation
Coaching Handbook Three
White Line Press, 1986

Physiology of Exercise
DE VERE H A
Staples Press, 1980   *Third Edition*

Safety First For Coaches
The National Coaching Foundation
Coaching Handbook Two
White Line Press, 1986

Stretching
ANDERSON B
Pelham Books

The Food Scandal
WALKER C and CANON C
Century Publishing, 1984

Sports Tester
Available from:-
Hampden Sports Limited
Bleasdale Court
2 South Avenue
Clydesbank Business Park
Glasgow G81 2LE

Video
Energy for Sport
Available from:-
National Coaching Foundation
4 College Close,
Beckett Park,
Leeds LS6 3QH.

Index

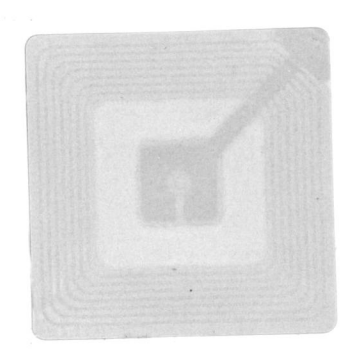

Lightning Source UK Ltd.
Milton Keynes UK
UKHW021147C21121
393255UK00005B/87

9 780953 081134

CLAIMING YOUR DIRECTOR'S CHAIR – REVIEWED BY RALPH E. MELCHER
The Journal of the Association for Humanistic Psychology

How do you get a teenager's attention and hold it? Vivian King has developed a course of activities that is both engaging and entertaining. Designed for those who are poised between childhood and adulthood, it helps and encourages them in facing this time of deep challenge and growth.

In *Claiming Your Director's Chair*, Dr King's programme applies the methods and metaphors of the theatre to bring teenagers in touch with their inner wells of creativity. The skills and insights unveiled in the chambers of the Inner Theatre can be of immense value in helping them to make the choices that will shape their lives and help them arrive at a true sense of self-awareness, self-acceptance, and self-mastery.

Dr King outlines her understanding of the sometimes overwhelming drama that modern teenagers must learn to face, and vividly outlines the possibilities of either Tragedy or Divine Comedy. Her stated goal is to support these amateur actors in producing an individual and collective drama that can be see as 'The Greatest Show on Earth'.

Plenty of resources are provided in both the Leader's Guide and the Playbook. Each lesson plan is carefully laid out, with a clear explanation of its purpose and a bit of theoretical background, followed by suggestions for props and setting the stage. The exercises themselves follow a series of activities that include readings, role playing, and the use of audio and visual aids. Scattered throughout are teaching tips based on the a author's extensive experience of working with similar groups. The segments are somewhat open-ended, offering numerous suggestions for optional activities and encouraging students and teachers to create their own exercises.

The Playbook is a workbook with text and spaces for writing and drawing. It is filled with illustrations and a feast of quotes, cartoons, and potent words of wisdom. Players who pass through this course will become acquainted with the depths and heights of themselves, and will have an entertaining way to handle the complexities of life. Those who continue to use these principles will develop a rich inner life, and will be able to contribute positively to the larger World Play.

Inner Theatre books only available from Inner Way Productions:
www.innerwayonline.com

BECOMING A STAR – REVIEWED BY RALPH E. MELCHER
The Journal of the Association for Humanistic Psychology

Vivian King has produced a wonderfully innovative tool for supporting the intrapersonal development of children from the ages of 8 to 12.

In *Becoming A Star* she addresses the needs of children on a myriad of levels, providing them with an entertaining way to develop self-awareness, self-acceptance and self-responsibility.

Based on the premise that children are inherently playful and creative, and that they respond readily to love, acknowledgment and understanding, the programme is designed to build a strong sense of self that includes the clear perception and acceptance of the child's unique desires, feelings, and talents. The child also gains an ability to contact inner sources of guidance and wisdom in order to express 'star' qualities.

The Leader's Guide involves as much trust in the child's own emerging 'inner curriculum' as it does a thorough familiarity with the material. The 'Preparation' is a careful walk-through to set the stage, involving the use of props, music, mood, and work materials. The 'Programme' is then carefully scripted, with each section annotated with the corresponding section in the child's Playbook. There is enough material to provide room for flexibility, and suggestions are offered for additional activities that children may pursue with the group or on their own. A set of illustrated visual aids completes the leader's package.

The Playbook is full of pictures and exercises, including many pages for children to engage their budding creativity. As the programme unfolds, new territory is continually unveiled as children explore first the theatre, then their inner actors, and eventually their own inner playwright and director. The programme touches on virtually all of the essential aspects needed to achieve self-reliance in a constantly changing world.

INNER THEATRE – UNMASKING THE HUMAN SPIRIT
Vivian King Ph.D.

On the corner of Imagination Street and Adventure Avenue, in the theatre of your mind, you will find a cast of characters as rich and varied as actors on a Broadway stage.

To produce a successful play – perhaps even a divine comedy – it is necessary to claim your director's chair, become acquainted with your players and playwright, and discover the secrets of directing.

Welcome to the rich and innertaining world of your inner theatre!

INNER THEATRE PLAYBOOK – Vivian King

Welcome to the Inner Theatre – the private world of your personality where you are the playwright, the director, and all the players; in short – the whole play.

Inside the theatre, you will be given an entertaining way to recognize and develop the many aspects of yourself. You can expect to explore the unknown regions of your mind, to broaden your emotional repertoire, and to strengthen your centre of inner authority. You can take off your masks and be your natural self.

In the beginning, you will meet a guide who knows her way around the Inner Theatre. First, she will take you behind the scenes and give you a tour of the set. Then she will encourage you to explore your director's sanctum and to find your director's chair. Your guide will introduce you to prominent members of your entourage, audience, and supporting cast She will reveal the profound, yet simple, secrets of directing and will stand beside you as you learn to recognize, accept, and direct your inner actors.

The principles you learn in this programme will not fail you. You will find them useful throughout life. By taking responsibility for your own act and giving the best of yourself, the world will become a better place to be – or a better play to see.

Rachel Spring and the Proclamation
Marilyn Barry

Part One of an exciting new trilogy written for teenagers and enjoyed by adults, dealing with family relationships, environmental issues and romantic love.

When 12-year-old Rachel Spring is sent from England to California to live with her cousin, Hetty Slymer, she does not realize just how much her life is going to change. She makes friends with Aaron, Hetty's son from a previous marriage to Spike, an eccentric inventor, who is attempting to solve the world's environmental problems. Her other friends include Pearl, a homeless teenager living on the streets of L.A., and Gideon whose large chaotic family bring warmth and Rachel's first experience of falling in love.

Rachel talks to nature spirits and her deceased mother who teach her the true meaning of life. Her inner world both nourishes and bewilders her as her outer world changes and presents her with many challenges, but this is no ordinary coming-of-age story.

On a camping trip with her friends to the mysterious mountain behind Spike's ramshackle house, their lives are changed for ever after an extraordinary encounter.

Some readers' comments:

'A wonderful world of fantasy mixed in with teenage and pubescent realities. Magical but with no sentimental slush, this is the perfect book for younger readers.'
William Bloom, author of The Power of Modern Spirituality, The Endorphin Effect and Working with Angels, Fairies and Nature Spirits.

A wonderful book filled with everything you would want your teenager to know: family relationships, environmental issues and the love of nature… all bound together in an engaging story that creates a really enjoyable read.

A great message for young people wanting to know how to help the earth and create a better future…

It's a whole combination of friendship, young love and some fantastic magical/ spiritual ideas that are totally believable and really well thought out and put across…the style of writing keeps you reading and I just loved the characters…

ISBN 978-0-9530811-5-8

SOUL PLAY
Turning your Daily Dramas into Divine Comedies
Vivian King, Ph.D.

Vivian King was director of the Psychosynthesis education and counselling programme in Pasadena, California. Inspired by Roberto Assagioli's monograph *Life As A Game and Stage Performance*, she created
the Inner Theatre approach to personality integration. *Soul Play* combines art, entertainment and personal growth in a unique and accessible
method.

*Vivian King's book is a great and thorough guide to our inner theatre and the
immense possibilities it holds within.*
Piero Ferrucci
Author, *What We May Be*

Soul Play *presents an entertaining and effective way to discover, develop and* inte-
grate the many archetypal energies that exist within us all.
Shakti Gawain
Author, *Creative Visualization*

*A masterful way to work joyfully and creatively with every aspect of your self and
to honour even your most minor aspects with clarity and insight.*
James Fadiman, Ph.D.
Co-founder, Institute for Transpersonal Psychology

*Who would have thought a self-help book could be so much fun and so profoundly
impactful? I highly recommend* Soul Play *to those committed to taking charge of
their lives.*
Jack Canfield
Co-author, *Chicken Soup for the Soul*

ISBN 978-0-9530811-8-9

THE EARTH AWAKENS
Previously THE AWAKENING PRINCESS
Marilyn Barry

The Earth Awakens was written by Marilyn Barry during her Psycho-synthesis training with Vivian King. In it she explores the higher, lower and collective unconscious through imagery. Conversations with her Higher Self reveal a vibrant, eternal spiritual world – temporarily forgotten between conception and death – which gently and lovingly prompts us to awaken and remember throughout our brief sojourn on Earth.

Described by its readers as enchanting, magical, and full of love, joy and humour.

This book will change the way you look at yourself and the world.
Vivian King, PhD
Author of *Being Here When I Need Me* and *Soul Play*

Readers' comments about *The Earth Awakens*
(previously *The Awakening Princess*)

"My heart jumps with joy! Just beautiful. So full of humour ..."

"Better than The Celestine Prophecy *– it contains many more insights."*

"What a joy it is! I just got swept up in the wondrous beauty of the writing, the story, and ended with a revelation, feeling blessed and enchanted by it all."

"Both powerful and delicate, this book will change the way you look at yourself and the world."

"... a delight to read as well as a learning experience. In it I found new hope for the planet as I shared the author's amazing spiritual adventure. Her illustrations are marvellous."

"Exciting and inspiring. This book is so important, it should be translated into different languages. Thank you for having the courage to write this book."

ISBN 978-0-9530811-9-6

BEING HERE WHEN I NEED ME – AN INNER JOURNEY
Vivian King Ph.D.

Inspired by Psychosynthesis, Vivian King invites us to take a journey into the heartland of ourselves where we will meet our inner healer, creative genie and beloved Self who is always here to love, understand and support us. With its unique combination of mysticism and science, this book helps to bring us home to the Self.

Vivian King writes: 'As you rest in the meadow by the brook, make your way through the forest, and climb the mountains of your mind, you will discover what is profoundly meaningful and holy.

'Learning to be here for yourself, you will no longer be dependent on material things or other people. You will have the inner strength to be with others without losing your sacred centre. You will never need to walk alone again.'

Described by its readers as down-to-earth, comprehensive, clarifying and powerful – a simple, pragmatic way to open up to the Higher Self.

"*Being Here When I Need Me provides a natural way to open to your higher Self. It is down-to-earth, comprehensive, clarifying, and powerful. Vivian King's approach to Psychosynthesis is both inspirational and scholarly. I highly recommend this book to those committed to personal and spiritual growth and to all humanity.*"
Edith Stauffer, Ph.D., Founder / Director of Psychosynthesis International
Author of *Unconditional Love and Forgiveness*

Some readers' comments about *Being Here When I Need Me*:
"*I began underlining with a marker until I realized I was marking the whole page.*"
"*A simple, practical, pragmatic way to open to the Higher Self.*"
"*Your writing helps me regain my faith in myself, in life and in God's presence.*"
"*A blend between prose and a literary novel. It doesn't have an arid feeling like most structured material has.*"
"*This book is not for wimps.*"

ISBN 978-0-9530811-1-0

Other books published by Inner Way

TRANSPERSONAL DEVELOPMENT
Roberto Assagioli

First published thirteen years after Assagioli's death, *Transpersonal Development* is a collection of his lectures, essays and notes. It would undoubtedly have formed part of the book he was writing which he planned to call Higher Psychology and the Self.

Transpersonal Development is divided into three parts: Part One describes the reality of the superconscious. Part Two delves into the problems and difficulties experienced on the spiritual path. Part Three deals with the everyday application of those insights gained in the process of spiritual awakening.

As Sergio Bartoli writes in the Preface, Roberto Assagioli was truly a 'scientist of the spirit' who dedicated his life to discovering the reality of phenomena beyond the evidence of verified facts.

The inspiring message of this book is that transpersonal development is not just for the exceptional few. It is possible for everybody. It contains practical guidelines to help people achieve the goal.

Assagioli's article 'Smiling Wisdom' has been added as a final chapter because when we step upon the spiritual path the quality that will help us the most is humour.

What a wonderful production! The new edition of Transpersonal Development is a great achievement. I had never liked the previous edition because the translation, for me anyway, made Assagioli's book seem rather uninteresting. Not so now! The new translation is fresh and brings the words alive in a new way, and there are real gems in here. Even though I've read it before in previous translations, it is like having a 'new' Assagioli book ... amazing!
Will Parfitt, Psychosynthesis Writer and Educator

ISBN 978-0-9530811-2-7

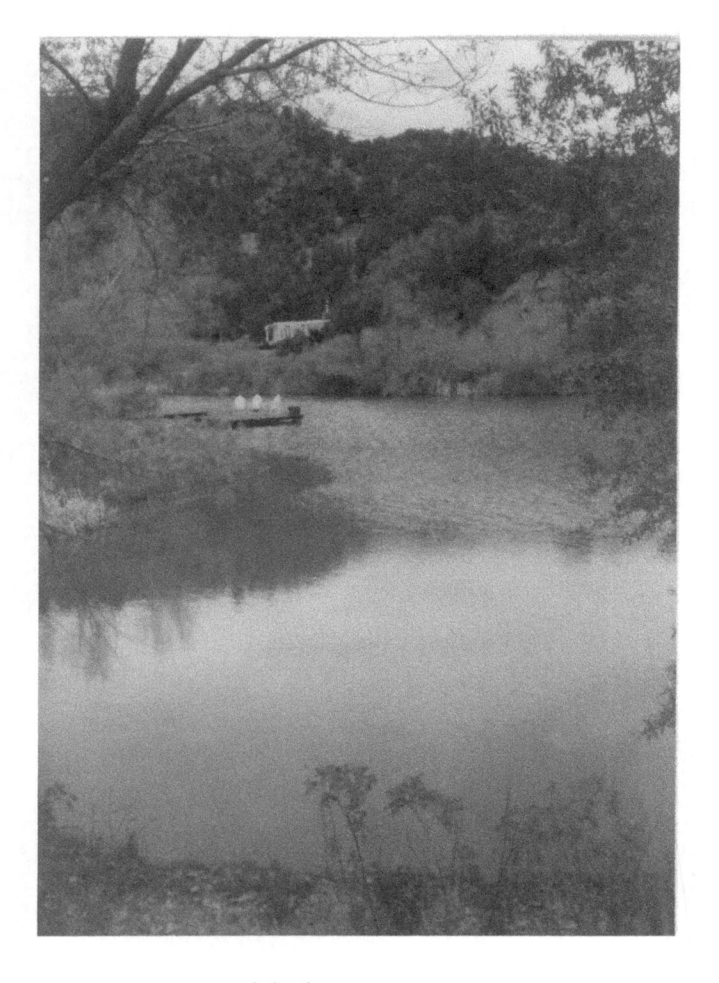

Vivian's adobe house on Spirit Mountain

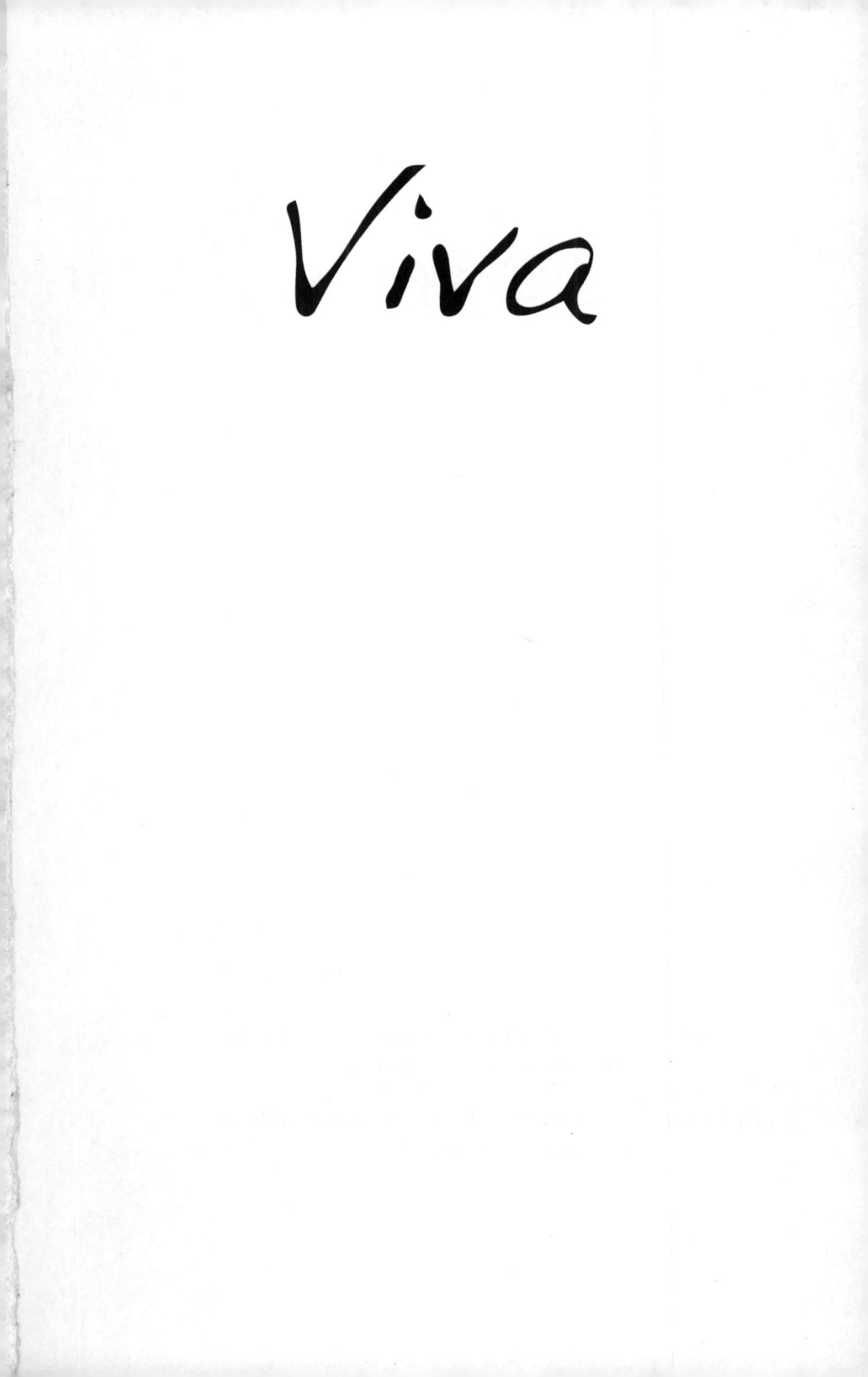

Viva

Front cover: *Vivian outside her adobe house with her dog Free – one week before the car crash.*

Back cover: *Vivian with her friends Patricia and Marilyn – one month before she died.*

Viva

*A promise made between friends is kept
in this detailed account of life after death*

Marilyn Barry

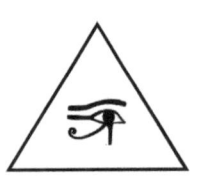

Inner Way
www.innerwayonline.com

Published by
Inner Way
77 The Park, Findhorn
Forres IV36 3TY
Scotland.
www.innerwayonline.com

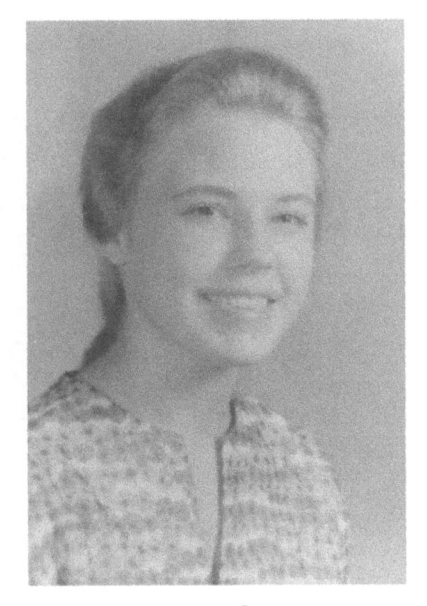

In Loving Memory of Vivian Kay King
18.2.1946 – 18.12.2000

Contents

Preface

In 2001 I was invited by Willem Reniers and Marilyn Barry to become the third point in their triangle meditation. They had been meditating since 1997 with Vivian King and, after she passed away, I was invited to take her place in the triangle. Little did we know that the link with her would continue for several years and be a profound experience for all of us. It was also a great comfort to Marilyn who had such a strong connection with this beautiful soul.

I had never met Vivian, though I was shown a photo of her, and later Willem showed me the moving poem she had written after her car crash called *A Man for All Seasons*. Yet in the triangle meditations I almost immediately felt her presence and gained a clear impression of her 'beingness'. I also saw the lovely adobe house where she had lived in Santa Fe and re-created on the astral plane. I recall the meditation in which she told us that she was moving on into the Ashram to become a teacher there.

In these triangle meditations she transmitted to us some profound teachings and information about her life after death. After a few years of connecting with her, I no longer perceived any kind of image or landscape, and realised that she had moved to a place of pure consciousness without form.

Having the opportunity to experience Vivian's journey after death was a huge privilege, as were the teachings that she gave us. I am so delighted that Marilyn has written this book about her dear friend Vivian whose soul name is Viva. I'm sure that it will bring inspiration to many who wonder what happens after the death of the body, and to know that telepathic continuity of contact with a loved one can sometimes continue after death for several years.

Frances de Vries Robbé
Forres, Scotland, 28th August 2015

Meeting Vivian

I first met Vivian in September 1985 when I arrived on her doorstep in Pasadena. The old Pasadena Psychosynthesis Centre, which I heard about in New Zealand, had recently closed down. Vivian was now teaching classes in her home, a beautiful detached house on the corner of South Arroyo Boulevard and Bellafontaine Street. I had travelled around the world looking for a training in which I could be steeped in Psychosynthesis and, against all the odds, I had found it. Vivian invited me to move into her house and become her secretary, cleaner and gardener. I typed up her classes, recorded onto cassette tapes, cleaned the house, and cared for the garden. In exchange I lived in her house, took her classes, and experienced her sweet presence on a daily basis.

It was love at first sight and for the next two years we were inseparable. She worked in the office in the mornings; I worked in the office in the afternoons. Sometimes she popped her head around the door when I was typing her classes and said, "Do you want to go see a movie?" We would sneak out of the house, giggling like naughty school girls playing truant, and take in a matinee performance. She was lovely to be with: a truly authentic and enchanting human being.

Our lives could not have been more different. Vivian had grown up on a farm with brothers. I had grown up in London, an only child with a widowed mother. Vivian beguiled me with tales of roaming the land and testing the cow-pats to see if she could stand on them. She told me so much about her childhood that I often felt we had known each other as children. Whereas I had been isolated and introverted, she had been outgoing and popular, becoming the Dairy Princess in Kansas, and marrying young. I had never married.

Vivian was the most integrated person I had ever known. Even when she was upset, she did not stay upset. She never had

mood swings. When her ex-husband wanted custody of their son, she told Mark she would always love him whatever he decided to do whereas Mark's father told him he would disown him if he chose to live with his mother. Mark went to live with his father and only saw Vivian in the school holidays.

When Vivian worked in the office in the mornings, I was either cleaning the house or working in the garden. Wherever I was working, I heard Mozart, which Vivian loved to listen to. Having had a traumatic childhood, I often questioned my sanity, but Vivian always reassured me by saying "You're a joy to be with."

On one occasion I pretended to be her English maid when she had visitors. I appeared wearing a white apron and carrying a tea-tray. I was always included when Mark stayed and we watched teenage movies such as 'Revenge of the Nerds'. Once he stayed up all night playing 'Dungeons and Dragons', much to Vivian's horror. He was a typical teenager.

Vivian told me that when Mark was four years old he said he had been her boyfriend but had been killed in an accident. She was shocked because she had never talked to him about reincarnation or mentioned the boyfriend who had been killed in a road accident before she met and married Mark's father.

I would have had a third year with Vivian if I hadn't fallen in love with a man I met in Scotland in the summer of 1987. However, at the end of 1989 I returned to Pasadena because the house was being sold and Vivian had to move out. I returned to help her and collect the things I had left in the house. I was back in my old room overlooking the garden. We were together the day the Berlin Wall came down which would bring big changes into Vivian's life. I encouraged her to buy the house, which we both loved, but she decided instead to move to Santa Fe in New Mexico. She moved there in 1990.

Vivian ended up living in an adobe house on Spirit Mountain where she was the caretaker of a beautiful piece of land which included a lake, woods, stream and even a waterfall. I visited her

there in 1991when she proudly gave me a tour of the land and shared her one-room adobe house with me. It was December and very cold. One night, after seeing a movie in town, the lock on the gate into the property had frozen, and we had to climb over it.

Vivian now taught Psychosynthesis in Russia, Latvia, Poland and Lithuania, which had been opened up after the fall of the Berlin Wall. Her friend and mentor, John Cullen, had taken Psychosynthesis into Eastern Europe and encouraged Vivian to teach there. She also worked on her Inner Theatre material for children, teenagers and adults. She told me the solitude on Spirit Mountain was something she had longed for when running the busy Psychosynthesis centre in Pasadena.

In 1996 Vivian visited me in Southern Spain. She had been teaching in Switzerland and had no idea how far it was from the Costa del Sol. She travelled on trains to Paris, Madrid, and finally Malaga. She arrived exhausted and spent a couple of days in bed. She had come to celebrate her fiftieth birthday. Having raved to her about the warm winters, it was unusually cold, and she wore her fleecy-lined slippers outside as well as inside.

On the early morning she left to catch her flight I remember her bursting into song in the deserted street as we waited for the taxi to arrive. She had a beautiful singing voice and loved to sing.

In 1997 she stayed with us in Scotland to visit and work with my editor on her book 'Being Here When I Need Me' which I was publishing. During the time she slept in the house I had nightmares in which I saw something crashing into me from the right. As I leapt out of bed to avoid it, I thought "I knew this was going to happen. Why didn't I do something to prevent it?" This nightmare repeated itself and I now believe it was a premonition of the car-crash Vivian would experience in less than a year when a truck turned onto the freeway without looking, and she crashed into it. I told her about the nightmares but neither of us realised they were prophetic.

Earlier in 1997 we had started to link up in a Triangle

Meditation with Willem, a man in Belgium. This involved linking in with each other once a week through meditation. We had no idea then what an important link this was going to be.

In May 1998 Vivian wrote:

I established a triangle from Santa Fe. It seemed really nice to have that three-way connection. As the light of the triangle grew brighter, I saw/felt Christ in the center, saying: "You are my beloved disciples. Live in my holy presence. I surround you, protect you, and go with you. You are never alone. I am with you always." I envisioned us all surrendering our human wills, and taking one step at a time – led by Christ. This was very reassuring and relaxing, since I didn't have to try and figure out the future for myself. I didn't have to worry. I just had to take one step at a time, listening to the inner directive.

I am aware of how much of the time I try to figure life out. It is so futile.

I felt a lot of appreciation for Marilyn for publishing my book. It is really a labor of love. I feel her love and accept it fully. I feel so supported. When no one else would take the risk on my book, she did. Now I hope it sells better than we can imagine. One of the nice things is that my book Soul Play paves the path for Being Here. As soon as I receive it, I'll be taking it to bookstores around. Since it is beautiful and the title is great, I think it will sell itself. However, I will do what I can to promote it also.

I feel appreciation to you (Willem) for holding the third corner for Marilyn and me. It just seems important that you do this, and also that you are a male. Thank you for adding stability and presence.

Love to you both, Vivian.

Vivian was never able to promote her books which were on the back seat of her car at the time of the car-crash.

Vivian writing about her life

I had the good fortune of growing up being seen, loved and trusted. My down-to-earth Christian parents provided the fertile soil in which I grew. True gardeners of the spirit, they nurtured the growth of me and my three brothers, and watched us blossom without trying to change our colours or patterns. They trusted our unfolding.

Even as a barefoot young girl growing up on the plains of Kansas, I knew that my family experience was unusual. In my contentment and gratitude, I wanted to give back to the world the gifts of love and caring that I had been given. I wanted to bring healing to those who suffered from not being loved.

In college, I entered nurses training because that was the healing profession about which I knew. Then, for the first time in my life, I experienced disillusionment. I didn't really enjoy my "training" yet I valiantly tried to fit into the structure that was intended to be healing. I graduated and worked in various hospitals, but I didn't feel that I was getting to the heart of the suffering people were experiencing; I was merely "binding wounds' – a "hand maiden" to the doctors.

At nineteen, I married a man to whom I was drawn by his good looks, intellect, and theological interests. In exchange, I offered love and emotional stability since he had grown up in a broken home and dysfunctional family system. (My heart was wide open and willing to give this man the love he never had!)

For ten years I worked as a psychiatric nurse learning to identify, understand, and "treat" mental illness. But while I became psychologically sophisticated in dealing with problems, I experienced a depression of my own spirit.

During this time, I supported my husband through seminary and he became a minister (which made me a minister's wife). But our marriage was tumultuous and unhappy, compounding my

existential questions: "Why, with my psychological and theological orientation, could I not make my husband happy? Why was my spirit numbed?" I knew my intentions were good, and my love was consistent, but good intentions and love were not enough. The thought kept coming to me: "I am just not myself." I longed for the equanimity of my childhood. I wanted to experience the freedom of my spirit that I had felt before, but what was wrong? Like Dorothy, I was on the yellow brick road with my straw man seeking clarity of mind, my tin man (who had an enlarged heart), and my lion looking for courage. We were searching for the Wizard who would help us find the answers.

Along the road, I took a weekend workshop introducing Psychosynthesis (a psycho/social/spiritual approach to the self) and recognized its importance to me immediately. Driving on the 210 freeway from Pasadena to Claremont in California, the thought occurred to me: "My self is always with me. I can stand by my self instead of standing alone or depending on someone else." Seeing two parts of my self standing side by side, I began to let this sink into my consciousness.

It further occurred to me that even if everyone I knew deserted me, my self would never leave or betray me. Laughter welled up as I exclaimed out loud: "I found it. I found what I have been looking for." What I had was the Wizard who was me at a higher dimension. I also found healing. I continued in this education of the self and was given gentle support in identifying and acknowledging my own truth. I began to discern the processes within the medical, psychological and religious institutions that had "educated" me away from myself. In a sense, I had unconsciously given myself away bit by bit to my husband, the doctors, the theologians, and the psychiatrists (male authorities in our society).

I realized that being medical did not mean being healing, being psychological did not mean being integrated, and being theological did not mean being spiritual. What was important was to stay in touch with my own (feminine) inner guidance moment by moment – to trust what was coming from within.

Feeling self-empowered, I left nursing and obtained a Masters Degree in Psychology, establishing my own program in Psychosynthesis counselling and education. I began to guide others in gaining access to their self in the most direct way that I knew. I also enjoyed nurturing my dear son, Mark, who was a very good teacher. At the same time, the illusion of my marriage became clear and our relationship dissolved.

As a girl, I had a strong sense of myself within my nurturing environment. Upon leaving home, I needed to independently develop a sense of who I was. Travelling down the Royal Road of the Self, I have at times slid in the ditch, I've taken wrong turns, and I've travelled down the roads of others, believing them to be my own. But, each time my inner voice calls me and I find the way back to my road more quickly than the times before. I have not found myself once and for all. Instead, I am continually discovering new aspects and dimensions of the person that I am.

Vivian's biography

Vivian had an interesting ancestry. Her mother, Fanny Yutzy, grew up in an Amish family. She had ten brothers and sisters, and left school early because higher education was not valued for a girl whose purpose in life was to marry and have children. Grandma Yutzy was important to Vivian because when she stayed they shared a bed and kept each other warm. When she was dying Vivian flew from Indiana to Kansas to be with her. She loved and admired her, seeing her as a "model of serenity"; someone she wanted to emulate because "she lived a life of integrity and joy." She taught her to say "Do you want to go to bed?" in Dutch which Vivian later had fun with. She kept Grandma Yutzy's Amish bonnet after she died.

Vivian's mother decided not to join the Amish church. Instead she became involved with a young man from the Mennonite church. After a short engagement, she married Alan King on her twenty-first birthday. Within three months she was pregnant with Vernon. Only thirteen months later Vivian was conceived "thanks to a defect in a condom." Her father joked that their only daughter was an accident! Three more boys were born: John, Nicholas and Kenneth. Vivian described her father, Allen King, as a "short, stocky, tanned, wind-blown farmer." His father, Levi Oliver King, was also a farmer and founded the Yoder Mennonite church where he was the first minister.

In the mid-1550s Menno Simons, an Anabaptist in Holland, acquired a gathering of people who believed in non-violence and baptism of adults upon confession of their faith. After his death his followers were called Mennonites by the surrounding community and the name continued to be used. The sect grew and the Mennonite church now has around 550,000 members throughout the world. In the 1600s a group broke away from the church because they believed it was becoming too "worldly" and this group called themselves Amish after a man called Jacob Amon. Their belief in non-violence and adult baptism continued, the only difference being in the way they dressed and lived.

In the 1770s many of Vivian's ancestors moved from Switzerland and Germany to America in search of religious freedom. The Anabaptist-

Mennonites were persecuted because they would not bear arms or baptise their infants. Vivian's Great Grandpa Erb married and moved to the plains of Kansas where a growing group of Mennonites migrated. There he established Heston College, and was a minister and bishop. His daughter, Anna, married Levi Oliver King. Of their seven children three sons became ministers and one daughter married a minister. They were sceptical about their son Allen marrying an Amish girl because they wanted him to marry a more educated Mennonite girl, but "his heart was set."

Vivian described her mother as "the most uncomplicated person I know. She says what she means and she says it simply. She grew up being honest about who she is, no airs, no need to be sophisticated. I appreciate and admire my mother, and love and accept her for who she is. To me she is a beautiful person and I'm proud of her."

Vivian's parents had a long, happy marriage, her father telling the children they had "the most beautiful mom in the world, and the most loved." He frequently asked them "Who has the most beautiful mom in the world?" and they replied "We do!" It was a ritual. Vivian wrote about her father: "He is a beautiful, rugged person, my dad. I love him."

The family farm was located by the Arkansas river in the middle of Kansas in Hutchinson. Large cottonwood and elm trees shaded the farm and the river's edge. They grew wheat, corn, alfalfa and soy beans. Vivian thought it was the most beautiful place in the world. She fed the baby calves from a bucket, giving them a lot of love and singing to them. She had a prophetic image of her future boyfriend being tall, dark and handsome. He would sing base, be a preacher or missionary, and be called John.

The family had daily devotions led by their father. This included reading the Bible, praying, and saying the Lord's Prayer. This took place after breakfast or supper. Vivian thought this was a natural thing for families to do. "God was just included as a part of daily life." Sometimes she was bored during "devotions" but she accepted it without question. They all learned to pray and had Bible stories read to them at bedtime. There was also a variety of religious records. One of them was called 'There is a balm in Gilead' but Vivian could not figure out why there was a bomb in Gilead "wherever that was."

Vivian attended Yoder Mennonite church, which had a rural

congregation of around two hundred people. It was in the country with a grave yard beside it where her grandparents and baby brother were buried. The church had been started by her grandpa who was the first minister. The church was traditional with the women wearing white head-caps called coverings. There was no jewellery, make-up or "immodest" clothes. The women and girls did not wear trousers or cut their hair. Long hair was thought to be "their glory and their submission to men." When one of the Sunday School teachers cut her hair, Vivian was concerned that she was getting too worldly, but her mother said that other good Christians cut their hair too.

At around the age of thirteen Vivian decided to join the church and was baptised along with other boys and girls her age. "It was with conviction and seriousness that I became baptised." She liked belonging to the church and saw the other members as part of her family. She now wore a covering on her head and received a new Bible from her Sunday School. She read the Bible from cover to cover and asked her mom what fornication and adultery meant.

When she was fourteen she talked to her family about cutting her hair. They said it was up to her, which demonstrated their open-mindedness, but that night she decided to "check it out with God" and made a deal: if it rained half an inch, she would not cut her hair. Otherwise she would. It rained three quarters of an inch, so she cut her hair. In high school her Bible teacher talked about heaven, not as a place, but another dimension of spiritual consciousness. Other literal concepts changed as she matured.

Vivian described her childhood as idyllic. She grew up thinking "there is no girl luckier than I." She was carefree, running barefoot on the farm, an "earth girl" with a sense of freedom. She thought she was "so lucky for having so many things that God has a special purpose for me. The purpose was for me to help people who are not fortunate like me."

As the second child, the only girl, she longed for a sister but compensated by thinking of all the advantages of being an only girl. "I didn't have to share woman-time with mom and being dad's little girl, I didn't have to share dad with a sister." Vernon, her older brother, thought she was "too talkative, irrelevant, trivial, and silly." He was critical and made her feel bad about her legs, which he said were too

big. She wrote "I wanted to please him, to have him be proud of me. I was proud to have an older brother."

Johnny was four years younger than Vivian and drowned in the water tank when he was only fifteen months old. His body was brought into the "folks's bedroom because they wanted him close to them. They used Kleenex tissues to wipe away the water seeping from his nose." Vivian figured "Johnny was playing with other little children in a grassy meadow where everything was lovely." She imagined "Jesus holding him and cuddling him." She and Vernon attended his funeral, their parents telling them "Johnny is not there any more, his spirit is with Jesus."

Nicholas was six years younger than Vivian. She described him as a "dry-humored, slow moving, quiet sort of person" who embarrassed her when he told her boyfriend she had made a cake and put mouse turds on top of it. During high school he was faced with the draft and wrote a paper on his decision not to be involved with the military. He wanted to live a simple life as a Christian.

When Kenneth was born two years after Nicholas Vivian was angry with God for not giving her a sister. Ken was more aggressive and picked fights with Nick, trying to tell him what to do, but they remained close. He went to college to study agriculture and became a partner in the family farm.

Vivian had the usual childhood fears of going upstairs to bed in the dark, of getting polio because a neighbour's child had it, of her "folks" dying. When she was nine or ten, she experienced blurred vision in her right eye, probably from being hit on the head by a ball at school. It caused only peripheral vision in her right eye for the rest of her life.

She grew up in a caring community in which Catholics and Protestants respected each other. Religion was a part of daily life. Most of the neighbours were farmers and the women worked at home helping their husbands who depended upon crops and animals for their livelihood.

The one-room one-teacher school remained an important centre until 1960. Vivian was in the last graduate class and cried when the school closed. "My grade school experience was rich. I learned to take my turn and to work alone. I learned to concentrate while other classes in the room were in process," Vivian wrote. "I worked in small groups

and large groups. Older children helped younger children. I was in the same room as my brothers so I knew more about them and what they were doing..."

When she was twelve her mother gave her a box of Kotex, a sanitary belt, and a letter about becoming a young woman. She wrote of her love and support, and hope for Vivian to develop "inner beauty" and to mature as "God had planned." She started menstruating on her mother's birthday when she was thirteen, and she wasn't sure she liked it. "I thought being a little girl was better."

Vivian made the top honour roll and decided to attend the Central Christian High School, a theologically fundamental school, which fed her need to help those "less fortunate". Being vivacious and gregarious, she quickly made friends. Her parents suggested she go to Heston High School for her last two years, and she agreed. Vernon went there and liked it, but it was thirty fives miles away. She was excited about living in a dorm. "I took a walk in our pasture one night and cried. It had felt good and comfortable to be a little girl. I wanted to be a little girl and I wanted to grow up. I walked home with my feet in the sandy dirt knowing that I didn't have a choice."

In high school Vivian was embarrassed about her "big legs and little breasts." She felt out of proportion. Her mother said she was focusing on the wrong thing, saying the "inner part of a person" is the most important and to ignore Vernon's teasing about her legs. Vivian was surprised when she "seemed to be attractive to boys" but her mother told her to "save her kisses for someone she really liked."

She became involved in music and the Christian organisation. She loved school and made the honour rolls again. Ellen, her new best friend, became her room-mate. "She had large breasts and wished they were smaller," Vivian wrote. "I had small breasts and wished they were larger." In her Senior year girls came to her regularly about their problems. "It seemed to them I didn't have any and they thought I could help them."

When she was seventeen her father came in from the milking and asked if she'd like to take part in the Dairy Princess contest. She was surprised, thinking the church would not approve, and she did not see herself as "real attractive." She worked out a humorous speech on milk, and out of nine contestants, she was a runner up.

Vivian was vivacious, witty and popular. She was involved in sports and school organisations. In the dorm she joined in sex conversations and ran naked from the showers. In the fifth grade she became aware of Carl Kauffman, who grew up in her community and attended Bible School in the summer. She wrote love letters to him but did not send them. He was her brother Vernon's best friend and did not encourage her. He was a good student and wanted to go to college, but told her she was the kind of girl he would settle down with when he was ready. He later decided to delay finishing college and volunteer at a hospital in Vietnam. He came to say good-bye to Vivian, hugging and kissing her, and said he'd write, which he did. He died two years later on his way home when he was hit by a car. Vivian had the same dream every year after his death in 1967 in which he returned and they planned to marry. She even had this dream after she was married.

Vivian graduated from high school with the Danforth award. She was chosen out of a class of forty three based on her character, leadership skills and scholarship. Although she hated chemistry, she decided to become a nurse because "it seemed exciting and romantic." Her mother thought it would be a good thing to do until she married and had a family. She "jumped head first into the nursing program somewhat anxious about whether I would make a good nurse." She soon rebelled against doing things because someone said so rather than because it made sense to her. "I didn't need to practise making a bed that often" she complained. She considered leaving nursing because she had not enjoyed the year and she hated her instructor. She disliked the medical roles: "God doctors and servant nurses." Her second semester was completely different. She liked obstetrics and paediatrics because she could relate to the mothers and children. She stayed in nursing for her final year, thinking the worst was over, but was told she had an "authority" problem. "I did have problems with persons who tried to control me. I had experienced freedom to grow and to be as I grew up and I didn't know how to handle someone who tried to dominate me. I didn't feel bad for having an authority problem."

"After having experienced so many positive feelings about grade school and high school, I was disappointed with my college experience. Instead of being enjoyable it had become an experience of endurance.

I wanted to be happy but I had a lot of angry feelings. I wanted to lash out at the persons I thought were responsible for my unhappiness. I remember having fleeting fantasies of murder. It distressed me to think how deep my resentment went."

That summer Vivian made high scores in her state nursing tests to become a Registered Nurse, but she was already thinking about psychiatric nursing.

Vivian had dated a variety of guys. "I was too good-hearted to turn anyone down. My policy was to date at least once anyone who asked me." In her junior year she met John Adams. He was a year older and told her his parents had divorced when he was fifteen after years of fighting and separations. His three sisters and brother, all younger, lived in a foster home. His family experience had been chaotic and his foster parents were dogmatic, authoritarian Mennonite people. He had finished his senior year at Heston and was out of school to earn money for college. "My heart ached for this guy. He was so sincere and attractive … I wanted to know him more and reach out to him. He sure hadn't experienced much love in his life."

On their first date he brought her a corsage which impressed her. Her parents suggested that, as she was young and planning to go to college for nurse training, she should date more than one guy. She told John and he started dating her friend Annette. She did not date anyone else because she wanted someone more "challenging and exciting". John was both and she kept thinking of him. When John came to say good-bye, she asked for a kiss. "I wanted him to be the first guy to kiss me even if I didn't see him again. He said he liked me but felt he did not deserve me, confessing he'd had intercourse with several girls already, including his foster sister." He said he would decide between Vivian and Annette that summer. "The two of us watched him from an obscure window as he left the next day. Both of us knew one of us would be chosen; both of us sensed it would be me."

At the end of the summer they dated regularly, both being in the choir and leaders in the Christian organisation. "We were considered a striking couple." When John said he did not know what love was, Vivian reassured him that he could love and feel loved. She thought "once I gave him enough love he would automatically give me a lot

back too." One evening he said he had been thinking and would like her to be the mother of his children. She realised that he was asking her to marry him but it wasn't the way she had envisioned being proposed to. She felt ambivalent.

"He was tall, handsome, had black hair, could sing bass, and his name was John. It fit my childhood imaginary boyfriend. In addition he brought to me a sense of mysteriousness. He was a challenge to me. He stimulated my thinking and my logic. He pushed me to consider new dimensions."

John was resentful and angry with his mother who was dependent and depressed. She had not been able to care for her children and needed to be hospitalised. She had moved to Heston to be close to John so he could help her make decisions.

He told Vivian that he had a bad temper but it was hard for her to believe since she had never seen him lose his temper. "He was moody at times but not overtly angry. I had a great trust that people could change to the point of being unrealistic ... I didn't understand the deeper meaning of his own struggle. I was unaware of the psychological significances of his relationship with his mother or other women."

John started talking about getting married before she had made a decision. She found herself going along with it because "I didn't want to make anyone feel bad but in the meantime I was not clear about what I wanted." He told her father that he wanted to marry Vivian because he wanted her to be the mother of his children and she would make a good home. Only as an afterthought did he say he loved her. Looking back, she remembered the "pained expression on dad's face."

In the Fall of 1965 they were both attending Goshen College and Vivian had sent out the wedding invitations when one evening John became angry with her. She thought "if the invitations weren't sent out already I would break up with him."

"I had a big need to give to him and he had a big need to receive, to have an all-accepting mother-type, nurturing, forgiving and supporting. With that we entered marriage."

They wrote their own marriage vows and planned the ceremony. "We felt together and had high expectations for our marriage centered in Christ. Our desire was to have a good Christian home. We were

young. I was almost twenty and he was almost twenty one."

After the wedding reception when Vivian's father said to John, "She is yours now. Take good care of my little girl" John was affronted and miffed for several years. Vivian was a virgin and did not enjoy their wedding night. She was "ambivalent about taking the responsibility of marriage. I felt very young ... I was afraid to trust him with my feelings thinking he would feel unloved and take it personally."

Their first year of marriage was busy. They were both at college and working one day a week to pay the rent on their one-room apartment and buy groceries. They were also active in the church. During their second year of marriage they moved to Westville for Vivian's psychiatric nurse training. Then John decided to take a year at Seminary college which Vivian was happy about. In the summer they moved to Florida to live in a type of Christian commune with two other couples and a single guy.

Then John decided he wanted to take a year of pastoral education in Ontario, Canada, so they moved there and Vivian worked as a psychiatric nurse in a large provincial hospital. They lived in a high-rise apartment with a balcony overlooking a meadow, woods and a river. She loved it and felt at home in psychiatric nursing, but their relationship began to deteriorate when she said she wanted them to spend more time together. She understood his need for space but she often felt left out and alone.

John was giving good sermons but was self-critical, asking Vivian "how can you listen to me knowing what I'm really like?" She loved "the strong, clear, purposeful John, the one who could preach and lead." She knew his intentions were good and ached for him, but he accused her of being critical. "No matter how good my intentions, no matter how I responded, things weren't working out."

Their American draft-dodging friends in Canada introduced them to smoking pot and Vivian experienced music visually, seeing the notes in colour. She loved "getting lost in music" but John was humiliated when she danced on a chair. He said he hated her goodness and her imperfections, and she sensed she was a scapegoat. Frequently their interactions ended with him giving her the finger and telling her to "Fuck off!" She tried to understand and love him no matter what he said or did. Then she tried to stand her ground but that ended in

physical fights. She felt lonely and powerless. She wanted to get away from him and the oppression. She had an image of a huge foot grinding her into the earth. She was sorry she had married him.

When they moved back to Goshen for John's final year in Seminary college, they saw a marriage counsellor. Vivian was the head nurse in a psychiatric unit and enjoyed her job. She felt more in control of her life. After John graduated, they sold their house and car, and went to Europe for fourteen weeks in the summer. They bought a VW in Germany and lived in it. "It was glorious," Vivian wrote. "We had a lot of close times and only twice did we get really angry with each other." However, she had a miscarriage on this trip which was disappointing to both of them. While in Switzerland they toured many of the places the Anabaptist movement had begun. "This summer was one of the highest points in my life. I was happy to share it with John."

They moved to Indiana in the Fall of 1971 after returning from Europe. John was the part-time pastor of a Mennonite church and an advisor to alcoholics at the Mental Health Centre where Vivian worked as a psychiatric nurse. They started buying another house. "I was feeling good about us. Being a minister's wife was a new role for me. We were a good team. I was a logical, feeling minister's wife yearning to find new avenues for spiritual integration."

Six months after they moved Vivian had her second miscarriage. They were again disappointed, but the following month she became pregnant. After three months she was optimistic about carrying this baby to full term. "We were happy. John talked about being a father proudly. I felt beautiful. I was so happy with a little baby inside." She started planning for a natural childbirth. "I had strong feelings about being able to experience the birth process and to share it with my husband. I thought it should be a couple experience." But John started to avoid her and said he did not like her "pregnant shape". He said it turned him off. She felt alone emotionally but luckily had supportive colleagues at work. Patricia was her supervisor and Marge had gone through a divorce. They patted her tummy and thought up names for the baby. John resented her friendship with Patricia but, as she wrote, "I didn't get any support from him so I found friends who supported me which made him angry so he didn't support me so much. I wanted

to be weak and I wanted him to be strong."

After seven years of marriage Mark was born by C-section in November 1972. Vivian realised that John was looking for a home and mother for himself, but she was not his mother and could not give him what he wanted from a mother. He struggled with dependency and independence. Vivian felt like "an empty cup". She had been "full and running over" at home with her family, but after giving all she had to John, she had very little replenishment.

"I was ecstatic with joy when Mark was born. I was determined to be a good mother. Mark and I came home on Thanksgiving day and it was a beautiful, loving day. We were happy parents. It was one of the best days of my life."

John helped take care of Mark, changing his diapers and bathing him, but he said he had fallen in love with his secretary who he said understood and listened to him. He was thinking about divorcing Vivian but wanted to be sure he had custody of Mark. He then decided to stay because he "really did love me, he said."

After the initial adjustment of having a new baby, their lives became more peaceful. Vivian stayed at home and was happy, but she became aware of how much energy was directed towards John in their marriage. "I tried asking for more things for myself. That was hard because it brought a resistance." She was determined to "make it good" with John and she continued her supportive friendship with Patricia who said her expectations of marriage were too high. Vivian had the hope that they could mature and create a warm, loving home.

In 1975 they moved to California. Vivian worked part-time at Pomona Psychiatric hospital, so she would have more time to pursue her interests. John, whom she described as a "walking encyclopedia" told her about Psychosynthesis and in 1976 she started studying at the Highpoint Foundation in Pasadena. "It combined education with personal synthesis," she wrote. "It also emphasised the spiritual part of man and I wanted to get more in touch with my spiritual part. It seemed to be just right for me."

She liked the idea of sharing the home responsibilities with John, who was open to it in principle, but in practise she had most of the home responsibilities! However, he did enjoy spending time with Mark

whom he loved. Vivian described Mark as her "delight". He was open, imaginative and creative, responding to affection, and in touch with his feelings. He loved to sing and made up tunes and words with his mother. As a family they acted out Bible stories and went on picnics. A Montessori school helped Mark to develop his skills and understanding in a setting with other children.

Vivian was coping better with John's anger although there were times when she longed for his support, affirmation and trust. "I am more hopeful than realistic," she wrote. "I do a bunch of denying to protect myself."

She started to meditate and keep a journal in which she recorded her dreams. She also started growing her nails after years of biting them. She planned and coordinated two adult Sunday School classes and sang with John in church. They were also hoping to have a second child. Vivian was looking at her problem of miscarrying and her ambivalence about having another child with John.

She knew that Psychosynthesis would be the foundation for her life's work because "it incorporates everything that's really important to me."

From 1977 to 1980 Vivian worked as a counsellor and teacher at Greenleaves Counselling Centre in Claremont, Highpoint in Pasadena, and the Psychosynthesis Association in Santa Monica, California. She also taught classes and worked as a counsellor at Synthesis in Kansas and was a part-time instructor at Hutchinson Community College in Kansas.

At some point during her Psychosynthesis training, Vivian realised that John was a narcissist and was only interested in having his own needs met. After a third miscarriage she left him and they divorced.

She worked at Highpoint until it closed in 1985. She then rented a detached house in Pasadena and set it up as a centre for counselling and teaching Psychosynthesis. It was a busy time for her, as she was also studying for a degree at Sierra University. Mark spent the week with his father in Claremont, where he went to school, and the weekends with Vivian.

From Vivian's Biography written during her Psychosynthesis training.

Paradise lost
Part one of A Divine Comedy by Vivian King

Welcome to paradise, say I to guests weary of the rumble of
daily life as they get out of the car in front of my casita.

A gift from the Goddess of Spirit Mountain,
my adobe dwelling cuddles up to the mountain
and opens to 1500 acres of pristine forest.

Come with me to the waterfall - a gentle hike by the stream
amidst wild flowers, ponderosa pines, and pinion trees.

If we walk further, we'll come to the walled-canyon-bedroom
where my love read his poetry as we lay beside the gurgling
stream; where Mr. Serr pitched the pup tent while I grilled
chicken over the open fire; where Gabriella's perfect sapling
was trampled to death by a trespassing bull; where my hermit
friend dreamed of hiding out to meditate for the world.

On the way back, let's wade in the stream
and pick aromatic mint for afternoon tea.

Home from our hike, the shade of the cottonwood is the
perfect place to sip tea and eat freshly baked apple pie.
If you have time, you can help pick apples
before the brown bear harvests the crop.

After resting, we'll paddle the canoe across the lake
to look for the family of mallard ducks in the cattails.
Let's go ashore to pick bouquets of wild flowers
for the kitchen table, and then sit on the deck
to watch swallows swoop for their supper.

It is so still. Can you hear the silence?

When ready to leave this Garden of Eden,
my guests breathe a prayer for the preservation of quiet places.

After waving goodbye, I pack one bag for a weekend trip,
lock the gate, and drive down the dusty road.

Mercifully, I do not know that I am being ushered out of the
Garden as gently as I was ushered in.

PART ONE

Vivian in hospital

I had just received an email saying Vivian had been seriously injured in a car crash and was in a coma in hospital in Texas. I immediately called my local travel agent and asked them to book me flights so that I could be there in a day. I flew from Inverness to Heathrow, Heathrow to Dallas, and Dallas to Amarillo. I was there by the end of a very long day.

I arrived in Amarillo on September 16th, ten days after the car crash. Vivian's friend Murial met me at the airport and drove me straight to the hospital where Vivian was on a ventilator with two tubes down her throat. The right side of her face, which had hit the steering wheel, was the size of a melon. Her face, eyes and legs were black and blue. She was in a coma and the doctors did not know if she had suffered brain damage.

I had been booked into a Ronald McDonald house which accommodates relatives of critically ill people in the nearby hospital. Yes, the MacDonald burger chain has subsidised houses attached to hospitals in America. They made a special concession for me because Vivian had no relatives in Texas. Her father had been taken ill, and she was driving from Santa Fe to Kansas when she smashed into a truck which turned onto the freeway without checking to see if anyone was coming. A trauma nurse driving to hospital saved Vivian's life.

I was given a comfortable room with an en suite bathroom and a telephone extension for the numerous calls I would receive from Vivian's friends and relatives in the coming weeks when I visited Vivian every day in the hospital. My accommodation was $10 a night and everyone contributed towards it. The staff were friendly and wrote notes about us in a book in their office. They wrote that I was a joy! I made them laugh when I asked why they did not have an electric kettle in the kitchen. Americans boil water for hot drinks in their microwave ovens. They had to show me how the microwave worked.

The only problem was that the air conditioning was on all

night and kept us awake. Hot air blew into our bedrooms if it was chilly and cold air if it was warm. We all complained about it but they refused to switch it off. So, I found where the boiler was and unplugged it every night. I had to wait until late, when there was nobody to see me, and plug it back in again early in the morning. One night I locked myself out of my bedroom and had to sleep on the library floor, but it was worth it to have a good night's sleep.

I visited Vivian every day in the Intensive Care Unit for brief periods. I was not allowed to stay for long and I sat in the cafe downstairs reading between visits. It was cold in her room and I had to wear my anorak.

A week later Vivian responded by blinking her eyes when she appeared to recognise me. When asked if she knew me, she made rapid eye movements. She started to make sustained eye contact with me and flickered her eyes when I asked if she wanted flowers and to listen to a music tape. She then agreed to lower her eyes for NO and roll them up for YES. Now we could communicate. She had been told about the car crash but I'm not sure how aware she was of not being able to move or speak. The doctors did not know if she was paralysed. I started to write a diary each day about our time together and her progress.

September 27th

This morning I told Vivian I would bring a Buddhist meditation tape in the afternoon. When I returned later I asked her if she wanted to hear Mozart: NO. Bach: NO. The meditation tape: YES. She had remembered. After we had listened to the tape I asked her about the various music tapes I had brought with me. NO. She wanted another Buddhist meditation tape.

Vivian loved listening to the tapes made by the Zen Monk Thich Nhat Hanh:

Pain, love and happiness

Like a pebble, allow the Self to rest at the bottom of a river.
Sink naturally.
Resting is the first part of Buddhist meditation.
Rest the mind and body.
Only through rest can we heal ourselves.
We are always struggling.
It is a habit!
When wounded, rest and fast.
We are restless.
Our consciousness needs to rest.
We know how to heal ourselves.
Being alive is a miracle.
Walk as if you are massaging the earth with your feet.
Don't regret the past or worry about the future.
"I have arrived, I have arrived, I am home. I am home.
I am here in the here and the now."
Smile at your eyes.
Smile to your heart.
To meditate is to be present.
Mindfulness is being here.
STOP.
Touch the foundations of your being.
God is the foundation of your being.
Love is available twenty four hours a day.

As I could not pronounce Thich Nhat Hanh, I called him Nick
Nack Noo!

The doctors were concerned because Mark, Vivian's son,
wanted her in New York where he lived, but her father wanted her
in Kansas where he lived. I led a meditation with Vivian so that
she could make her own decision. She then slept all afternoon.

The following day she was delighted to receive a photo of her dog Free whom she had left with neighbours. This photo is now on the front cover of *Viva*. It was taken a week before the car-crash.

September 30th
Vivian was very attentive and her eyes were moving together for the first time. I played a meditation tape which she really enjoyed. Her eyes were going up a great deal showing pleasure. Her chest was still congested but the stuff coming up was now a lighter shade. She started to feel being touched although she still could not move.

October 1st
Vivian was alert and responsive. I asked her what she wanted and she chose another Thich Nhat Hanh tape, 'Dharma Talk', to which we both listened. I was now placing a warm wash cloth on her face, sprinkled with fragrance, which she loved.

October 2nd
We listened to another Thich Nhat Hanh tape during which she drifted in and out of sleep. I left her with the dawn bird song tape she had recorded when we lived together in Pasadena. In the afternoon I asked her if she wanted to listen to a music tape: NO. A talking tape: NO. Guided Imagery: YES. The Guided Imagery I did with her was not written down or rehearsed. It merely flowed through me when I sat beside her bed and looked into her eyes.

The stream of love

Imagine yourself in a beautiful meadow, feel the grass beneath your bare feet: cool, springy and a little damp with morning dew. The grass is like a green carpet stretching out to a stream with mountains in the distance. Look at the red and orange poppies growing in the

grass at your feet. You can pick some if you want to. They look so vibrant and alive. You notice that they are all turned towards the sun which shines down upon your head, its healing rays warm and vibrant. It feels SO good.

Walk to the stream which flows down from the mountains. It flows from heaven to earth. It is the Stream of Love. Step into the cool clear water and let yourself float. You feel SO light, and as you float, the sun shines its healing rays on your face and body, and all around you. There may be some beings embracing you in the Stream of Love.

Each day I visited Vivian in Intensive Care I asked her what she wanted and gave her choices. She always knew exactly what she wanted. She could now sit in a chair, but not for long, as it exhausted her. If she spent a morning sitting in the chair, she slept all afternoon in bed. What she loved more than anything else was the guided imagery I did with her. A nurse asked me what I was doing to cause her to look so enthralled.

The Rose Garden

We are going on a journey to the rose garden. We will start in the beautiful green meadow where we are running hand in hand through the damp grass and bright red poppies. Feel them on your feet and legs.

Now we are beside the Stream of Love where there is a small rowing boat. We are climbing into the boat and I'm rowing us up the stream towards the mountains. Can you see the snow on the mountain tops? Around the next bend you will see a sandy beach where we are going to leave the boat. Now you can feel the water and the sand on your bare feet. It feels SO good.

Beyond the beach is a wood where tall trees reach for the sky. Fallen leaves cling to our bare feet as we walk beneath the trees. Choose one of the trees and put your arms around it. Feel its strength

and patience. This tree took years to grow. It just IS. Taking up moisture and nutrients from the earth, it reaches for the sky, offering shelter to birds and small animals. It does not move unless blown by the wind and it does not weep when its leaves drop off. It knows that new leaves will grow again in the spring. It teaches us to be patient and strong.

Beyond the wood you notice an ancient stone wall with a gnarled wooden door. Feel the cool stones and the grain of the wood with your fingers. The stones are as old as the world and nobody knows who built this wall. Beyond the wooden door you will find yourself in the rose garden. It is filled with roses of all types and colours. Their fragrance fills your being as you search for your rose. How is your rose? What does it need? Ask the gardener for help if you need to. Then stand back to admire its beauty and inhale its fragrance. Become the rose.

October 5ᵗʰ

Vivian appeared to be sad. Her brother and his wife had just visited and left. We listened to a tape in the morning and she slept all afternoon.

The following day she smiled when I read a card from a friend who described herself as "Vivian's soul-mate". I acted 'possessive' which caused her to smile. Most of the friends who called said Vivian was their best friend, and indeed I saw her as my best friend. She then began to nod her head, which does not sound much, but it was a major step for her.

I continued with the guided imagery whenever we were alone.

The Healing Pool

Beyond the Rose Garden is a Herb Garden where every type of herb grows. You can smell the lavender, rosemary and basil as you approach. Their fragrance fills your being. In the middle of the Herb Garden is the Healing Pool where lotus flowers grow. You can step

into the healing pool and stand with your feet in the mud where the lotus flowers have their roots. With your head above the water, you can feel the sun on your face and head. Let it penetrate your being with its healing radiance. Smell the herbs and look up at the eucalyptus trees which surround the pool. They are all rooted in the earth. Let the gardener pick some healing herbs for you.

October 9th

Vivian was obviously pleased to see me and indicated that she had slept well the night before, but she was in pain with her left arm. I was only able to massage her hands and feet, which she loved me to do, and she did not want me to leave.

When I spoke to Vivian's doctor, he said she could be stuck here in the hospital for months if a decision was not made by her family. Mark still wanted her in a care facility in New York but her father wanted her in one in Kansas. A care facility is a nursing home usually for the elderly. I told him that she could communicate and make her own decision. He was amazed to hear this because he thought she had suffered brain damage. I explained that I was communicating with her every day. She looked down for NO and up for YES. I told him that I had taught physically disabled children, some of whom could not talk or move, like Vivian.

I visited Vivian every day offering various tapes, a foot massage or guided imagery. Bill, who had fallen in love with her just before she had the accident, sent her a music tape called Celtic Woman, which I pretended to forget about, but which she remembered. She still could not speak but she responded when I asked her what she wanted. Guided Imagery was her absolute favourite.

The Healing Temple

High in the mountains is the healing temple. It is in the middle of a beautiful garden where every type of flower grows in abundance. There is a stream nearby and a winding path leading up to a door. We are going to walk through this door into the healing temple which is circular with beautiful stained glass windows. As you walk in, the sun shining through the windows casts pastel shades onto your face and body: pale pink, turquoise, yellow, blue, lavender. Let these healing colours penetrate your being. Now you notice an altar in the centre of the temple. It is your altar created for you by your Soul. Walk up to it. In the middle stands a gorgeous golden candle holder. It is tall, graceful and intricately carved with exquisite designs. In it stands a white candle, its light encircling the altar. This white candle, set in its golden container, is your Spirit. Around it, in a circle, are six candles. The first one is red and symbolises your physical body. Around it are gifts for your physical body. Examine the gifts before moving onto the orange candle which symbolises your emotional body. Look at the gifts for your emotional body. Next is a yellow candle symbolising your mental body. As you examine the gifts for your mental body, you feel a new presence by your side. You look up and see your Soul radiant and wearing an exquisite gown which appears to shimmer. She is giving you a beautiful golden bag which she says belongs to you. It is covered in pearls symbolising times of suffering in your life. There is a great secret within suffering. It is this: our suffering creates pearls which are our gift to the world.

You are asked to choose a gift from beneath your red, orange and yellow candles. Take these gifts for your body, emotions, and mind, and place them in your golden bag. Now look at the green candle, which symbolises your heart, and choose one of the gifts placed there. Then look at the blue candle symbolizing your throat/voice/ creativity, and take one of the gifts beneath it. Now you have five gifts in your golden bag, but there is one more candle: a beautiful

*lavender candle symbolising your intuition. When you have chosen
your gift from beneath it, look at the white candle in the golden holder.
Beneath it lies the largest and most gorgeous pearl you have ever seen.
It is placed in your hand as a symbol of your current suffering and it
symbolises the great gift you will one day give to the world.*

*Now with the gifts in your golden bag, you are led to the Inner
Sanctum where you stand in the Golden Fountain of Eternal Life to
be healed and to see what your life purpose is.*

I had no idea where this guided imagery came from. It just
flowed through me when I sat beside the bed and tuned into
Vivian. Although she could not communicate, she was obviously
deeply moved.

October 11ᵗʰ
We had a quiet morning listening to a music tape as I massaged
Vivian's hands and feet with a lot of eye contact. In the afternoon
she was strapped into her shoes and chair. She was upset about
Mark's insistence on taking her to a care facility in New York.

That night I dreamt she was in a refrigerator and I was
concerned that she would not survive. Then she climbed out and
walked. In another dream she was searching for silver.

Vivian had a tracheotomy in her throat, which is a surgical cut
in the windpipe with a tube inserted into it, to enable her to
breathe. This prevented her from talking, but she had been
promised a special valve which would enable her to speak. As she
still had stuff coming up from her lungs, the nurses and I suctioned
through the tube in her throat using a special suction device.

October 12ᵗʰ
Vivian was obviously upset. She wept with tears rolling down
her cheeks. It was the first time I had seen her cry. After some
questioning she indicated that she was upset about Mark. In the
afternoon a nurse arrived with the speaking valve which we

hoped would enable her to speak. We had both looked forward to the arrival of the speaking valve. She tried desperately to talk but only managed to growl. We were hugely disappointed. Then her heart rate went up because she was on her right side causing spasms in her stomach. She was more comfortable on her back but the nurses were concerned about bed sores.

The following day social workers arrived to see if Vivian could choose between New York and Kansas. She could not decide and indicated that she wanted to stay in the hospital. She then slept all afternoon with a high temperature. She looked depressed when she woke up. Her father called and told me he did not know what to do. He sounded upset and close to tears. The hospital wanted Mark to visit Vivian and talk about possible solutions.

Bill came for the weekend and felt that she was depressed. Who wouldn't be? Her father and brother visited on the Monday but left on Tuesday. There was talk of moving Vivian to Dallas. She was fed up with being in intensive care and should have been moved two weeks ago. Dallas was probably chosen because it was the nearest rehabilitation facility.

In the middle of our Triangle Meditation, which we had been doing every Monday for a year, a nun called Maria, who had been involved in a car crash a year ago, visited Vivian. She had totally recovered and was able to walk and talk. She had come to reassure Vivian.

I continued to go to the hospital every morning to spend time with Vivian. I had lunch in the hospital cafe and walked back to my accommodation through a park. I returned later in the afternoon and remained until supper time when I walked back. Volunteers often arrived at the Ronald McDonald house in the evenings to cook meals for us even though we each had our own fridge and could cook for ourselves. I spent the rest of the evening emailing and talking to people on the telephone about Vivian's progress.

Vivian's Dreams And Memories From Amarillo:

I am in a grey place. I don't know how to get out. I look up and see Marilyn with a book. She has one foot on a step leading to an arch. I look past the arch and see the City of Gold, and I know I will be O.K. if I follow Marilyn. So I do not worry."

I remember dad's hand on my leg, and it was comforting. He asked if I could feel his hand and I said yes. He said 'Good. That means you can feel.'

I thought I could write. I was upset they never gave me paper or pen. I kept asking for both. I thought I would ask for pen and pad. That was the shortest word for both that I could ask for. Then Bill came and I thought he would understand what I wanted. He had a gold pen between the second and third buttons on his shirt. He sat beside my bed and I kept looking at his pen, hoping he would give me the pen. He sat and cried. I thought he was crying because our future was destroyed. I wanted to reach over and comfort him but I couldn't and I was mad at him for not giving me the pen.

I thought I was collecting pens and pieces of paper people left behind or pens I took from their pockets. I decided it was not stealing. I would hide them in my bedside drawer but I never could find a pen and paper at the same time.

One male attendant gave me paper and a pen and asked me to write my address. I wrote a full page letter and put it on the bedside table for him. I never saw the paper again. I thought they changed the bed and threw away the paper. I was frustrated.

I thought I could move my arms and legs. That's all I remember from Amarillo.

Then I started having memories in Dallas. I remember Marilyn telling me that I was in an accident.

Vivian's Inferno
Part two of A Divine Comedy by Vivian King

With sirens and flashing red lights,
I am transported on a stretcher to the House of Suffering.
For weeks I sleep, unmindful of where I am.

Friends, family, and angels gather round to uphold me
on a red, velvet pillow. Their prayers sustain me
as I descend into the deep.

My life is upside down on the other side of light.
I who love beauty, fun, privacy, freedom, ease, and laughter:
I am now bereft of these in the House of Suffering.

I suffer ...
... thinking I am in a dark attic maze.
... being unable to talk or ask for help.
... being unable to walk or to move my arms.
... being unable to change positions in bed.
... wanting to call for help but the call-bell is out of reach.
... thinking I can write but no one gives me pen and paper.
... discovering that I can't write after all.
... fearing something is wrong with my will because I don't move.
... believing something is real when it is not.
... being handled like a bag of potatoes by some of the attendants.
... feeling like a frozen fish in a room kept cold for 'brain patients'.
... watching my lover cry without being able to reach out to him.
... tasting no food because I am fed through a tube in my stomach.
... drinking no water because I am unable to swallow.
... living with disorder in my room.
... letting others comb my hair and put on makeup – their way.
... living by the timing of others.

... having double vision and thinking I have three eyes.
... seeing my face in a mirror.
... sounding like a swamp monster as I cough, wheeze, and gurgle.
... fearing I am losing my grasp on life.
... knowing that my family and friends are suffering because I am.

Gradually I grasp the fact that I am ...
... an independent person now totally dependent.
... a communicator without a voice.
... a writer without the use of my hands.
... a lover without the ability to caress.
... a mother unable to pick a birthday present for my son.
... a daughter unable to assist my aging father.
... a nature lover confined to a wheelchair and bed.
... an orderly person in a chaotic situation.

Still I don't feel this is a tragedy.
Yes, I have lost my home, my work, my dog, my car, my health,
but I have not lost my self.

I remain, whether dependent or independent; grieving or joyous;
confined or free; misshapen or beautiful; pitiful or dignified;
disorganized or organized; frustrated or peaceful;
handicapped or normal.
In life or death, I cannot be destroyed.

PART TWO

Rehab in Dallas

October 22nd
We flew to Dallas in an air ambulance just big enough for the pilot, Vivian, a nurse, me and our luggage. We left at 8.30 a.m. Vivian was transferred to the Baylor Institute in Dallas to a ward with four beds. We were disappointed that she did not have her own room, and there was nowhere to put her Get Well cards so that she could see them. I tied her angel balloon to the end of the bed and stuck her angel picture on the bottom of the TV screen where she could see them. I was given a temporary apartment nearby. Vivian was put back on oxygen and appeared to be down-hearted.

A week later she was moved to a corner bed in the ward between a window and a wall on which I could display her cards. We both preferred this location.

Valentina, a Russian healer, and a local healer called Janice visited Vivian regularly. We also had a meditation for Vivian every Wednesday evening in Janice's house in Dallas. I did not know how these people knew about Vivian but she had a large network of friends especially from her teaching in Eastern Europe.

At Baylor Vivian was dressed in loose trousers and baggy T-shirts during the day when she had her various therapies which included physiotherapy, speech and occupational therapy. When I first gave her the T-shirts, she looked horrified. They were big because I had been told to buy big ones. It was painful to see her in a wheelchair with a urine bag strapped to her leg.

In the Assessment it was revealed that Vivian had a fracture close to her pituitary gland. We were told she would be in Dallas for two months and then have to choose between New York and Kansas. I had already told her that there needed to be a point of synthesis, a third option. It was not either or. I was busily creating projects to help Vivian communicate and arranging her many Get Well cards. When her brothers visited they said I was

wearing colours their mother would have chosen. I often felt I was there in place of her mother who had died in 1995.

I was installed in a self-contained apartment in the Ark House, which had been set up by a charity for families visiting critically ill patients in the local hospitals. Some of the people staying in the Ark House had sold everything, including their homes, to pay medical bills.

I walked to Baylor in the morning to spend time with Vivian. I had lunch in the hospital cafe nearby, and in the evening I called for a free lift back which was provided by the Baylor Hospital Police. As I had a telephone in the apartment, people often called in the evening to talk about Vivian's progress. I was also able to email updates on my laptop to a long list of friends and family.

Vivian was exhausted by the various therapies and slept a lot. The left side of her face looked normal, and that eye closed when she was asleep, but her right eye always remained half open and was not tracking. She was seeing double and often looked above my head as if she was seeing me up there. Her lungs had cleared and she was dressed during the day. She was pleased when I told her I was staying. My return flight had already gone!

She started communicating with her eyes, using a big alphabet card, and spelled out a letter to Mark: "I love you. I miss you. I'm still here. I'd love to see you."

On Sunday November 1st I took Vivian exploring the building in a wheelchair and we ended up in a chapel where we prayed. It was a small chapel with stained glass windows and an altar. I have never prayed for anyone as passionately as I prayed for Vivian. I was desperate for her to recover. If anyone talked about the possibility of her not recovering, I went into denial. I could not entertain the thought. Of course she would recover. How could such a wonderful person not recover?

The following day we were meditating together in our Triangle

Meditation when a young man arrived to take Vivian to another hospital for surgery. He told us, as he pushed her on a trolley through a long underground tunnel, that he had been involved in a serious car crash in 1991 and had made a full recovery after nine months in rehab. He showed us the tracheotomy scar on his neck. This was the second time someone had appeared during our Triangle Meditation and told us they had made a full recovery. The first time was when the nun appeared in Amarillo. I saw it as a positive sign for Vivian's recovery.

Vivian's CT scan had revealed fluid on her brain. The surgery was to insert a shunt in her brain to drain off the fluid. I waited with her and left when she was taken into surgery. She looked scared. She was brought back the following morning looking like the Last of the Mohicans with the right side of her head shaved. She was pleased to see me but slept most of the day. Her right eye had been stuck shut with tape because she could not close it. We were praying that the shunt would help her to move and communicate. In my dreams she walked and talked.

Vivian was looking very distressed as her growing awareness revealed the full extent of her injuries. She was unable to move or talk. What a horrible shock. She looked at her cards as if she had never seen them before. She had looked more dreamy and peaceful before surgery.

November 6th

Vivian's friend Penelope arrived in the evening and saw that Vivian was visibly distressed. Although she was pleased to see Penelope, we were not sure that she recognized her. It took a long time to calm Vivian who was anxious with rapid eye movements. Penelope started rubbing a homeopathic remedy for shock onto Vivian's elbow because the doctors would not allow it in her mouth. Penelope replaced me over the weekend, as I was by now exhausted.

When Penelope read emails from friends, Vivian was visibly moved. A beautiful bouquet of flowers arrived from Adam, a friend in California. Vivian chose to listen to the Sacred Garden tape and then the Gregorian Chant tape which appeared to calm her.

Penelope lay on Vivian's bed and sang to her, but when she tried to lead a guided meditation Vivian was not responsive. Penelope tried again and asked if Vivian wanted her eyes open or shut. She was thrilled when Vivian mouthed "Open." She also stuck out her tongue a few times, obviously attempting to talk.

By Sunday Vivian was mouthing the words yes and no, and was nodding her head. Her eyes were tracking together and the right side of her face was relaxing. They had a wonderful day reconnecting and gazing through the window at the treetops.

Penelope asked if Vivian was sad or angry. "No," she mouthed. "Scared." She also mouthed "No" to being bored. She loved it when Penelope climbed into bed with her. She whispered into her ear that if anything ever happened to her, she wanted Vivian to promise that she would climb into bed with her. Vivian nodded vigorously. When Penelope cried, she asked if it was O.K. for her to cry. Vivian nodded a vigorous YES.

In her diary entry Penelope encouraged other people to hold Vivian and give her physical support. I had attempted to write in Vivian's diary every day since I arrived in Amarillo, and this explains why I can recall dates and details.

After Penelope had gone, Vivian wanted to communicate using the big alphabet card, eye movements and mouthing words. She clearly formed the word "love" with her lips and tongue. She dictated another letter to Mark: "I hope that we can talk on your birthday. I will call you. Love, Mom." I'm not sure how she thought she was going to be able to talk to him.

I had bought several birthday cards for him and she chose one that said:

"A great person is one who has not lost the heart of a child."

Vivian mouthed seven kisses. She was now much more alert but did not remember being in Intensive Care. With the birthday card we sent a copy of 'The Diving Bell and the Butterfly' by Jean-Dominique Bauby, who could not move after a car-crash, but was able to write a book about his experiences, using eye movements and an alphabet card, likeVivian.

At this time I attended the Assessment Conference on Vivian. Dr Barnett, the neurosurgeon who had put the shunt inside Vivian's head, had found a blood clot on her brain-stem but said it was too dangerous to operate. She had experienced a brain-stem haemorrhage. He also said her 4th ventricle was blocked, causing facial droop, and her 7th cranial nerve was damaged. It had been decided that an ocular plastic surgeon would either sew up her right eye, which would not close, or put a gold weight on her eye-lid. Her hearing had also been affected. She could not swallow because the cuff balloon was still inflated in her throat to prevent mucous from her sinuses going down into her lungs. This inflated cuff prevented Vivian from talking which by now she was desperate to do. It also prevented her from eating. She was fed through a tube directly into her stomach.

Vivian commented through the alphabet card: "Spirit down."

I no longer had time to write in the diary every day, as I was now attending Vivian's therapy sessions. She showed me how she could move her head from side to side, and up and down. She could also move her tongue. I wheeled her around the building and often to the chapel where we prayed. During this time I looked at the people in wheelchairs, who could move their arms and talk, and I longed for the day when Vivian would be able to do these things. In her condition she was totally dependent. Before leaving I always asked her which music tape she'd like me to leave playing for her. I was thrilled when she mouthed "Mozart" which she had played almost every day when we lived together in Pasadena.

She commented through her alphabet card: "Hopeful."

November 19ᵗʰ
Vivian breathed through her mouth and nose for the first time since the crash, and she swallowed three times. I wrote it on her wall calendar.

November 21ˢᵗ
I rented the video 'Fly Away Home' for us to watch in the Quiet Room which I booked ahead of time. The weekend nurse made a big fuss, saying the night nurses would refuse to put Vivian to bed, but the Receptionist said the nurses were there for Vivian and insisted that I take her to the Quiet Room as planned. The Supervisor joined in and said he would make sure she was put to bed. Vivian was spell-bound watching the video. Then all the problems started.

As I wheeled Vivian back to the ward I saw Sandy, the day nurse, rushing to the elevator in order to avoid putting Vivian to bed. The night nurses, who had just arrived, obviously did not want to put her to bed. The Supervisor had totally disappeared, so the aide yanked Vivian out of her wheelchair and dumped her on the bed without supporting her head, which jerked backwards. This is extremely dangerous for someone with brain-stem injury. I subsequently reported the aide and Sandy, who was friendly but lazy, spending most of her time playing card games on the computer.

The following day Vivian's friend Cait arrived and I went into the city to the place where J. F. Kennedy had been shot. It was the anniversary and I thought it unlikely that I would ever be in Dallas again. I also went to the Book Depository which is now a museum.

A private concert by Stephen Levine, who channels angelic healing music, was arranged for Vivian, and afterwards she communicated that she felt "Blessed and loved."

She was now communicating through the alphabet card every day and spelled out "I hope that I will be normal" when we were talking about the future. She was understandably concerned about her physical condition.

Vivian showed Carlos, the Occupational therapist, what the pink sponge he put in her mouth tasted like. She pulled a horrible face indicating that it tasted disgusting.

The following day Vivian's chest was congested. She had an eye test which revealed that she needed to wear glasses. She also swallowed twice which was a great achievement.

At the end of the week Vivian was moved into her own room. We were thrilled because the ward was full, noisy and busy. She was often left sitting in a chair until quite late in the evening. Vivian had always been a lark: early to bed and early to rise.

A new healer called Varena arrived. She worked on Vivian using Toning, which had healed another woman after a serious car crash, who could now walk and talk. The woman who had been healed appeared on Sunday evening when we were watching a video. She had been brought by Anne Marie, Varena's friend, who made Vivian feel tired because we had to "listen her talk" which meant she talked too much. Vivian wanted her to visit less often, and I had the task of telling her.

Vivian now wanted to communicate using the alphabet card whenever I visited. On Thanksgiving Day she spelled out "Bored. Would like to read. First let us call Mark." She often wanted to call Mark, but dictated a letter instead: "How was your birthday? Did you get my letter? Tell me about your life. I love you."

Sometimes her messages were hard to understand, like "Head bed" when she wanted her bed raised and "Down" when she was feeling down.

She had a water mattress in her new room to prevent bed sores but it caused endless problems. "Get nurse" Vivian spelled out. "Upside down – bump – turn side." The nurse explained

that the water mattress would prevent bed sores. "Move upside bum make bed sheet water bed put the bump side turned a fix" which I interpreted to mean the water mattress was hurting her. "Turn section wrong side water mat" she continued. I called the nurse again but we could not figure out what the problem was. Vivian would not stop complaining about it for over an hour and I felt like throwing it out of the window. I even lay down on it myself to see if I could feel any bumps.

Thanksgiving weekend was a bad time for both of us. I had run out of money, food and energy. On the Sunday I arrived at 5 p.m. and the nurse said, with obvious judgment, "She was up and dressed ALL day." I had rented another video but Vivian wanted to communicate first. We finally watched the video at 8 p.m. and the Bailor Police failed to collect me until late. I must add that this minor problem was nothing compared to Vivian's!

Vivian remembered sending an email about going to Kansas but did not remember leaving home in Santa Fe before the car crash. She did not remember leaving Amarillo but remembered being there. She did not remember going for surgery or returning, but she remembered Penelope's visit.

"Come here when I did fly?" meant "When did I fly to Dallas?"

"Rested tired bed laying" meant "Tired of laying in bed."

At the beginning of December I found Vivian sitting in her wheelchair on Reception. She looked depressed and later told me she was worried and needed prayers. A new person had been to see her. "New person" she spelled out. "Strange speech therapist." I never found out who it was.

December 3rd
Vivian returned from surgery with a gold weight inside her eye lid. She could now close both eyes and was thrilled to get it done before Bill arrived for the weekend. I did not have the heart to tell her that she now had a black eye!

Carlos, the occupational therapist, told us a communication specialist was coming to explore the technology involved in bio-engineered environmental control. We had NO idea what it meant but it sounded good.

Vivian confided that she'd had wonderful dreams when she was in Amarillo and was going to write about them in her next book. I wondered if she was remembering the guided imagery I had done with her. She whispered my name and I had her practising "Hi Bill" and "I love you." We fell apart laughing when I tried to imitate her voice. I missed her voice, with its wonderful Kansas accent, and so did she.

After the weekend with Bill, Vivian told me it was an "amazing weekend" and they had been able to go outside. "I love Bill" she shared through the alphabet card. "I felt loved" and "Bill is patient."

As I'm dyslexic, when we used the alphabet card I had to write down every letter she spelled out, which was laborious. I was impressed when others knew what she was saying without having to write down every single letter, as I had to do.

December 8th

When I arrived Vivian was using, with great dexterity, the laser pointer Patricia had sent her. It was attached to an elasticated band around her head and enabled her to point to the letters on the alphabet card with more accuracy.

Her father, brother and sister-in-law arrived to attend the Case Conference at which we were told Vivian would definitely be staying in Dallas until January 7th because she was making good progress. She had motor functions in her arms and legs, and was able to communicate with the laser pointer. Her doctor hoped that she would stay until February 4th. The shunt and gold weight in her eye lid were both successful, and she could now close her right eye when she wanted to. Her speech therapist was

working on talking and swallowing, which Vivian was responding to, and she would be getting a special mouse to use with a computer. She was also going to a Wheelchair Clinic to get an electric wheelchair she could operate herself.

Mark was on the conference phone and asked about TBI units. He was told they are the same as rehabilitation facilities. The point of the TBI unit was to get Vivian to Kansas to be close to her family. In Dallas she only had me and occasional visits from friends and family. This was the only time we heard Mark's voice. He did not call, write or visit Vivian.

I wrote her Christmas cards and she told me what to say to each person. "Marilyn there's a note angel" she spelled out. It took ages for me to figure out what she meant. There was a note beside the angel. Then I lost the cards and we laughed as I searched for them. They were underneath the Christmas decorations. To Mark she wrote: "Another Christmas and we are not together except in spirit. I love you, Mom." To her family she wrote: "I won't be in Kansas this Christmas but all of you are in my heart. I love you, Vivian."

I massaged her feet and put on the long warm socks I had bought for her. She was always complaining about being cold at night. I put extra blankets on her bed every night which the nurses took away because they said Vivian had to be kept cool. The disappearing blankets really upset her and I was constantly searching for more blankets to put on her bed.

At dusk I often took Vivian outside in a wheelchair to hear the birds singing in the trees. She missed nature and being free. Earlier that day I had been for a long walk along Swiss Avenue, an historic street, to look at the beautiful mansions decorated for Christmas. I wished that she had been with me because I knew she would have loved it. In the evening we watched the video "As Good As It Gets".

Patricia came for the weekend and stayed with me in my

apartment where we were kept awake by rats. It sounded as if they were in the sitting room but they were probably only inside the wall trying to get into the sitting room!

Patricia put notices up everywhere about Vivian's needs. She wrote in the diary:

I was so excited by her progress in four weeks since I last saw her. When I arrived the respiratory therapist was giving her a treatment and then he placed a speaking valve over her trach and she said 'Pat can you hear me?' I jumped for joy. She was whispering really clearly. It's amazing how a little air coming up the windpipe can make so much difference. One can also read her lips much better especially when you know the context of what she is saying. She was able to keep the speaker valve in for an hour, with the therapist checking the oxygen concentration in her bloodstream, and it was saying 100%. Later in the day around 5 p.m. she again had the valve in for about an hour and 15 minutes. We were able to talk about several things that were on her mind. She wanted to talk about how cold she has been since she has been here. I had brought her cotton camisoles to put on under her shirts, also a long-sleeve cotton shirt in one of her favourite colors. I got permission from the supervisor to keep the air conditioning turned off at all times. She is in a small private room which can easily be cooled by hallway air. With brain injury they keep them cooler. She was given two blankets, knee socks which Marilyn had got her, camisole and long sleeve shirt, and no air conditioning. She had her first warm night at Baylor. I spent much of the two days negotiating with supervisors and nurses to get the continuity of care she deserves. Evening shift is the weakest link in the system because they have all part-time help and Vivian has to orient someone new every day to what she needs. They were not taking the time to try and read her lips or do the letter board. A week ago I woke up with the idea of affixing a laser light to a headband, so she could put the light on the letters making the process quicker. I shared the idea with her speech therapist and she encouraged me

to send it. I proceeded to sew velcro on a wide stretchy hair band. My husband had a small 2" square laser light with a switch in his workshop. It was perfect. We put velcro on it. The lithium batteries that last a long time are $9 each. Delva found it to be very suitable for Vivian and said they were impressed with her progress since they saw her on her second week at Baylor.

Vivian is swallowing better but her speech therapist is the decision-maker on when she will be able to try food. They usually start with apple sauce which goes down better than water. 'I don't have anything to swallow,' Vivian had told the respiratory therapist.

She has strength in her legs. She pressed down against my hand. She can't apply enough pressure in her hand to ring the call light. A pressure bar was put right next to her head, so she can roll her head onto it, and get the nurse.

Marilyn had suggested she needed a headset telephone, so for Christmas I got her a headset telephone, so when she is talking to someone, she does not have to hold the 'phone. It also allows for a three-way conversation. We put an adaptor on the wall which allows both 'phones to be hooked up at once. Vivian can listen and tell the person on the second 'phone her response, and they can repeat it. I thank my husband, Radio Shack and Marilyn's idea that she can more easily communicate with the 'phone system. Someone has to be in the room to help set it up for Vivian.

A neurologist has said Vivian is capable of making her own decisions, and she wants to. During the time I was there I found her sharp, on top of events, time and her care. She was watching the clock to make sure I didn't miss my shuttle to the airport. Her mental state was completely normal during the time I was there.

She has a sense of humour still, especially when she coughs and blows off the trach sponge cover, which is called a nose, and everyone is trying to dodge it. She said her presentations were not always a polite process.

When I told her I hoped I could see her every two weeks, she

spelled, 'Pat that is too much of a sacrifice.' I said, 'You would do it for me, wouldn't you? Wouldn't you?' and we both started laughing. On a semi-serious note she said she is tired of hearing from us that we couldn't go through what she is going through. 'I would rather not go through this at all,' she said. 'OK Viv I hear you,' I told her.

When you are first with her there is a learning curve or rhythm to get into dealing with equipment, lip movements etc.

Marilyn has set up Vivian's room so well with her bulletin board of cards, a small Christmas tree, and I brought a stocking. She is preparing to have a non-traditional Christmas with Bill, brother Kenny and his wife, and others I may not know.

She said she loves her freedom and this is such a polarity. 'Sometimes I don't know how I will do this whole thing but I try to stay positive.'

I really believe, after this weekend, that she will be able to talk, eat and walk again. I believe it will take time, but I believe it is possible.

We need to keep the prayers and energy coming for a long time but it will happen. I hope this gives you a glimpse into Vivian's experience and progress.

After Patricia had gone, Vivian told me she had made a Living Will which was in her house in Santa Fe. She said she wanted to give it a year. She also wanted me to call her neighbour and ask her to look for some apricot jam she had made last July.

On Tuesday night the aide stormed in, obviously in a bad mood, and ripped off Vivian's clothes. She then left Vivian in an uncomfortable position, and it took me an hour to get help. The Receptionist told me to move her myself but I had already tried to move her. Then the Respiratory therapist came in. "Hi baby doll," he addressed Vivian. "You look gorgeous tonight."

"I'm having difficulty breathing," she mouthed, and I repeated it to him, but he was deaf and did not wear a hearing aid. I said

it louder but he was too busy fiddling with the respirator. "She's dead!" I exclaimed, and Vivian cracked up laughing.

On Wednesday Vivian's friend Carol came with her husband who took me shopping. This was a rare treat for me. My nearest shop was a 7.11 convenience store a block away from the Ark House. It was a poor area and I had been told not to go out after dark.

December18th.
Vivian had surgery for a blood clot in her leg. She had an 'umbrella' inserted in her groin to prevent the blood clot from reaching her lungs.

December 20th.
I was leading Vivian in the Healing Temple imagery when her cousin Larry walked in. He had brought an email from Bill and some cookies. Larry described himself as "the black sheep of the family". Vivian's family were Mennonites, and her mother had shocked her parents when she cut her long hair. Larry had rebelled against the family's strict religious beliefs and had no contact with them. I loved hearing about Vivian's childhood, and as he talked she squeezed both our hands. Larry said Vivian was as sweet-natured as her mother, but when he told her she looked good, she pulled a hideous face and made us laugh. I often wondered how she kept her sense of humour.

On Tuesday Vivian moved her toes, feet and legs. I was thrilled and she was elated.

Bill arrived on Wednesday and was delighted with Vivian's progress. We opened our presents together on Christmas morning. Then we both sang to her as she sat on the bed-pan. I would have been embarrassed but she just smiled. She hated the bed-pan because it hurt her. Although she could not move, she was not paralysed. Bill slept in the bed with her over Christmas.

I had a quiet time on my own preparing for my departure, and grieving. I had been with Vivian for over three months and felt bonded to her like a mother to her child.

It was busy after Christmas. Vivian's friend Jenny arrived and lectured us both on "being grounded in our bodies". We ate together in the hospital cafe and, after giving me a long lecture, she tripped and fell flat on her face which I thought was an act of divine justice!

Valentina, the Russian healer, gave Vivian a healing session, and then offered one to me. She told us both to go to California, and then gave us some advice: "Don't kiss your honey when your nose is runny. You may think it's funny but it's not." She was amusing and I preferred her to Varena who did not appear to have a sense of humour. That night I dreamt I gave birth to twin girls on June 11th. When I told Valentina she said June 11th was her mother's birthday. This is interesting because her mother almost became Vivian's carer when she later moved to California

On Wednesday an Attorney arrived. He specialised in personal injury claims and wanted to claim damages from the person who had caused the accident: a 21-year-old driving his father's truck. He had been out shooting prairie dogs and drinking with a friend, and was not paying attention. I thought it was tragic that Vivian, who taught and wrote about consciousness, should be hit by someone so unconscious. Unfortunately the truck was not insured and Vivian decided not to prosecute the young man who had ruined her life.

After Christmas I developed 'flu and spent a week in bed with Patricia's electric blanket which she had left for me in the Ark House. My friends called from the UK and were concerned to hear me croaking and coughing. At some point I crawled out of bed and went to the 7.11 store to buy cough sweets and a tin of soup. When I had recovered I returned home to Scotland, with special thanks to British Airways who allowed me to change my

non-refundable return ticket. It was painful leaving Vivian, but she had a wonderful new nurse called Joan, and Bill and Patricia were going to make regular visits.

Email from Patricia

Vivian's mood and physical condition continue to improve although she is still hampered by her respiratory condition. Tomorrow morning Baylor will do a fiberoptic endoscopic evaluation of her swallow.

Vivian still has weakness on the right side of her face. An ENT will do a high resolution CAT scan on her temple bone where facial nerves run. Also a nerve conduction study to see if more can't be done for her regarding this.

It still looks like February 4th for her discharge date. Baylor will strongly recommend a short stay in a sub-acute (Long Beach Memorial) before recommending her to a skilled nursing facility. When I talked with her insurance company this morning, her case manager indicated that they would probably approve this move with Baylor's recommendation.

I spent this Tuesday, Wednesday and Thursday with Vivian and found her to be in good spirits. She had been battling some depression but still trying not to give energy to it. The Zoloft is kicking in and she feels better. Dr Carlisle tells her she is quite a trouper and she is trying to be that.

I went to all of her therapy sessions and saw how much she has gained in overall strength. She can push down with her legs well and pull them up so knees are approximately ten inches off the bed. She can move her arms from her side so her hand can reach her navel. She can touch thumbs to each of her fingers and her grasp has strengthened. She can stand momentarily when being moved from wheelchair to bed or to physical therapy mat. She is working on mouth exercises. Her volunteer friend Beth from Dallas, whose husband had a similar injury, has been visiting and she told Vivian

about how her husband increased his swallow strength by sucking, so Vivian said what about a pacifier? Beth checked it out with the doctor and immediately purchased a dummy from the hospital gift shop. We gave it to Vivian and she latched on well. We all broke into laughter! It was too funny but we agreed she could do it in private! I removed the pacifier after a minute and placed my hand on the right side of her neck and asked her to swallow. She had a strong swallow on the right side of her throat but it felt less strong on her left side. Having a one-sided swallow still puts her at risk for secretions to go down her windpipe. We are hoping this will help to strengthen the 368 muscles it takes to swallow.

She is making tentative plans to leave Baylor but Dr Carlisle explained they never know exactly because as long as she is making progress they may O.K. her stay at Baylor. I am hoping to visit the facility in Long Beach on the 29th January on our way to Kauai for a week's vacation. I told Vivian I would fly with her if I get back in time. She believes she can fly commercially but the airline would have to agree to it, according to my United Airline Captain husband. A plane just for her would be the best. A respiratory therapist would also be important to have along.

She is very alert and on top of situations. When I visited she told me George Winston would be having a concert at 3 p.m. at Baylor. We attended and it was good. She later said she wanted to watch Clinton's State of the Union speech at 8 p.m. We did and she was listening intently. She is interested in all that is going on. We went through one battery in one day but of course she said I should turn the laser off more to save the batteries. Usually a battery lasts four days. We had lots of laughs. She worries about the distortion of her face as it is now, with left side animated and the right side much less so, but better than it was a month ago. I encouraged her to reframe this in her mind and pretend we were at a workshop making masks, and this mask is not the wholeness of Vivian. She is remembering her wholeness behind the present distortion instead of taking the

distortion into her heart.

The weather was warm while I was there, so she got some veranda time outside in the sunshine. It was great for me as well, having left the snowy cold of Indianapolis.

I read her several cards that came while I was there. She is going to the eye doctor on the 26th. She needs glasses to read.

Murial suggested we do something collectively for Vivian's birthday. I thought Vivian would like a personalized quilt. She currently has a quilt on her bed that her father made. He is a quilter. Vivian loves quilts in general. Several people have responded to this idea, so I will put it out to the larger group. I know we won't be able to have it finished by her birthday on February 18th but we could tell her about it or keep it for a belated surprise. If each person sent a square of material that is unique to what you want to say, I will engage a professional quilting friend to put it together and quilt it. You could have a picture of yourself or family scanned onto the material or make a collage of symbols, words or pictures. The possibilities are endless and knowing a little about this creative network of people, I am sure you can come up with something special. Let's make the squares 9" x 9" because Vivian has 41 people on this email list alone. The Blanket of Love will be large on her bed.

Marilyn asked if I would spread the word that Vivian's book 'Being Here When I Need Me' is available in smaller New Age bookshops through New Leaf Distributors.

Email from Bill

Vivian is definitely going to Long Beach memorial on 3rd February and her insurance has approved of everything including the air ambulance. Vivian will probably have Varena accompany her. I intend to meet her at the airport and ride with her to the hospital and stay for most of the week to see to it that she is set up in the most loving way possible.

Vivian's mood is much improved from the Zoloft but she is

beginning to feel homesick at the thought of leaving loving people like Joan (her nurse) and the healers who have given of their time. I'm sure it won't take her long, with all the friends she has in Southern California, to be inspired all over again to keep working at her rehabilitation, especially the swallow, so she can begin to talk. Of course she will have a communication device but I'll bet within three months she'll be talking on her own.

Marilyn, you love Vivian like a mother her child and it has helped Vivian very much. Now you need to rest while we take over for you until you can come back renewed.

Vivian continues to make steady progress and I really do believe she will be talking within three months. She gets very frustrated because there are so few who take the time to really listen to her. She leaves the morning of the 3rd and will spend a week on the acute side of Long Beach Memorial before being moved to the sub-acute side. Again, angels are clearing blocks and making her way easier. I plan on meeting Vivian at the airport for the ride over to the hospital, and will stay through the weekend to see to it that everything is to her liking.

PART THREE

Vivian in California

Vivian's letters to me from California

I have been thinking of you a lot. Thanks for your letters and card. I had a good birthday with friends. I forget my condition when I am with friends.

I am liking being in California again. I feel like it is easier to heal. Baby steps are my speed.

Sometimes I fall down. Like now I am recovering from pneumonia and have been all weekend. Yuk!

Bill has been here the past two weekends. He even gets in bed with me and spends the night with me. Night nurses like having him because he helps out and jokes with them. They have labelled me Ms Rehab, besides being Dairy Princess, I have this identity. Bill is easier for me to love and understand. Not that he wasn't easy before but we keep going deeper. He is emotionally intense and passionate. I am more cool emotionally, but I am stimulated by his feelings. He is similar to Penelope. I wish I could take him in my arms. He is very sensuous and touches me just right.

When do you think of coming? I am thinking of living close to here and coming to rehab. Valentina's mom may be my caretaker. If not we will find someone. If you come we can begin writing.

So for now I will say goodbye, and I love you much.

Dear Best Friend,

I love getting your letters and before too long I will be able to email also. It takes me a long time and my hands get tired fast. So the message is short. I'm looking forward to your journey to Mecca in sunny California.

Bill bought me a great boom box so you can have the tape recorder I had. Don't bring one. Mine has a great CD player. Until you get here I send my love.

Visiting Vivian in Granada Hills, California

I flew to L.A. at the beginning of July to spend a month with Vivian, who had joined New Start, an organization run by an English woman called Mary Williams. The aim of New Start was to enable disabled people to live an independent life. Its intention, it stated, was to offer affordable, accessible housing, specialized equipment, physiotherapy, transportation and carers.

New Start Medical Evaluation

Referral Source: Vivian King was referred by her private speech-language pathologist and her occupational therapist.

Medical History: Vivian King is a 54-year-old female with a diagnosis of traumatic brain injury with spastic quadroplegia, secondary to brain stem injury, which she sustained in a car accident on September 5th, 1998. She has had daily occupational and physical therapy for the past year and a half, and speech therapy on a weekly basis. Vivian's prognosis is medically stable.

Social and Educational History: Vivian used to work as a psychologist with a Ph.D. in psychology, and has authored several books. She desires to continue her vocational pursuits in the way of writing via computer access, but currently physical limitations interfere with efficient typing. She has a large family and friends support network, from whom she receives regular visits. She currently lives in a one-storey bottom-level apartment with a live-in attendant. She requires an attendant for self-care and meal preparation.

Motor Abilities:

Seating/positioning: Vivian is non-ambulatory and independently uses a powered wheelchair for mobility.

Head/trunk control: Vivian has good head control and uses back support and armrests for trunk support.

Upper extremity coordination and functional abilities: Severe

impairment of the upper extremities precludes the ability to write or use manual sign-language. Vivian is able to access computer keys with the use of a mobile arm-support on her right side. She currently uses her index finger with a rubber-tip splint to type on the keyboard. This is a slow and tedious way for her to type, in that she is limited by having to visually look back and forth at keys, and at the screen, and is only able to type one letter at a time. Additionally, her finger/hand extensors fatigue easily.

Secondary to vocal cord paralysis, Vivian has a difficult time instructing her attendants of her daily needs and on how to be positioned appropriately in her bed and in her wheelchair. She currently uses an amplified speaker system which is not functional in all her settings. The person that Vivian is communicating with must stand close and often needs her to repeat words/phrases. Vivian has expressed frustration in not being understood and more frequently resigns to not speaking secondary to this problem. Additionally, she is at risk of decreased safety secondary to time-consuming communication methods which could be life-threatening.

Musculo-skeletal: Vivian demonstrates minimal to moderate flexor tone in bilateral upper extremities, especially in her forearm pronators and wrist flexors. She has minimal wrist extension and finger extension. She has good grasp in bilateral hands. She is able to extend her right index finger and push/pinch with her fingers. She is able to easily use adaptive switches.

Sensory Abilities:

Vision: Vivian requires glasses to read. She occasionally reports having double-vision with difficulty focusing. She is able to engage in computer tasks and reading if print is enlarged.

Hearing: No formal audiological test results were available. Vivian responds to speech at conversational levels, with occasional need for repetition.

Cognitive/linguistic abilities:

Ms King is alert and oriented to time, place and person at all times. Her attention span is within normal limits. She exhibits very mild short-term memory inconsistencies and high-level cognitive diffi-

culties, but only in high-pressure, multi-task situations. She usually demonstrates good basic problem-solving and reasoning skills.

Present System of Communication:

Ms King's primary mode of communication is by mouthing words without any phonation. She uses facial gestures and silent spelling to get the listener to understand the main topic. She also uses tongue clicks to get attention when the listener's back is turned. With no functional use of her upper extremities, she is unable to use body language or physical contact to enhance the message.

Expressive Language:

Ms King mouths words, phrases and short sentences. She uses mainly a true whisper (no air or sound). She can use a stage whisper (some audible air current) but only on the first 2 to 3 words. If the listener is present, her amplification system enhances these few words, and they are then audible. If the listener is more than 10 or 12 feet away, however, the message is unclear. The amplification system has limited use for phone communication and usually is not picked up by her speaker phone.

Receptive Language:

Ms King understands all communication of any length in complexity, both written and verbal.

Pragmatic languages skills:

Ms King initiates communication and attempts turn-taking as needed. But because phonation is absent, the finite inflectional changes, timing, and other prosodic features that allow us to show sarcasm, humor, anger, etc. are all absent.

Communication Function:

Ms King is highly intelligent and a gifted writer/lecturer who had demonstrated her skills worldwide prior to this auto accident.

With the appropriate communication device, she can again write, edit, lecture and begin to take more control of her own life with telephone access to hire aides and companions, make appointments, etc.

Now that chews, swallows and the drooling/mucus retention problems have been addressed and resolved, she can present herself in a variety of communicative situations, taking charge as

necessary. She can be productive professionally and more personally independent. Her present communication is inadequate for these kinds of interactions and is an obstacle to moving to the next stage of her life.

System Features Needed:
Representation system: Vivian has no difficulties with reading and writing. She can spell messages that she wishes to communicate and easily utilizes abbreviations/expansion and word prediction features of electronic devices to enhance communication rate.

Vocabulary Encoding: Since Vivian has appropriate reading and spelling skills, she requires a text-to-text system, which will enable her to create new and novel sentences to express herself.

Rate Enhancement Techniques: Vivian selected items using direct selection with a switch button. In order to improve Vivian's speed and accuracy, a program is recommended which utilizes word predictions thus reducing the number of "hits" necessary to produce the desired word.

Access Techniques and Strategies: Vivian was successful independently using a switch button without her mobile arm support, and the touch screen with the use of her mobile arm support.

Overlay Organization and Features: Various keyboards and overlay configurations were used in the evaluation and Vivian was successful with icons of half an inch in size and on a 128 key arrangement. She will need access issues regarding key rate and delay or dwell time to be addressed in order to maximize accuracy after she acquires her communication devices.

Portability Concerns: Vivian will require the device to be mounted on a swing away folding wheelchair mount so the device can be accessible at all times.

Integration with other Technologies: There are no other technologies used at this time.

AAC Systems Considered:
Over the course of her communications/dysphagia therapy, Ms King has been assessed using a variety of communication devices. At her prior rehab in Long Beach, the Alpha Talker, Billfold and Ultra

Voice were all attempted and were found to be ineffectual for her.

The Cooper Rand (intra oral) electrolarynx, the AT&T electrolarynx (extra oral) and Servox (extra oral) all proved non-functional. A second person had to hold these mechanical sounding devices, turning them on and off for phrasing with the listener only guessing when to do so accurately.

Ms King was fitted with a Chatter Vox with a high-gain headband microphone to allow her to communicate her immediate needs with her new home-care aides and with the therapists at the rehabilitation center. At that time, it was the hope of a consultant (ear, nose and throat specialist, Dr Marc Kerner) that collagen injection treatments would assure enough adduction of the vocal cords for more of an audible air stream, which would then be picked up by the Chatter Vox microphone. However, after several collagen injections, functional tone was only maintained for 12 to 15 hours, after which time her body rejected the foreign substance and she became aphonic again.

Ms King was then referred to the chief of head and neck surgery at UCLA Medical Center (Dr Gerald Berke) for possible placement of prosthesis to enhance vocal fold closure, but this too proved unfeasible. Neither physician has recommended a follow-up re-evaluation.

Given the fact that vocal fold adduction is non-functional for phonation and her diaphragmatic muscles do not allow her to use the compensation techniques necessary to abruptly push up the air to force vibration, it is the opinion of this therapist that it is time to consider an alternative augmentative communication system that will take her to the next step and help her again become a productive human being.

The system that possesses the features that Vivian needs is the Freedom 2000 with EZKeys from Words+ Inc. The Freedom 2000 provides both spoken output produced through a speech synthesizer as well as written output on the screen and is capable of printing a hardcopy. The Freedom 2000 provides rate enhancement through abbreviation expansion and word prediction techniques. A large number of messages can be stored for later use and recalled

through abbreviation/expansion for quick production of critical or lengthy messages regarding health issues. With the use of "Side Talk" the user can easily transition between speaking and writing functions, and can compose messages while the Freedom 2000 is "speaking" the previous message. Since the speech synthesizer is an internal component of the system rather than a separate outside component and, as the Freedom 2000 is portable, it can be mounted on her wheelchair with a Simplicity wheelchair mount.

With the use of the Freedom 2000 Vivian will be able to direct her own medical care because she will be able to communicate her needs to her caregivers. Her caregivers will be able to understand her needs regardless of their ability to understand spelling on the communication board or their ability to see the board. Vivian was able to access the Freedom 2000 during the evaluation. She immediately understood EZKeys for Windows and was able to create novel messages.

The Freedom 2000 with EZKeys system should be purchased, as it is clear that she can both use it and urgently needs it. A trial period is not recommended, as Vivian has explored many types of communication devices up to this point. The Freedom 2000 will overcome the disabling effect of communication impairment through the restoration of normal communication activity to a level appropriate to Vivian's linguistic and cognitive abilities. The system will allow Vivian to get the help she might need in emergency situations and would allow her to communicate with others regarding medical issues and other needs.

Recommendations for an Alternative Communication System:
The Freedom 2000 with EZKeys for Windows is recommended for purchase for Vivian.

The following equipment is required for the development of a complete communication system for Vivian. It can be purchased through Words+, Lancaster, California.

Freedom 2000 Tough book Extreme with Touch Screen
Training for up to 4 hours
24 volt Adaptor

Jelly Bean Switch
Environmental Control Unit
Wheelchair Mount

Dated 21ˢᵗ April, 2000.

As I never saw the Freedom 2000, I can only assume that Vivian's insurance company refused to pay for it. It was probably how Steven Hawking communicated and would have really helped Vivian.

Vivian was living in a one room cottage in Granada Hills close to Van Nuys near Los Angeles, and I stayed in an empty cottage next door. Vivian had improved since I last saw her. She was now able to whisper, swallow and eat. She had an electric wheelchair she could operate and she was starting to feed herself. She could lift her bottom and shoulders off the bed and was beginning to walk between parallel bars in physiotherapy.

My concerns were that there was nobody on site and she had NO way of calling for help. There was NO buzzer and nobody to buzz. A series of carers came in each day to get her up and put her to bed. As July 5ᵗʰ was a public holiday, nobody came between 10.30 a.m. and 9.30 p.m. Luckily she had me, and two other friends visited, so we were able to make her comfortable. The evening carer always spent the night with Vivian.

There was a third cottage where two young men lived. One of them had been paralysed in a car crash and spent all day in bed watching television. The other one could get himself down the ramp outside but not up it again because it was too steep. He spent the day in the garage lifting weights to develop his arm muscles. He explained to me that he had been injured in a shooting accident. He loved going to the beach but could only go on the days he'd had a bowel movement. Disabled people, who are unable to get themselves to the toilet, usually have their

bowel movements scheduled in the morning. He could not go out without having had one in case he had an accident. This also applied to Vivian, who knew when she needed to go to the toilet, but could not get herself there. She had sensations in her body but could not get the messages through to move because of brain-stem injury. Unfortunately Vivian's bathroom had a step up into it and she was often put on a commode in the sitting room, where people frequently passed through, including a maintenance man. Vivian, sitting on the commode with her panties around her knees, merely smiled.

The heat was unbearable and went up to 110 degrees during my visit. I moved my bed under a ceiling fan in an effort to cope with the heat at night.

Just before my birthday Vivian dictated a letter to Mark:

"It is like a circus. We either laugh or cry. Tuesday is Marilyn's birthday and we'll have a low-key celebration. She is so organised that she moved her birthday gift from its hiding place. It is good to be together. She is an eccentric delightful English actor."

We celebrated my birthday with a Chinese take-out and a chocolate cake. Vivian could now feed herself but had difficulty lifting the food from the plate to her mouth. She gave me a bottle of bubble bath and a tube of KY Jelly as a joke, which someone else had bought and wrapped. After eating we watched a video called "Talks With Angels".

In my birthday card she had dictated this message:

"My dear friend Marilyn, We have been to hell and heaven together as we live on earth. Being 54 takes you into the new century. I hope we start a new trend of good living with little frustration. I'm glad we are celebrating together. Thank you for all you do for me. You have a lot of good karma saved up! Love from the bottom of my heart! Vivian."

When Bill visited he slept with her but communication with Vivian was tiring. It was difficult to hear what she was saying

and she wanted to talk a lot. I could see that Bill was also finding it exhausting, although he had loved talking to her before the accident, when they spent hours talking on the telephone.

Varena, the healer, often arrived late at night with her entourage of healers for a healing session.

Fortunately on the day I left Murial was there to keep Vivian company. It was painful leaving.

Letter from Vivian on Thanksgiving:

Be thankful for little things like making messes. Some people will never make a mess because they can't move. I'm glad I'm learning to feed myself. Ate lobster last weekend with Bill. Very good. Like writing a book, healing takes as long as it takes. Patience is a virtue so I must be virtuous. Surrender. Trust. Faith. What a DIVINE COMEDY. Crying and laughing at the same time. How long is long? My trach is out but I still can't talk. I'm going to see a specialist at UCLA. A new procedure to connect nerves may work. I still can't lift my legs to walk. A new contraption-like-walker-harness may help. Hope I am asked to move again. Will let you know details. Six times in 15 months. They call it progress, but it's business. Still takes time to type. Going to Kansas for New Year.

I keep forgetting to thank you for the apron. I use it every meal. Good idea. Love, Viv.

Letter from Vivian Christmas 1999:

I'm wordless – literally and figuratively. Seems like an awesome time. My life is so puny and so important at the same time. More aware of the puny now. I am glad we are going together into the next

millennium. I hope the New Year is truly good for us all.

I'm slowly progressing. By now you would expect me to be about recovered. I thought I'd be walking and talking this Christmas. Not so. I'm still completely dependent. I can feed myself if someone puts the food in the right place. I talk in a quiet whisper and don't often talk about concepts or ideas. I have learned not to joke because humor includes inflection and timing. I have my private humor though. Even my expression when I laugh and cry looks a lot alike.

My vision is better but I still see double. I thought I had three eyes for several months after the accident. I asked the doctor how I got the 'third eye' and she said I just had two. It is hard for me to read unless there are big letters on the computer screen. I type using one finger with my arm in a mobile arm sling.

I can move my legs and arms some, but I can't turn over or reach for something. I stay alone at night and I sleep quite well unless I am not positioned right. I can stand for a short time if the therapist balances me. I live in a small place but will be moving again soon. I don't worry about housing because angels in human clothes have made worry unnecessary. I feel gratitude.

I still don't understand this but I am learning to trust the divine mystery. On some level it makes sense. This is not where I thought I'd be the end of the millennium. So much for thought. Nadu, my nurse, says she isn't where she thought she'd be either. I wonder how many people are where they imagined they'd be?

If you want to read the poem I wrote for Bill's Christmas, it is attached. It is one page. Our relationship changed direction, but we remain close friends. I am very grateful to him.

I don't know what the next year holds. I just ask that God's will be revealed to us. I am so glad we have been together the past century/ies. I value our connection.

Eternal love, Vivian.

A man for all seasons

Her voice, like spring rain, soaked the thirsty ground of his being
and refreshed his soul.
Blossoms and buds of every hue and fragrance burst forth
arrayed more elegantly than King Solomon in all his glory.
Cultivated for half a century,
he arranged his flowering character into voluminous bouquets.
Sweet William graced each arrangement,
accentuating blossoms of Acquired Wisdom, Reliable Truth,
Brilliant Expression, Poetic Creativity, and Masterful Listening.
Another spray was abundant with Pure Heart,
Buddhic Compassion, Loving-Kindness, Precise Resonance,
Private Passion, and Shy Sensitivity.
A third bouquet displayed Skillful Will, Musical Magic,
Gracious Generosity, Entrepreneurial Spirit, Ordered Life-style,
and Sane Simplicity.
His arrangements were impeccable,
yet she kept her enthusiasm in check.
Would summer bring more beauty and abundance,
or would it bring weeds and allergies?
"I want to know your bearing each season,"
she admitted cautiously.
Undaunted, he assured her that he was a man for all seasons.
Summer never came.
Wreaking havoc with the seasonal flow,
a fierce blizzard blew in, leaving their souls on ice.
She lay nearly frozen and mute; he, grief-stricken and wilted.
Winter, long and bitter, threatened to destroy their lives, yet his
crocus-self pushed through snow to assert his strength and love.
Only warm tears kept him from freezing.
Fall came next.
Falling, falling into the dark Mystery.
Falling into God.

She fell into the void, surrendering all she held precious.
He fell into the moment, surrendering his expectations.
Stripped naked, they breathed the holy scent of Essence.
And summer? Would the lazy days of summer ever come?
Knowing there is order in chaos, they trusted the God
of all Seasons and entered the Mystery of the new millennium.
Vivian King, December 25, 1999

Vivian had started to write beautiful poetry including *A Divine Comedy* in three parts.

Letter to Free

Dear Free,
After 22 months of absence, I know what I want to say to you. It has been a long time since I dropped you off – and promised to pick you up in a few days. Did you know then that something would happen?

You came to me and touched my heart. Everyone who met you recognized that you were special. You were perfect in my eyes and I loved/love you. Thank you for coming to me.

My spirit is still the same but my body works only about 15%. Instead of taking care of others, I need care myself. I considered bringing you out here to be with me – to help me, but for three reasons I won't.

I want you to be my ambassador in Spirit Mountain canyon. You are the part of me who runs free and chases butterflies and lizards. I want you to be free in nature.

I know you are happy with the family there. You have comfort, companionship, and plenty of exercise. I want you to be healthy and happy.

There are no pets allowed where I am moving. Even if they were, I don't think you'd like living confined. It would be nice for me to have you but not at your expense.

So I want you to stay with Whitney and Will and to represent my

presence there. You will always be my beloved dog and you will live in my heart. Remember that everything physical changes but our spirit lives on.

Your human mother, Vivian.

Email from Vivian dated 28.4.2000

Got the gifts. Dress is great for summer. You are always in thoughts and heart. The new computer will make it easier. I can talk on phone with it when/if I get it. MMA is considering now.

Since I don't go to rehab, I will have someone come 3x a week to help with exercises.

For Easter I stayed home and had TV church. Prayer special for family and friends.

Jenny is pulling together all my financial needs for Whittens who asked her. She is looking for a house with realtor. Maybe next week? Lot of issues.

Love spring. Good weather here. Love your letters on email.

Love you, Viv.

As Vivian's Social Security payments did not stretch to a live-in carer or a decent place to live, the people who owned the land where she had lived as caretaker in Santa Fe, offered to pay for a house where Vivian could live with a carer.

A house was found overlooking the ocean in Long Beach and Vivian was able to move in with a carer. She now had an office where, when set up in her wheelchair with her arm in a mobile sling, she could write on her computer. We still meditated together every Monday in our Triangle Meditation and we wrote to each other almost every day, but she still could not move or talk without an amplifier. In August she wrote a letter to all of us:

Letter to my physicians, healers and helpers:

On the stage of life, I had a crash Sept. 1998, which left my physical vehicle disabled and beside the road. The headlights didn't focus, the horn didn't honk, and the wheels didn't turn. Many mechanics and body workers came to help and to do what they could. After almost two years, the vehicle looks better and the fuel line and carburettor run easier, but the car splutters, it doesn't move, and the horn doesn't have a sound.

The driver and the passengers (self and personality) were stunned and perplexed after the crash but they were OK. They changed their destination to "nowhere" and lived in the moment. What else could they do?

Now, with about 15% function, I am here to thank you for the part you played in doing what you could to make me better. I had the best traditional and non-traditional medicine and I am still left with the Mystery.

We are not God, so we are not infallible. Yes, it's humbling to be human. The 1ˢᵗ year I deeply believed I'd walk and talk again. I thought that if it took others two years, I'd do it in half the time. Energy medicine would accelerate my progress. And besides, people all over the world were praying for my healing.

I have a clearer idea now of the difference between 'curing' and 'healing'. Curing is to go back to the way I was before the crash. Healing is to get closer to God. I am not cured, but I am healing. You in the 'helping professions' do and do not have a lot to do with this. You do make it easier and some make it harder.

When my heart smiles and sings, I know I'm healing. When I feel like crying, I'm not. More Zoloft doesn't help – as much as you'd like to believe it.

Most of my life I have focused on developing the intelligence, love,

and will of the Self, and more specifically, good, and strong will. Almost all my care providers have goodwill – the will to do good.

When all three aspects are balanced in spirit, the result is effective and effortless. Where there is too much effort (strong will) without skill, chaos reigns. Burnout occurs in those helpers. I have watched this happen and have tried to pull back and enter the silence to get perspective.

Because it is difficult to communicate (this takes enormous effort) I observe more than I speak. As a result, I am a sitting duck for others' interpretations. Most are wrong. It is a hard situation for us all.

I do what I do for a reason. Most of my decisions are 'catch 22', They may seem 'bad' to you, but not if you consider all. I have given up trying to explain, expound on, or defend my actions. Too much energy. This requires a lot from us all, but it can be an opportunity to see deeper.

I am not afraid to die. I have written a Medical Will – attached for your information. This is not depression or weakness. Relax. I will live until I die – to quote my mom.

Since I am going through this, I can share what is helpful and what is not. Don't assume that you know what is helpful and what is not. Don't assume that you know what is best/ right for me. Come to me with an open mind. Discover; don't interpret. Connecting with my deep Self makes the difference.

Two books I recommend:

Still Here *by Ram Das.*

The Role Death Plays in Life *by Robert Leightman.*

Vivian King's medical will

I have lived a good life and this is my will in case of 'medical emergency'.

> *Do not resuscitate, ventilate, or give IV's or antibiotics.*
> *Do not call 911 or hospitalize unless I instruct to do so.*
> *Do not attempt to prolong my life.*

I have instructed my family to file a law suit against anyone who does not honor my will.

It had become clear that Vivian did not want to continue living in her present state, and who could blame her? She could not move – not even to scratch her nose, reach for a glass of water, or go to the toilet. She looked at websites recommending dehydration as a way to exit. I sent an email asking Vivian to wait for my arrival. I had two thoughts: that I may be able to talk her out of ending her life, and if not, I wanted to be with her. It did not occur to me that I could be prosecuted for being involved in an "assisted suicide". All I cared about was Vivian. No, I did not want her to die. I wanted her to recover.

PART FOUR

My visit to Long Beach

I arrived at the beginning of November and stayed with a friend of Vivian's who lived just around the corner. He had also been affected by Vivian's car crash. His wife had run off with Varena, the healer from Dallas, and taken most of the furniture from the house.

Vivian was living in a lovely house overlooking the ocean which she could see from her double bed in the sitting room. She had canaries in a cage beside her bed. I recognized the furniture from her house in Pasadena. She had a carer from Belize, who lived there, and a nurse who came in every day. She had everything except the ability to move and talk. I could live without speaking but Vivian was a communicator. She spent a lot of time observing those around her and learnt a great deal about human nature: the good, the bad and the ugly. Although she had an electric wheelchair, she rarely went out in it. Long Beach was wheelchair-friendly with ramps, and was one of the reasons why she had moved there. There was even a local bus with a ramp for wheelchair access.

Although her fridge was empty when I arrived, Vivian had instructed the carer to mail a big chocolate cake to Mark for his birthday. The nurse, the carer and I discussed whether this indicated some brain damage from the accident. They informed me that they often had to buy food for Vivian with their own money. They obviously loved her. The carer from Belize later named her first child Vivian. I filled the fridge with food which Vivian and I ate, but feeding herself was a laborious process and most of the food fell off the fork on its way to her mouth. I wanted to help but the nurse said she had to learn to do it herself.

Everything had to be set up for Vivian. I spent hours trying to help her use the remote control for her television, but the use of a remote control involves subtle hand movements, which she did not have. Other people switched on the television and she was stuck with whatever was showing. We watched the American elections and were shocked when Al Gore appeared to have won but George Bush became President.

I arranged for us to go and see the film 'Billy Elliott' at the local cinema complex. This involved booking a special van to accommodate Vivian's wheelchair. We had to take an elevator up to the cinema and were stuck in it until someone came to release us. After seeing the film, with Vivian sitting at the end of a row in her wheelchair, we waited ages for the van to arrive and take us home. It showed me how difficult her life was. A simple outing became a drama.

Then the Big Drama began when Vivian decided she could no longer live with her disability.

Email 27th November, 2000:

Dear Family and friends,
We have chance to practice PEACEFUL PRESENCE in midst of busy life.

Issues:
  1. how to live in world, not get stuck (not of world).
  2. how to dance with personal will and God's will.
  3. how to be point of peace in contemporary world.

We're in this together (so is Bush/Gore/nation).
I am going to Kansas Nov 28 – Dec 4.
Relax. Enjoy holiday preparation.
I stand steady in Light, Love, Will of God.
Vivian.

Letter from Vivian after returning from Kansas:

I returned from my good trip to Kansas. Am resting now. The faith of my father and family bolster my spirit. Kids keep life moving ahead. Visited uncle – 80 years. Can't walk or talk either. We just

looked at each other.

Some wonder about Mark, my son. Some of his actions appear to be rejecting. So many hard things to deal with, and inability to affect my health, cause him to focus on one person he can affect – Nicole (his girl-friend). Keep doors open to him. This situation is bigger than us. We need each other. He does too.

This is hard for all of us. I love life, family, friends, food, etc. NO, I am not giving up on life. YES, I am releasing my limited body. Like a baby in the womb, I am preparing to enter a new, bigger world. Focus on More life, not less. I don't want to die, I want to live fully. Please GET THIS DISTINCTION.

I wish I could protect all from suffering and grief. This is the hardest thing for me. My life as-is and my physical death both cause grief. Only promise is that deep feeling of grief is preparation for great joy. Human highs and lows are part of the drama. For Christmas, I will, in some way, bring a sense of peace and joy to you. You will recognize it coming from me and you'll know it's OK.

In Dad's complex, people got together to trim-the-tree while I was there. The good time we had transcends the loss – and all had losses.

Joy comes in the morning.

Love, Vivian.

Letter 6th December 2000:

My actors are cooperating and are working together with me. No one is depressed. As the Director, I am not willing to spend more time on this production. If the playwright wants us to continue on the earth show, there will have to be major changes in the script. We are partners and I'm not willing to keep this show on the road. I don't believe that the soul hands the script down in a dictating manner. So it's now in the playwright's lap.

Problems are in the interpersonal play. Other people are upset and are creating a lot of action. I am trying to hold still in the midst

of chaos. If everyone worried about their own performance instead of mine, it would be better.

We may or may not get this interpersonal act together.

Vivian's friends were split between those who supported her and those who opposed her. Whereas I did not want her to die, I saw how difficult her life was, and knew I could not bear it. I often wake up in sleep paralysis, unable to move or call out, and I know how scary it is. However, before Vivian stopped eating and drinking, she became ambivalent. When her nurse asked if she was willing to pay $2000 to have the bathroom modified to meet her needs, she said yes. The landlord had shown and offered me a small cottage at the back of Vivian's house. I promised to stay with her if she agreed to stay alive! I talked to her nurse who said there was a good chance of a full recovery if she continued with physiotherapy. I shared my dreams in which she walked and talked. I was convinced my dreams were prophetic.

Vivian argued that there was no purpose to her life. I argued that there must be a purpose otherwise she would have died. She said she did not want to suffer and God doesn't want her to suffer, but I pointed out that we DO suffer on this planet. She said she wanted pleasure, and I told her she was on the wrong planet. I pointed out that if it was her soul's purpose to die, she would die. If she ended her life, it was her personality having its way. At the end of this conversation she asked, "How come you're so smart and I'm so dumb?" I felt terrible. What did I know of her suffering? What could any of us possibly know? We weren't trapped in a disabled body.

Patricia visited and tried to talk Vivian out of ending her life. Varena, the healer, was angry with her for giving up. The esoteric group Vivian had belonged to did not support her at all. Their leader wrote:

In my opinion developing continuity of consciousness falls under the rubric of self-development, personal growth and integration, for they prepare you to become a better disciple. But this is only one side of living the life of discipleship. The other side, which is the most important, is to provide service regardless of life circumstances. You have demonstrated your talent as a writer and could find purpose in writing a book in which you share your life experiences before and since the accident, including your hopes and disappointments, your despair to the point of contemplating suicide, and your life-affirming decision to contribute to the world despite your physical condition. It would be a very inspiring book, and a gift from your inner being to many people.

He invited her to attend their monthly meditations, saying they would welcome her with open arms, not only for what they could give through love and support, but also for what she could give as a radiant soul, simply through her presence. I wondered if he realised how difficult it would be to transport Vivian and her wheelchair to the monthly meditations.

Another friend looked at end-of-life options but these only apply to the terminally ill. A severely disabled person does not have the right or the ability to end their own life. We talked about it and Vivian asked me to write a book about her struggles to escape the body which had become her prison. It would take another fifteen years for me to write this book because of the pain I knew it would stir up. Another option was to go to Switzerland for a life termination, but that was only an option for the people who could lift a lethal drink to their lips and drink it. Vivian could not do that. Her longing for freedom depended upon her friends. At this time assisted suicide was illegal in California.

When the people paying for the house and carer found out about Vivian's intention to end her life, they sent in a Suicide Prevention team who would have taken her to hospital if a

doctor friend had not agreed to make sure she ate and drank. They left and Vivian retained the right to end her life. It was her decision. If a person cannot reach for a glass of water or put food in their mouth, is it suicide if they do not want to be fed or given water to drink?

Vivian was upset with me because I had sent an email telling everyone of her intention to end her life. This is how the people who sent the Suicide Prevention team had found out. I was locked out of the house for almost a week feeling terrible about sending the email. It was only when her friend Jean came to say good-bye that I was allowed back in. Jean drove me to a beautiful Bach concert during which we held hands and cried.

We had not been able to talk Vivian out of it and, although we had the power, being able-bodied, to force-feed her, we surrendered to her wishes. She stayed in bed, the nurse visited once a day to make her comfortable, and the carer returned to Belize. I bought huge pink lilies and filled her room with them, so she could both smell and see them from her bed. I sat with her and held her hand, we meditated together and listened to beautiful music. I moistened her dry lips with a wet sponge. I massaged her feet, which were very cold, with lavender oil. We talked about her life and her loves. I asked her to stay in touch with me after she died, and she promised that she would: a promise she kept.

In the final two weeks of her life she told me she dreamt about fruit and sex, which amused her. I was sleeping on a mattress on the floor near her bed when late one night her two brothers and sister-in-law arrived. I could no longer stay with her but I visited every day and sat beside her bed. It was not what we had planned, and I did not appreciate the way they bustled about, eating meals close to where Vivian lay in bed.

On Sunday night, December 17th, I sensed Vivian's mother in the room and told her she would probably die that night. She was still alert but was drowning in the fluid building up in her

lungs. The doctor friend had brought some cough mixture containing morphine but it only caused her to choke. He could not stay with her because it would have ruined his career to be in any way involved. The nurse also risked her career by volunteering to come in every day. By now Vivian could not swallow. She asked me to stay. I told her brothers that she wanted me to stay but they said no, I was not family. I regret that I did not insist but I did not want to create a scene. I left and they said they would call me.

Vivian died at 4.30 a.m. on December 18th, exactly a week before Christmas even though I had begged her to stay alive for Christmas. This was because my father had died a month before Christmas when I was six.

I went to the house where her body was still in bed, eyes turned to the left as if she had seen someone standing beside the bed. I knew it was her mother who had collected her. I sat beside the bed and closed my eyes. The family were preparing breakfast and offered me some. I declined. A van arrived from the Coroner's Office and some men put Vivian's body in a black body bag, and drove away with it. When I left, her family were loading her furniture into the van they had driven down from Kansas. I returned later in the day to find the house stripped of everything but her clothes, papers and books. They had not approved of any of Vivian's decisions and complained to me about the books she had written in which they felt she had put herself up there with God. They said I was lucky not to have spent the night with her because of the horrible gurgling noises she had made and the time it took her to die, but I would spend the rest of my life wishing I had stayed with her. These God-fearing people then left me to deal with what was left behind and drove off in the van. I sat on the floor and wept.

We moved what was left of Vivian's possessions to her friend's house around the corner. It was then that I remembered the

dream I'd had when I first lived in Vivian's house in Pasadena in 1985. In the dream I was in the basement of a house belonging to a man who cut up bodies. The dream had repeated itself but I had not seen its significance until now. The house I was staying in had a basement and belonged to a pathologist. The dream had shown me where I would be staying when Vivian died fifteen years in the future. It was prophetic.

Vivian had left instructions about her funeral, which clothes she wanted to be dressed in, and what to put in the casket. I called the Funeral Home and was told her body would be put in an incinerator. There would be NO funeral. In America there are no crematoria with chapels attached to them, as there are in the UK. There was no funeral to attend where we could grieve and say good-bye.

On January 6th 2001 we held a Memorial Service to celebrate Vivian's life. It was held in the Pacific Palisades Presbyterian church. Vivian had written the Eulogy before she died and her friends read it out loud for everyone to hear:

Reader 1.
"Thank you for coming to celebrate my new adventure. Death is not a tragedy really, but it takes time to realise this. I am still here – without my body, yet fully in spirit.

I entered the earth stage February 18, 1946 in Hutchinson, Kansas, born to Allen and Fannie King. Growing up, I believed I was the luckiest girl in the world. There were three reasons: I had the best parents, lived on the most beautiful farm, and had the best brothers. Love was evident in my family and community.

In high school, I met John Adams and married him just shy of 20 years of age. Later, when he was ordained, I became a minister's wife, fulfilling a childhood dream. The best gift of the marriage, however, was Mark, our beloved son. I simply loved being a mother. We

divorced after 13 turbulent years.

In 1980 I married Wilhelm Solenthaler, a beautiful man from Switzerland, the country of my ancestors. This marriage lasted two years.

Education was always important to me and to my family, but not just to get information or knowledge. I wanted wisdom as well. In college I graduated with a BS degree in nursing (1968). Ten years later, in 1978, I tried to get closer to the source of people's suffering by obtaining my MA in Counselling Psychology. Licensed as a Marriage, Family and Child Counsellor, I guided others in personal and social issues, and taught classes in Psychosynthesis – a psychology of mind, body, spirit integration. In 1988 I completed a doctorate in Counselling Psychology and created teaching material for personality and soul development. I later created an entertaining way of making this material more available to people. I called this 'Inner Theatre'.

Essentially, in the 1950s, I was an innocent, trusting girl growing up in a rare functional family.

In the 1960s I explored education.

In the 1970s I focused on mothering, wifing, nursing, and teaching parenting skills.

In the 1980s I focused on teaching Psychosynthesis and counselling people.

In the 1990s I developed the Inner Theatre approach to integration, wrote books, and taught in the USA, Poland, Latvia, Switzerland, Russia and Lithuania.

In 1998 I was in a car accident that sent me on a 'crash course' in letting go of my attachment to all things – and eventually to my earthly body. Christ showed how death has no hold on us, and the power of eternal life. He said 'Let not your heart be troubled...' I know what He means. I am excited about this adventure and know first hand the limitation of physical life. Today, celebrate who I was, who I am now, and who I shall be."

Reader 2

"This is not the end. I pass this on.

1. When we judge and criticize, we say more about ourselves than the other person.
2. People who don't understand give us an opportunity to develop more compassion.
3. Accumulate fewer things, so you have less to dispose of.
4. Spend time developing qualities. You have many opportunities.
5. Nothing can destroy us ultimately. Go through the fear, sadness, or grief until you come out into laughter. It's the belief of separation that makes us cry. When we see deeper, we laugh at the illusion. But, both have their time and place. Just don't get stuck in one.
6. Think of me abroad, getting the next act together. We'll be together again – just different costumes and props with an ever better performance. It keeps getting better because we improve with cosmic age.

A story is told of twins in a womb. The 1st one is born and enters a new world of light and sound. The 2nd, not knowing what happened to the first, grieves the loss. Shortly after, the 2nd is born and joyously joins the other in the grander, new dimension. Grief is temporary and is minimized when we know the truth of exits and entrances. Joy underlies the transition from the appearance of death and birth.

Reader 3 – I was reader 3 and remembered when we watched the movie *Gladiator* in which, as the main character is dying, he moves towards the door into paradise. Vivian had loved this scene and the accompanying music.

Paradise regained
Part three of A Divine Comedy

Welcome to Paradise, says Viva – my soul – as I enter The
Gate and stand in front of my glorious Home. A gift from God,
my mansion spreads across heavenly terrain and opens to
the backyard of infinity.

Beside us, an Angel asks what I have discovered while on
the earth stage. Reviewing my life, I reply:

I have learned that Intelligence, Love, and Will must be
developed and balanced to have an integrated
personality. The soul can only infuse a personality that is
open and receptive. Much of my adult life was involved in devel-
oping and teaching this process of integration. I founded a new
and entertaining way to bring this about and I wrote books on it. It
was creative and joyous as Viva and I worked and played together.

I have discovered that to love is not enough in a relationship.
This was important because I thought love alone would
make everything work out all right. I knew genuine love
as a child and as a mother, but it wasn't until I was fifty
that I experienced love with wisdom and power in an
intimate relationship as well.

I allowed my ex-husband to intimidate me and I have seen the
painful effects on our son ever since. I regret that I did not refuse to
be intimidated, especially in our mediation process.

With humility, I let go of the need to fully understand events
and to trust the divine Mystery. Life is complex and only
God knows the real Reason behind circumstances.

I have learned how to forgive and to live without holding grudges. This has brought real freedom with others.

I have learned to relate to the inner self instead of to the outer personality of others. Since everyone is different, I looked for what was unique instead of expecting others to be like me. Psychosynthesis and Integral Psychology have helped me with this.

After further review in which my earthly production is looked at in detail, Viva thanks me for having given her physical expression on the earth stage and for directing the human play for over half a century.

Viva says enthusiastically: come with me to the waterfall and to the healing pool filled with fragrant flowers. There we will meet The Great Healer.

We have always been one reality, but when on earth, we were on two dimensions – physical and spiritual. In the healing we become one again.

She continues: Afterwards, we shall celebrate restoration With your mother, relatives, friends, and the hosts and Hostesses of heaven.

Not just those who have left the earth will be here for the festive occasion, but also the souls of those still on earth – family, friends, colleagues, students, clients, caregivers, therapists, healers, doctors and all those who wish to attend. It will be the biggest and best celebration you have ever known.

There will be celestial music by those who inspired Mozart, Handel, and Vivaldi, and who presently inspire Robert Reiher, Deane Hawley, and Marcey Hamm.

The feast is prepared by those who inspire Martha Stewart,
Julia Child, Peter Osbourn, Mirial Buller, and Nadu
Lawson. It is divine food and fills your spirit completely.

I am ready, say I, anticipating the presence of Christ, my Master,
and the fragrant healing pool.

Stripped of everything physical, I step into the Water,
take the out-stretched hand of Christ,
and in the presence of infinite Love,
am healed completely on every level.

At-one with Viva, I bathe in the sacred scent of essence
and luxuriate in Heaven's blessings.
I emanate these fragrant blessings to my loved ones on
earth and see through the illusion of our separation.

Ceremoniously, I am escorted into the Hills that are alive
with Music to sing and dance and celebrate my beautiful life...

Vivian King
February 2000

Vivian had written letters to her friends. Mine was dated the 22nd October 2000:

My Dear Marilyn,
Rare friend, thanks for sharing life-times – the highs and the lows.
Now we can continue on as ever. Ah the mystery of it all. Death no
longer has a sting.
Let not your heart be troubled.
Eternal Love,
Vivian.

Although Vivian had prepared me for her death, I missed her terribly. I returned to the UK with ulcers in my mouth and throat. Vivian left me the full rights to all of her books and writings, and I decided to spend the rest of my life publishing and promoting her work.

PART FIVE

Vivian writing about death

The illusion of death

The phone rings. My sister-in-law in Kansas informs me that my beloved mom just had a heart attack and is unconscious in the Intensive Care Unit in Hutchinson. Totally unprepared for this, I tearfully scramble to pack some things then drive ten endless hours through the night to be at her bedside.

Not knowing what to expect, I enter the room and gently hold her hand – the hand that has been here for me all of my life. Arousing from unconsciousness, she opens her eyes and squeezes my hand in response. Unable to talk with the tubes in her nose and mouth, she looks deep into my eyes, smiles, nods her characteristic nod, and closes her eyes for the last time. Trying to be strong for her, I whisper that if this is her time to go, it's okay, because our love for each other is eternal and our souls will live on together.

The family gathers in the room. I caress Mom's hair and face and kiss her forehead. My youngest brother notices that each time I kiss her, the EEG registers a blip as the line decreases, then becomes straight. Silently and gracefully, she slips out of her human costume and leaves her body behind with us.

As I stand by her in grief, I recall a dream I had two years earlier. In the dream, Mom is talking to me as we sort through old clothing. On a table lies a piece of cloth that looks like her body. She says, "Fold it up and put it in the Goodwill box." I follow her instructions and we continue to sort.

Now, holding her lifeless hand, I'm aware of how attached I am to her physical body. I don't want to lay her costume in the Goodwill box. She's only seventy-three and I had planned to have her in my play for another twenty years. She was such an important, loving player in my life. I wonder how I can possibly live without my mother.

In subsequent days, my daughter-self grieves deeply, missing

Momma and feeling the wrenching pain of separation. On another level, my director-self feels love and compassion for the daughter-self, and is with her in her agony. On yet another level, my playwright-Self is deeply connected to Mom's spirit and knows she is not dead. Mom says to me, "It's only my body that isn't with you anymore. I'm still here." Our souls laugh at the outrageous illusion that she could ever die.

Death feels like a tragedy to those who forget that they are the soul playing a masquerade. I guess for them, it is a tragedy. But for those who remember who they are, death is the grand finale on the Earth stage, not the finale of the Soul's Play.

Part of the Divine Comedy is the pain of endings. And while pain and grief are deeply significant experiences, they are transient emotions. They come and they go. What is ultimately reliable is the soul behind all the masks of emotion and human experience. The soul remains ever stable, steadfast, and radiant!

Dark comedy
From *Soul Play*

Sometimes we suffer too much. In such times, The Divine Comedy turns dark and the pain is intense. In Inevitable Grace, Piero Ferrucci talks about the crippling effect pain can have on us. "When suffering becomes too strong, it imprisons our attention with its impersonal brutality, kills our enthusiasm, turns our hopes into empty dreams. Its incomprehensibility undermines the psychophysical structure we have come to know as ourselves. In pain, be it mental or physical, we are faced with the concrete possibility of our own annihilation."

We could die! We could be engulfed by our difficult situation. If, in our pain, we give up our dreams, our hopes, our faith; if we become bitter or hateful; if we betray our self or deny our

soul – that is real tragedy! It's a tragedy because pain doesn't have to destroy us. As we teeter on the ragged edge of destruction, we can remember that we are more than our body, more than this situation. We will not be destroyed.

Furthermore, we are not alone in our suffering. During dark times we can find comfort in two ways. One way is to step back from the actor who is distressed or in pain, then take this suffering one in our arms and hold it close. As director, we can come into resonance with the depth of misery this part of us is feeling.

Another way is to remain in the pain, but to relax in the embrace of your playwright-soul, (or your angel or Christ) and together go deeper into the fear, pain, or grief until you move through it to the other side. Yes, there is always another side, because pain is not permanent. We can make it through the darkest of nights if we know we're not alone. We can go through hell if we know that the presence of the divine is leading us through. Once, when I experienced great emotional pain after the breakup of a relationship, I wanted the whole universe to understand my feelings of agony. So without using my physical voice, I screamed inside so loud that the farthest galaxies got my message. (In the inner world, making a noise that terrible is possible!) After I shook the whole universe with my cry, I felt a wonderful relief. At that moment, I realized how important it is for our pain-racked cries to be heard and understood.

Yes, we can walk with our inner cast and with each other through times of suffering and loss. We can be carried on the wings of divine love. And when we make it through, we'll know the meaning of triumph over tragedy.

Even death won't part us
From *Being Here When I Need Me*

To live forever in our physical body is not the goal of our journey. While it is true that we do not need to suffer or become ill in order to die, it is also true that disease is one way the Self may choose to be released from the body. If we feel we have done our very best to be well in the midst of a life that is very complex, we can maintain dignity as we prepare to die. Mahatma Gandhi reminded us that satisfaction lies not in the attainment but in the effort.

At this point in time, few people consciously choose the time and way they want to die. But there are those who do, and like them, we can prepare for death as part of our on-going adventure.

Many people fear death because they believe that "Death" comes without their permission or choice. Like symptoms, they believe death "just happens". Such a belief generates a feeling of powerlessness. For many the end of life is a time of suffering; a time to reluctantly let go of physical existence.

We generally don't think of death until we have a personal encounter. My first experience with death was when I was seven years old. It was late one afternoon and I was helping my mother prepare supper when I heard my father's frantic calls from the barnyard. I dashed barefoot out the door and saw him trying to resuscitate my wet, limp, fifteen-month-old brother in his arms. Johnny had climbed onto a bucket and toppled into the cow's water tank. My father had found him floating face down.

I watched as my mother drove wildly out the lane with my father in the back seat trying to bring my brother back to life. I was dazed and tried not to think of what was happening. My brother and I tried to entertain ourselves by playing a game until our parents returned after dark.

Johnny was dead. The next day his body was brought to our house where the casket was positioned in my parents' bedroom. My

*mother and father wanted him to be close to them until the funeral.
The lid was left open and a box of tissues sat on top to wipe the
moisture that seeped from his nose. It was also there for us as we
came often to touch and kiss him, gradually letting the truth
penetrate that he was no longer in his body. My parents said that he
was still alive with Jesus, which made me feel better. At the funeral
my father lifted me up for one last kiss before closing the coffin lid.
Then it seemed OK for dirt to be shovelled on the casket in the
ground because Johnny was no longer there.*

Since that time, I have experienced the deaths of relatives,
friends, patients, students and strangers. In the book, *Death: The
Great Adventure*, Master Djwhal Khul assures us that "Death is
essentially a matter of consciousness. We are conscious one moment
on the physical plane, and a moment later we have withdrawn onto
another plane and are actively conscious there." Djwhal Khul
explains that death, like sleep, marks the transition from one state
of consciousness to another. The difference is that in sleep, we come
back to our physical body while in death, we don't.

For those who have no relationship with the Soul, death seems
lonely and final. Death loses its awfulness for those who are aware
that consciousness is not limited to physical reality. When we have
completed our purpose in coming to earth, we can allow our Self to
withdraw the life force from our body as we consciously cross into a
higher frequency dimension.

Our Self does not desert us in our final hour of need. In dying we
can consciously allow our Beloved to hold us as we let go. It is as
though our Self says to the cells of our body: "It's OK to let go now.
You have been faithful to me while I needed you on earth. Thank you
so much. Your work is complete now."

And to our mortal self, our immortal Self may gently say, "I have
always been here for you in life, and I am here for you in death. I
hold you, dear one, even as you now leave your body. You are not
alone. Now let go and come home. Feel my presence and come

forward to our Oneness. Relax into my arms. Feel our peace. Welcome home."

Plato said, *"True philosophers are always occupied in the practice of dying."* Perhaps you can discuss death with your Self and let go of your apprehension. I have communicated to Viva that I want to live a healthy, long, fulfilling life for us on earth. I want us to decide together when my work is done. I want to be *"awake"* as I come home. But for now, *"I have miles to go before I sleep."*

Death is a bridge whereby the lover is joined to the Beloved.
Abd al-Aziz b. Sulayman

PART SIX

Even death won't part us

When I lived with Vivian in Pasadena I quickly discovered the Alice Bailey books in her office. These books were written by a Tibetan called Djwhal Khul and channeled through Alice Bailey. They are about spiritual growth, the spiritual planes and the beings who dwell there. Even though the books are extremely esoteric, I found them fascinating, and read them whenever I had time. Vivian belonged to an esoteric group which met in her house once a month. They were developing a Psychology for the 21st Century based on Psychosynthesis, a spiritual approach to psychotherapy developed by the Italian psychiatrist Roberto Assagioli. Robert Gerard, the leader of the group, had helped Assagioli when he visited California and wrote his book about Psychosynthesis.

Roberto Assagioli was one the disciples DK wrote to in 'Discipleship in the New Age'. Assagioli's esoteric back-ground is quite controversial but Vivian was one of the few Psychosynthesis teachers who was open about it. In other trainings it is rarely referred to.

I had been meditating since I was twenty two and had progressed through Spiritualism and Anthroposophy when I discovered Psychosynthesis in the 1970s. I am also psychic and often have prophetic dreams. During my training in Psychosynthesis I was told I could make a lot of money as a psychic, but this is not how I want to help people. Being psychic often made me question my sanity. It was reassuring to find a message for me in one of Vivian's books after she died. She had written my name in the margin with an arrow pointing to this quote:

"If you can co-experience mystical reality and material reality - if you know the difference, yet can integrate and use the force of this awareness - then you are not merely sane, you are super-sane. I don't really think there is a soul that exists in the world today that does not know at its deepest level about divine things. These feelings seem to be 'built into' humans.

*When you touch such knowing, it is as emotional as going
home to a place that has always been yours, a place that you
know fully but only glimpse occasionally."*
Infinite Mind by Valerie Hunt, page 292

It is important for me to explain certain terms because of what
happened to Vivian after she died. I have included a Glossary of
Terms to explain and clarify references.

Our most important point of contact was the Triangle Meditation we had entered into with Willem, a man in Belgium, the
year before Vivian's accident. The three of us had meditated
together once a week, usually in three different countries.
Willem and I continued to meditate with Frances, a friend of his
who had also been meditating for many years, and we were
delighted when Vivian appeared in our meditations. The fact that
the three of us saw and heard her confirms the connection we
had with her. This connection continued for more than a decade
and was faithfully recorded.

In the meditation reports I use dates to convey movement
through time. In the higher realms there is no time but without
dates the reports would run into each other. I also use capital
letters for Soul, Earth and Sun because of their importance in
our lives.

Before Vivian died in December 2000, she promised to stay in
touch with me, as a friend would before embarking on a long
journey. Vivian kept her promise. The following is an account of
what happened after her physical body died on 18th December,
2000.

Vivian had asked me to light an orange candle when she died,
which I kept burning until she woke me up in the middle of the
night and told me to extinguish it and light a white one. I kept
the white candle burning for three days and three nights.

Four days after Vivian's physical death I had a dream in which

she was singing. She always loved to sing and often burst into spontaneous song. This had ended with the car crash, after which she could barely whisper. In the dream she was singing from her heart and telling me telepathically that it was a song John Lennon had written after he died. It was a beautiful song that I did not recognise and cannot now remember. I do not know how she could have heard this song or known that John Lennon had written it. I can only conclude that it was in the ethers.

Four days later I had another dream in which I was searching for Vivian in a watery place but the water was not wet. Esoterically this is called Cosmic Liquid which Vivian would have passed through immediately after death. It links the physical and the astral plane as well as all the other planes. The Buddhists call it the Bardo and it is where we face our fears and missed opportunities. Vivian did not spend long in the Bardo because she had spent the last two years of her life in it. I arrived at a house and was invited in by a young woman whom I later recognised as Vivian's mother from an early photograph. Vivian was waiting for me inside and we had an ecstatic reunion. We were thrilled to see each other and embraced. Another friend arrived but he could not see us. It was as if we were hidden behind a veil. We both thought it was hilarious that we could see him but he could not see us. The friend later shared that he'd had a dream about travelling through water which was not wet.

Usually after death we go to a familiar place to recover, where we are reunited with our guides, who gently break the news that we are no longer in a physical body. Sometimes this place appears to be a hospital or convalescent home. Vivian had been preparing for her own death and therefore did not need a guide. Instead she was reunited with her beloved mother who had died five years earlier. So it is not surprising that I found her with her mother whom I had sensed in Vivian's room the night she died.

A week later Vivian was doing her Life Review which she

found fascinating because she could view any event in her life as if it was a movie. She could even rewind it and review significant events. She could also see how she had affected others and how she had appeared through their eyes. The Life Review is final proof that the physical form and its life on earth has ended.

After the Life Review Vivian started to detach from her personality.

2001

Two months later Vivian appeared in a meditation. We had been in the Triangle Meditation with Willem since 17th February 1997 in which we meditated together at the same time once a week but usually in three different countries. We sent reports to each other, the point being to synchronise our inner experiences. This became an important link and point of contact for us. We usually met in what we later knew to be the Ashram gardens. The Ashrams or Halls of Learning are where many of us go to in our sleep and continue to attend after we die. We all saw Vivian who was wearing a white robe with a pale blue sash. She looked radiant. We sat with her in a quiet corner of the gardens amongst the fragrant flowers. She said she was working with a group being prepared for entry into the Ashram. They were making their transition from the astral to the mental plane. She asked me to stop grieving for her. I'm ashamed to admit that I grieved for Vivian for far too long. It felt as if a light had been extinguished in my life. Although we had lived in different countries, we emailed each other almost every day and knew the intimate details of each other's lives

In a meditation on the first anniversary of her passing, Vivian silently communicated her sense of freedom, which was in sharp contrast to my feeling of being in exile. I wanted to be where she is.

In a later meditation Vivian took me away with her to a quiet corner of the gardens where we could be alone. What is interesting about this experience is that Frances saw Vivian taking me away. When two or three of us in the Triangle shared the same inner experience, although we were often in different countries, it was a confirmation.

All three of us saw Vivian when she moved into the Ashram. In the same meditation we all saw her sitting on the grass under one of the trees with a small group of students. The grass, flowers and trees were vibrant and we all felt that they are blueprints for the ones we have on earth.

In another meditation Vivian told me that what happened to her was a test. "How it makes you feel is your test," she said. "Working through your grief is your work."

My grief was so intense that in a dream she called me on a telephone and said, "Grieve for what happened to me. Don't grieve for me." It was such a vivid dream that I woke up crying.

A meditation, which began with the song "Let It Be", continued with Vivian's appearance holding a Tibetan bowl. She sounded a note on the bowl and said, "Each life is a note which the Soul makes into a song." Her life had just been a particular note that her Soul needed to make. Every life sounds a note which only makes sense when it is incorporated into the Soul's song.

'Let it be' is a song Paul McCartney wrote about his mother who died when he was only fourteen. It set the tone for his life and inspired him to create beautiful music out of the tragedy of losing his mother.

2002

It was two years since Vivian's passing when I found myself again in the Ashram gardens, which I can only liken to the gardens of

the Alhambra Palace in Granada, Spain. There are flowers, trees and pools of running water. The Ashram buildings are a cluster of circular structures, which are classrooms surrounding an inner sanctuary, all overlooking the gardens. I looked into a chamber with a golden couch, which I recognised. Vivian had spent a lot of time on the golden couch in this chamber immediately after the car crash when she was in a coma in intensive care. When I sat by her bed meditating, this is what I saw. I knew then that she was going through some kind of group initiation because it involved so many other people: her family, friends and students. We were all affected by this tragic event.

A month later we were standing outside a building with soaring columns and a triangular roof, which is called the Hall of Higher Learning and Service. Above the entrance it says: "Abandon hope all ye who enter here." There were many people milling around outside. Not many of them were able to "abandon hope" which is letting go of attachments and desires. Vivian was there to greet the three of us, but only two of us entered the building. The third person could not relinquish a relationship.

2003

At one point I asked Vivian to find a friend who had recently died. She said it was not part of her work to find people who have died but she later told me he was with another deceased friend of mine who was helping him. He had died at the age of forty two from drowning in a river. The older deceased friend had been a therapist and was able to help him in his transition.

Vivian described her work as "liberating people from the astral plane" and it demonstrates how important it is to do our inner work when we are on the physical plane, where it is so much easier. This is why Roberto Assagioli placed so much emphasis on it in Psychosynthesis, and it is why people reincarnate.

Problems and psychological blocks do not automatically disappear after death. They can intensify when we no longer have the distraction of a physical body. Repressed emotions are more difficult to deal with after death. Addictions are even more difficult when we can no longer satisfy them on the physical plane. This is when entities can seek to attach themselves to those who are still alive and addicted to alcohol or drugs.

Between birth and death we "internalise" the external world. After death we "externalise" what we have internalised. In other words our inner world becomes our outer world. We are therefore responsible for how we react to outer circumstances. Religions speak of heaven and hell, but these states are self-imposed and are not inflicted upon us.

Vivian recreated her adobe house on Spirit Mountain with its lake, stream, waterfall and 1500 acres of pristine forest because it was a place she had loved and missed during the final two years of her life when she had no freedom of movement. It is very common for people to recreate a place they have loved and occupied on earth. I often visited Vivian in her adobe house and she would take me out on the lake in a boat where we could just be together, share our lives, and enjoy the scenery. Yes, Vivian has a life. It is a life lived beyond time but it is in constant motion. She told me she does not need to sleep any more but she can choose to. She knows intuitively when she needs to be somewhere else. She is still evolving and growing. Inner growth is not just in time and space. As we grow in consciousness, so does our awareness of higher realities.

Vivian told me that the adobe house is her inner sanctuary where she finds peace and rejuvenation. She also visits her mother who lives somewhere else. She studies in the Ashram which is a reflection of the main Ashrams on higher planes.

When Frances saw a swan flying over me I knew its significance. It was Vivian's totem. Maybe in this meditation Vivian trans-

formed herself into a swan knowing I would remember its significance. I once embroidered a swan onto one of her pillowcases.

In another meditation we saw a column of angels extending from the Earth to the Sun. They were in constant motion and were uplifting us. They were singing "We ARE the Light" and I realised that the light from the Sun is alive. I was lifted up but would then fall back into the void. I heard "Do not be disheartened. You are going through the Burning Ground." Vivian appeared and reminded me that I had felt like this before. Frances felt Vivian's presence and saw that she was supporting me through this phase, and will watch over me for as long as it takes.

A week later we again felt Vivian's presence. She wanted us to do something with the knowledge that we now have about Reality and Essence; on living Spirit and being in Spirit; not reading about it or writing about it. Willem heard Vivian say, "Marilyn is able to do it, to manifest this."

On December 15th I heard: "Do not wait until you die to experience the cool clear light. Stand in it now. Transcend the illusion of the finite physical world and know that you are infinite. You judge your experiences as good or bad but they are merely lessons in this school of drastic discipline. Wake up!" In the same meditation Willem saw me stepping into a fire and reaching out my hands behind me, so that he and Frances could hold them. It felt like a Baptism of Fire burning away the dross. Frances heard "Be Whole-hearted."

2004

In January we attended a meeting in the Inner Sanctuary of the Ashram. Vivian was there and smiled at us with her eyes. Huge double doors were closed and a gong sounded. Willem heard an invisible choir singing and could follow the Speaker's thoughts. The state of the world was being discussed by beings who, like

gardeners, discuss world problems as if they are ailing plants in a garden. We saw angels dancing. They told us "We are outside of your world yet intricately linked to it." Frances felt Maitreya's love and heard: "Be outposts in the world - outposts of the Great Mother. Let her compassion flow from you to all beings." In this meditation I sensed that Christ would return as a great Islamic teacher to unite all religions and nations.

(Maitreya is the eastern name for the Christ who often appeared in our meditations. See Maitreya in the Glossary.)

On April 5th Frances heard: "Develop the clarity of the Diamond Mind. Are you prepared for the shattering of concepts about yourselves? Start by stepping into the void. Your only compass is the Light of the Soul." In this meditation Willem saw me receiving a text in golden letters. He heard "It is the language of the heart." I also experienced receiving a text about containing the suffering of the world within the heart. We all experienced Vivian's presence in this meditation.

On April 26th Vivian told us to start building a bridge through creative visualisation. The building of the bridge continued for several years with all of us building it in our meditations. It now connects us to the Far Distant Shore where the Golden City is located.

In a later meditation I asked Vivian why she had the car crash. She told me she had incarnated with a "sharp edge", which needed to be made smooth. She asked me to look at my "sharp edge" and then to reflect on the time after the car crash when I flew to Texas to be with her in Intensive Care. What did I learn? I knew the answer: patience and self-discipline.

Our meetings with Vivian in the Ashram gardens continued. The gardens are always fragrant and in flower. We are reminded that this is where we really are. Frances asked, "What is needed to create such beauty?" She was shown a dark place under the ground where hard work is going on. "Work is needed in dark

and difficult situations to create beauty."

On another occasion Vivian took my hand and led me to a healing pool, which was hidden away in a corner of the gardens. It was surrounded by rose bushes and had lotus blossoms floating on the surface. I walked down some steps into it and could breathe under the water, which was not wet. Vivian told me to visualise this healing experience at night before falling asleep.

"I always look forward to connecting with you in the Monday Triangle," Vivian told us. "Open and align your consciousness to the immensity of your multi-dimensional being!"

Vivian showed us many egg-shaped auric fields of different colours, one within the other, like Russian dolls. Each aura is in a different dimension, which makes it look like an inter-dimensional vortex or doorway. She told us: "Broaden your perspective still further and learn to live lightly on the beautiful Earth plane you inhabit. You see the evil that men do, and you despair, but do you not see the beauty and the wonder; the many deeds of sacrifice and courage? Remember to stand at the midway point and let the light and joy of the Soul permeate the personality. In the Ashram we live in joy. This is the reality of being. All else is illusion. I feel such joy that we can communicate through the veils. Tell Marilyn to let go of her sadness. It is misplaced. I am still with her, though I cannot reach her if she does not lift her consciousness to where I now am. Where I am there is only peace even though there is also an intensification of focus on precipitating the Plan of our Teacher. I wish you could experience the unity of purpose that there is in the Ashram!"

On October18th Vivian took me back to the healing pool. I tried to climb out but she insisted that I remain there. She reminded me of the times in Intensive Care when I guided her into the healing pool and how much it helped her. She also reminded me of the trees outside Rehab in Dallas which I took her to at dusk to hear the birds singing.

On November 15ᵗʰ Vivian appeared and said, "The Ashram is not a comfort zone. The level of Soul tension is intense and there is ongoing rigorous training. Create your own ashram where you are and help us build a bridge from the mundane to the subtle world."

A week later I had a profound meditation in which I met Vivian and she talked to me about being "born again" which is letting go of our belief systems and opinions. I felt free and light as I experienced what this would be like on a daily basis. Vivian said we perceive life through filters. She told me to be like a new-born baby without preconceived ideas of how life should be. Life is a process, full of changes, which we cannot understand with our personalities. We cannot feel Europe and Africa moving towards each other, but they are, and will one day collide. World events and our lives are long processes, taking aeons to complete. In this meditation Frances saw Vivian taking me away. She and Willem remained in the gardens and were told by a teacher: "Do not give way to despondency and discouragement. In the Mantram of Unification it says: "Let the Soul control the outer form, and life, and all events, and bring to light the Love that underlies the happenings of the time.

"Let these words speak for themselves, and embrace their truth in your life. Through Vivian as an intermediary your Triangle is invited into the Ashram. But your work is bridge-building: within yourselves and between the kingdom of Souls and the human kingdom. You have to do the work, but many are there to aid and support you."

Frances saw Vivian bringing me back and noted that I was wearing a white robe with a pale blue sash and a golden circlet around my head. She said I looked happy.

Willem looked up the meaning of "born again" and discovered it is an important Masonic term. When initiates are accepted into the temple, they are referred to as "twice-born" or "born again."

2005

At the beginning of 2005 I asked Vivian why she was 'called home' when she was doing such useful work in the world. She said it was part of the 'polishing' process, and added that I am also being polished.

In a later meditation we were standing on a bridge with people walking in both directions. I heard "If you perceive the spiritual world, it is your duty and joy to bring that perception into the physical world. It is humanity's next evolutionary step to access and integrate knowledge of the fifth kingdom and bring it to the world. If you have any doubts about this, look around you. How many people have knowledge of the spiritual world? You have that knowledge. Use it. Share it. You are like the early explorers who travelled to far off exotic lands and returned to tell others about them – and how to travel there."

I found myself climbing a mountain in another meditation. At the top of the mountain was an enormous monastery like the ones in Tibet. There are many different departments within this monastery where people are serving the planet. For example, in one department people are praying. This is their field of service. In another department people are receiving instructions for more active service in the world. We were asked to choose our field of service. As I passed through the various departments I saw that people are totally committed to what they are doing. They are not caught up in emotional reaction nor are they disheartened by the enormity of their tasks. They see the suffering in the world and are totally focused on serving the planet and the evolution of humanity. This monastery appeared often in our meditations.

In a later meditation I saw two mountains, each with a citadel on its peak. There are two paths leading to the two mountains. One is smooth and easy and is called "the path of least resistance". The other path is difficult and rocky with many obstacles.

Between the two paths humanity is struggling with its many problems. These people are either too poor or too immersed in matter to choose a path. The people on the rocky path reach out to them but the people on the smooth path are in too much of a hurry to stop and help. They are heading towards the citadel where all of their needs will be met and where they will be able to survey the world from a superior position. Those on the rocky path take long diversions in an effort to help the struggling masses. They are not in a hurry even though the citadel they are heading towards radiates light and compels them to return to the rocky path with is many boulders and obstacles. They often meet others who have given up on this path and are retracing their footsteps in order to find an easier path. Some of these people are angry and bitter, feeling that their efforts have not been rewarded or recognised. They are going to take "the path of least resistance" which glitters with fools' gold, glamour and grandiosity. I saw Jesus in the wilderness, where he wandered for forty days and nights, and where he was tempted to take the easy path, which would have elevated him to a position of power. He chose the rocky path because it took him closer to humanity and ended in crucifixion. I saw that each one of us has to choose between the two paths and the two citadels, which symbolise the two Lodges.

In March Vivian appeared and spoke directly to me. She said: "Remember how we worked together and shared our innermost feelings and thoughts. The intimacy of the Soul is never lost. Fiery hearts yearn for union. Heart connections need to be shared. The Greater Heart in Whom I have my being wants to extend. It wants to encompass and vibrate in unison with your heart. Reach out. Let us create a bridge of glory."

In a meditation in April I found myself in a hot air balloon with Vivian who was pointing out how beautiful the Earth is and how lucky I am to be here. I could see the curve of the Earth and

I had a feeling of absolute joy and optimism as she pointed to the future. As I type these words five years later in my house in Southern Spain, from where I can see the curve of the Earth in the ocean, I know this was prophetic. Vivian can see into the future!

I found this quote years later:

"The Higher Self, on its own plane, is not trammelled by time and space, and (knowing the future as well as that which is past) seeks to bring the desired end nearer and make it more rapidly a fact."

Letters on Occult Meditation page 33

In a meditation just after Easter we were transported to the Ashram gardens where we met Vivian. There was an atmosphere of unusual stillness and everyone was walking in a state of silent contemplation. They were preparing for Wesak which starts with the Easter festival. There was so much lightness of being, peace and joy. Frances heard: " Step into the joyous light of your own Soul and let it clear negative thought forms, old patterns of thinking and living. There is no need for inner conflict. Just open yourself to the light of the Soul and follow where it leads. Past karma has been cleared. Do not cling to redundant thought forms. You are free, believe it, and move on. Take care not to create any more karmic situations, for you will find the result is instantaneous, but the opportunity for clearing karmic debt is also instantaneous."

(See Wesak in the Glossary of Terms.)

In May Willem saw Vivian standing behind me. He saw that our deep connection has created a bridge facilitating our contact with the Ashram. We are a Living Bridge. Our link is fiery and will help me to write. Vivian will be looking over my shoulder.

In a meditation in June Vivian appeared and spoke to each of us. She told me to raise my awareness from my 4th Ray (harmony

through conflict) personality to my 7th Ray (order and ritual) Soul. I must stop seeing the glass as half empty, but most important of all, I must stop missing her and start working with her. "We have much work to do together," she told me.

(See the Rays in the Glossary of Terms.)

In the same meditation Frances was told to raise her awareness and hold a higher frequency: "Energy and manifestation follow thought. What is the nature of your thoughts?" Vivian asked. "To enter the Ashram you must be in the realm of inspiration or intuition. The Soul has a causal body and transmits via the personality. The Monad is its Soul. Observe your thoughts, raise them to the Triad and help bring Heaven to Earth. Be an oasis of Soul light where you are now. There is no 'ideal' place to be. Create it now. Then you will not be wishing your life away. Now is the only time you have. The past is past and the future is the result of what you are creating now."

In the same meditation Willem saw me sitting on a rock trying to decode a sign. It looked like the three sphere symbol Roerich saw on his trip to Tibet, which inspired him to create the Banner of Peace. Vivian appeared and said, "It is the language of the heart." Willem saw her link to each of us in a different and specific way. He felt completely refreshed. In this meditation we all saw that Vivian has gone through a shift. She now has more authority and is obviously respected within the Ashram.

(See Roerich in the Glossary of Terms.)

In another meditation Vivian encouraged us to hold our awareness as high as possible. We now form a chalice holding a finer frequency, which can be poured forth into the world. We were told: "When you are radiant you positively influence the environment around you."

Later in June we all experienced meeting Vivian in the Ashram gardens. She told me to "step out of the drama and do the work." When Frances thanked her for the privilege of taking

her place in the Triangle and still being here, Vivian thanked her for coming into the Triangle and said, "Incarnate the purpose your Soul is holding." To Willem she said, "Do not wait for things to happen. Make them happen. Use your focused thought." To all of us she said, "You will recognise when you are under the influence of your Soul when you feel joy. Where there is joy, there is the Soul."

Frances asked Vivian if she could ask a question about her niece's son who is an Indigo child. This was her response: "Indigo children have great difficulty fitting into the present world reality and its low vibrational frequency. They are often exceptionally gifted and specialised in one area, and can therefore display what appears to be obsessive behaviour. They are coming in to build a New World. They need a single-minded focus in what they have come to manifest. Their very strong will power is a challenge for their parents. The Indigo child's strong will and focus must be tempered but not suppressed. They can appear to be almost autistic but that is because we do not understand their reality. Some of these so-called Indigo children, incarnating now, already carry the frequency to which the planet and humanity is ascending, and they have difficulty coping with the lower and slower frequency. They can react to this with frustration and even rage. Many of these children have tantrums and express their extreme frustration at our slowness and lack of etheric sensitivity. Their sensitivity is acute. There is a definite 'generation gap' and a sense of dislocation between their reality and the 'old dispensation' or energy we are still conditioned by."

(See Indigo Children in the Glossary of Terms.)

In a meditation at the beginning of July I experienced the three of us in a wide valley surrounded by mountains. We were attending a Ceremony of Dedication. Masters and teachers were presenting discs attached to ribbons. Bronze, silver and golden discs on different coloured ribbons were being presented. We

were each given a disc. We all repeated: "I dedicate my life to the unfolding of the Plan." Frances and I, whose silver discs covered our throat chakras, promised to be "true of voice" and to practise "right speech and harmlessness." Willem's disc was on his heart chakra and he was in a different group. We were taken inside the large monastery where a group of Tibetan monks were chanting in deep resonant voices, which 'vibrated' our discs. I could feel it in my throat even after the meditation.

In another meditation Vivian was guiding us through the Halls of Time. She showed us how we can walk through the thin veils that separate our present lives from our past lives, and how we can also cross the veils that separate the dimensions. Thus, we become Time Travellers. We have always been Time Travellers but the heaviness of the old world's frequency kept us imprisoned within the illusion of separation. "With the veils getting thinner and your expanding consciousness, you can detach yourselves from the physical-emotional-mental sucking force of the old world," she said. "The New World is ready to ascend with you. Only the outer shell needs to crack open." This helped us to understand why we often climb mountains in our meditations and find ourselves on top of a mountain where heaven and earth touch – where the highest and the lowest meet. Vivian explained that the vivid memories in our meditations, often from ancient Egypt, remind us of who we really are. It shows us our power, transcending the Egyptian reality, and leading us back to our connection with Home. "Open yourselves to what is coming," she said, "Be ready!"

Vivian advised us to maintain the Triangle link outside of the Monday meditation time. We were told to "seek out and destroy all that hinders our ascension into the higher realm of the Soul."

On July 18th we met Vivian in the Ashram gardens. She invited us, as our sponsor, to enter Lord Maitreya's council chamber. Frances caught a glimpse of Maitreya sitting on his

golden lotus throne radiating golden light in all directions and out into the world. We were standing in front of huge golden doors, Willem on the right wearing a white robe with the insignia of a book with crossed quill pens on his chest (a symbol of the scribe), around his neck a ribbon with a disc, and next to him the symbol of a red living heart. Frances and I were wearing priestess robes in a light blue/green colour with golden belts, discs on ribbons around our necks. Frances had the symbol of a lyre; mine was an open book. We were standing at the door of initiation and Vivian was one of our sponsors. The guardian of the door told us we would not be permitted to pass through the door until we had worked at expressing and mastering the areas our symbols represent. Frances was told to sing her song and "Speak forth the Word". She must use her voice to sing and transmit divine wisdom. Willem's symbol and mine were obvious. He is a scribe and I am a writer.

(See Lord Maitreya in the Glossary of Terms)

On July 25th I saw Vivian teaching in the Ashram gardens, looking radiant and animated. We sat down on the grass to listen to her. "There is so much more to learn and explore," she said. "You are on a path leading to planes even more fragrant and exquisite than this one. You are fortunate to have reached this far. Reach back to those who follow and forward to those who wait for your arrival." I started to weep and Vivian said, "You can always meet me in the Ashram gardens. We are not separate."

In the same meditation Willem felt the incredible unlimited unconditional support coming from Vivian, the Elders, the Masters and vast Beings. This kind of love and solid Brotherhood is beyond mundane thought and feeling. It is real Heart Energy.

At the beginning of August I experienced sailing in a small boat across a vast expanse of totally still water. It looked like Benares. An Indian dressed in a white robe and turban was waiting for us on the shore. He handed each of us an urn containing the

ashes of the glamours we have burnt away in the 'burning ground'. We scattered the ashes on the water and they floated away. Then we sailed away in the boat. I felt elevated – as if an enormous burden had been taken away and disposed of.

(See Glamour in the Glossary of Terms.)

In the same meditation Willem experienced us being brought before an Elder, an ancient teacher older than the Masters, and a Transmitter of divine energy. Willem wondered if it was the Ancient of Days. There was no communication. We were being uplifted. All of our irritations, frustrations and unconsciousness vanished. We became as solid as rocks.

At the end of August Willem saw Vivian present us with a crystal chalice in the form of a lotus flower. "You are the chalice receiving dew-drops from heaven," she said. "You should be overflowing with joy, but what is happening? Can earthly pre-occupations and worries be so strong that they throw huge shadows and blot out the Sun?"

In the same meditation I saw the bridge we have built in previous meditations. I also saw many bridges connecting stars, planets and star systems throughout the universe.

At the beginning of September Vivian invited us to connect with her heart. It connected us to a higher frequency. She said she appreciates our connection with her. "It's a joy," she said. "You forget how important your work is for the Ashram. You are the pillars we need. We are co-workers. If you could but know how important it is to be fully integrated within the One Work. It will make the connection more fluent and it will help you to overcome the difficulties on Earth." Vivian is the heart of our fusion, which is Love.

On September 19th I saw Vivian sitting on the grass teaching in the Ashram gardens, as she did in the garden in Pasadena, under a great old tree. I heard her say "As in Heaven, so on Earth." I felt nostalgic about out time together in Pasadena, and

she gave me one of her smiles, which told me to let go of the past and live in the present.

In the same meditation Willem heard Vivian explaining how to extend our auric fields. They are much wider than we imagine. We need to extend the field through the power of the heart. The aura is impersonal, yet powerful.

At the end of September we were given a new colour. It was placed in our auras and is a beautiful salmon pink colour. Vivian was watching as the colour was added.

In a later meditation Willem saw a beautiful thick book with a golden cover and gilded pages. It looked like the Book of Doves painted by Roerich. In a meditation at the beginning of October I saw the book bound with gold leaf. I opened it and saw that the pages are beautifully illustrated. It is called 'The Book of Deeds' and contains the daily random acts of kindness we can so easily miss. We were told: "Pay attention to the little things and the big things will take care of themselves."

In another meditation I saw a sturdy door with engravings but no knob or handle with which to open it. Vivian was smiling and standing nearby. The door was at the end of a long corridor above an abyss. It was a problem I had to solve. Vivian knew the answer but she could not tell me.

A week later the problem was solved when I realised that the power of a group, working together, reaches higher and achieves more than an individual. I saw the door and how a group can open it by helping and supporting each other. They can 'bridge' the abyss and easily reach the door. Beyond the door was a large circular chamber with groups of people joining together in meditation in order to create a global network of dedicated people. I suspected that we had been admitted into an Inner Circle.

In a meditation in November Frances saw Vivian waiting for us in a beautiful building in a valley beneath high snow-covered mountain peaks. She took us to meet three beings wearing white

robes and waiting on a terrace. They took us to a room and gave us teachings. I saw a swirling unfolding matrix of light emanating from our higher bodies. I was told that meditation causes the connection between our brains and our higher bodies to expand and grow, enabling us to achieve higher states of consciousness. I also heard the song 'The windmills of your mind.'

In the same meditation Vivian showed Willem how, through our unity of hearts, we touch electric fire. This touch is like the touch of a wand. It creates what earth people call 'magic' but it is the opening of the fifth dimension. He heard "Widen the path of magic and remember that you are Magicians." It often happens in our meditations that each of us has a piece of the experience.

On November 28th Willem saw Roberto Assagioli addressing me. He said, "Draw the fire from within yourself instead of hoping for warmth and heat from outside. You know what kind of fire it is. You are the fire!"

I often receive this message because I go to Southern Spain in the winter to avoid the cold.

At the end of December Frances saw Vivian with other beings in deep unity and communion. We were reminded to keep our etheric bodies clear and vitalised, so that our physical bodies can absorb, contain and radiate the greater intensity of pure light being transmitted to all light workers over the Christmas period. "Remain connected to the intensity of light. You are light beings. You are filled with light. The light volume control is in your hands. There is no need to be affected by the winter climate and lack of light. Truly the light is within you."

2006

At the beginning of 2006 in our Triangle meditation I was standing before the Great Mother, but I was also inside her. I experienced a vast, compassionate, unconditional love and heard

"The Great Mother is being unveiled."

Vivian and many others were there.

In this same meditation Frances saw us in the Ashram with Vivian who said, "You may have noticed that the mundane world has become more remote to you and that you dwell more often in the frequency of the Ashram. Try to remain connected as you go about your daily routine. Find a routine that helps train you as a disciple. Discipline = discipleship. You are almost part of the New Reality."

In another meditation Frances saw the Pythagorean Mystery School where we were students in a previous life. She heard, "Past and present are converging but in a different way. The consciousness is new but the training you received in the past is being activated now."

A week later in our meditation Vivian gave me a glorious smile, obviously delighted that I have finally stopped grieving for her! We were in the Ashram gardens and she took us into the classrooms arranged like the petals of a lotus flower around an Inner Sanctuary. All of the rooms look out into the gardens surrounding them. There were many people and a feeling of joy and celebration. Frances and I were given beautiful blue robes and were told we are priestesses of the Great Mother. Others were given blue belts or scarves in the same scintillating shade of blue. Willem was given a blue belt. We were waiting for the Mother in great anticipation but were told that we are already inside her. We are her hands and feet. We live in her aura. We walk in her body. We are expressions of her love.

In our meditation at the beginning of February I saw a mountain with a jagged peak. I heard "All must climb the jagged peak" but it appeared to be too steep and dangerous. I saw Vivian at the top looking down at us. Then I realised that we can only climb the jagged peak when we have dropped our baggage, burdens and limitations. We have to be light. When my mind was

empty I found myself soaring, but quickly descended when thoughts returned. Only by becoming empty and light can we ascend the jagged peak.

Two days after what would have been Vivian's sixtieth birthday we had a long conversation about her papers. I was in California clearing the four-drawer filing cabinet, which had stood in her office in Pasadena. It had been the first job she gave me to do – and now it was the last. I had to decide which papers to keep and which to throw away.

In our meditation in May I found myself in a vast circular library with a transparent domed roof. There were millions of books and manuscripts on shelves extending up to the domed ceiling. There were corridors off the central area with small circular spaces for study. I suspected I was inside one of the Great Libraries. Vivian was in a study area and said she was studying. She showed me an ancient manuscript bound in leather with a lock. She said it was called 'The Saving Celestial Constellation' and indicated that I would enjoy reading it.

Two weeks later I was attempting to read the book. "The Saving Celestial Constellation" refers to a sisterhood of which the Pleiades and our planet are members. Our planet is part of a sisterhood concerned with cosmic salvaging beyond our comprehension. Isis and the Hathors belong to this sisterhood - also known as the Seraphim Sisters.

In June we were inside a chapel with stained glass windows. We were each receiving guidance. Vivian showed me the areas of my personality that need to be transformed. It was painful to see the areas where I am stuck, solidified and unyielding. We were shown the rugged edges of our diamonds that need to be polished and made smooth. It was very revealing. Frances also experienced receiving inner guidance in this meditation.

A week later we were with Vivian and a teacher on the veranda of the building with the columns overlooking the moun-

tains. "Spiritual practice is about embodying and radiating every minute of your life, and includes within your sphere of activity the people you meet in your daily life," I heard. "It includes the cashier in the supermarket, the bus driver, and all the Little Ones you meet in your daily life. You have NO idea how you may be influencing these people. Do not exclude anyone. This is true spiritual practice. You are IN the world. Bring Heaven to Earth."

In the same meditation Frances experienced being welcomed by Vivian and a dignified man in a white robe. She heard "Your Path is the Path of the Mother. It is the mysterious path about which little is known. Veiled in secrecy is the power of the divine feminine. There is much unconscious misogyny even from the most enlightened of your brothers on the Path. It wounds you deeply as you pick it up with your sensitive equipment. Do not make yourself vulnerable but clothe yourself in the raiment of the Mother, and stand in radiant being. In this Triangle and in your daily life it is not through what you do that you serve, but by the radiance of being that you transmit. This should not be undervalued."

At the beginning of July Frances saw Vivian waiting for us. She was wearing a white robe and looked serious. She took us to the Halls of Higher Learning where we also wore white robes and symbols on our foreheads. Willem's was a double triangle. Frances and I had Vesica Pisces and were dressed as priestesses of Hathor. We were then taken to a room with a flat blue screen along one wall on which we could see parts of the world and beyond.

In our meditation at the end of July Willem felt very close to Vivian and heard: "Develop synthesis even more and continue your search for simplicity and truth. Marilyn creates magic with her words. May words reveal the light – may they BE the light." It entered the pores of his being like a summer breeze.

At the beginning of August Vivian advised us to establish a

permanent link with her and confirmed that we are on the same frequency. In the same meditation Frances saw her leading us through darkness holding a lantern. "Learn to see what's in the moment," she said. We walked through the darkness with the lantern lighting the way. We entered an underground cavern where the Great Mother was enthroned. She was veiled but her power filled the space. We knelt before her, our arms crossed in the ancient Egyptian way. A great angel holding a fiery sword was guarding the entrance to the cavern. We heard "The raiment of the Mother is the sweep of all created forms." The Mother gave Frances a chalice of fire, Willem a chalice of water and me a chalice of earth. Frances assumed these are the elements we each need the most.

I found a photograph of Vivian in a book called 'Passage to Power'. I had no memory of putting the photo there. In our meditation I found myself in front of a fluted column. It was part of a doorway with a fluted column either side of it. Vivian appeared and said, "It is time to hold the Rod of Power. It is a time of decision. You can only hold the Rod of Power when you are clear about the decisions you have to make and the nature of those decisions." I was too indecisive to hold the Rod of Power - and I was not the only one!

In the same meditation Willem heard Vivian say, "Discover the limitless array of our connections." He did not understand what she meant, so she helped him to see it as spiritual radar, an inner knowing – maybe the diamond mind. It functions when mind, heart and Soul are aligned.

At the end of August Vivian took me to the home she has created which resembles her adobe house on Spirit Mountain. It was the place where she experienced the most peace and where she had time to be creative. Spirit Mountain is now the place where she relaxes and refreshes herself. She explained that she does not need to sleep but she can go into a deep witnessing state

where she accesses higher levels of being. She took me in a small boat out on the lake in front of her home where we relaxed and enjoyed each other's company.

At the beginning of September Vivian took us into an octagonal building with a particular function. Around a central circular chamber, where the Masters meet, there are seven smaller chambers where the various teachers meet with their students. When the Masters meet in the central chamber it is a special time for us to gather in order to link in with them in the smaller chambers. The radiation from the Masters speeds up the process of opening our chakras. I felt my crown chakra vibrating. The outer chambers form the petals of a lotus with the eighth chamber as the inner bud of the lotus. With most aspirants this inner bud is closed but the Masters have opened their inner lotus buds and are therefore beneficial in helping us to open ours. In the same meditation Frances heard a bell ringing, calling people to a particular eight-sided building.

On September 11th I found myself in a vibrant blue room. As I looked into the now familiar flat blue screen, I heard "A useful server is a detached server. If it is not eternal, it is not real. You are involved in a process. Even 9.11 was a process – a collective process which appeared as a tragedy. Do not be polarised by global events. They occur to help you grow in consciousness. Tragedy is a process helping you to awaken. Nobody died but many were awakened." It was the five-year anniversary of 9.11.

In the same meditation Vivian asked Willem if he could encompass all the people he has met and known in his life. Could he embrace all of them, take them into his heart, setting aside his likes and dislikes?

At the beginning of October I saw an octagonal open-sided building with columns and steps leading up to it. It reaches up to the Sun and is a solar transmitter. Dancers appeared and danced inside the building transmitting the dance of the solar

angels. It was like a dancing rainbow with heavenly music. Then we entered the building and were able to transmit prana from the Sun to our physical bodies on Earth.

Vivian reminded us that we are now a part of the Ashram, building both ends of the bridge. Through our bodies we are rooted in humanity; through our spiritual heritage we are rooted in Hierarchy. She said, "Leave your worries behind and join the stream of Love Divine."

(See Hierarchy in the Glossary of Terms.)

A week later in our meditation Vivian took us to her inner sanctuary and told us how important it is to create an inner sanctuary. Spirit Mountain was her home for eight years and it is still her inner sanctuary. She asked where ours are. I realised that my inner sanctuary is still my room in her house in Pasadena with the golden Californian sunlight streaming in through the window. Vivian suggested I create a new inner sanctuary. She attempted to tell us what it's like to live in eternity. It is an inner experience of timelessness. She knows intuitively when to be in the Ashram, and took us to where others were gathering. I heard, "Create Heaven on Earth within yourselves in order to create it externally on Earth."

In another meditation I saw monks meditating on a natural stone platform in front of the Tibetan monastery. Dancers in colourful costumes were dancing on the platform to an accompaniment of horns and cymbals. They were dancing around the Mother of the World, who was veiled, but the veils were falling away as the Sun rose in the east. She was bathed in light and her eyes were luminous. She said "I have come for my children" and there was fierceness in her voice, the way a mother is fierce if her children are being hurt. Maitreya knelt in front of her. She lifted him to his feet and turned him to face the world.

A week later I heard "Elevate! Radiate!" and saw a huge golden statue of the Buddha with many beings surrounding it.

Maitreya was at its feet. We were on the outer rim, each of us holding a candle. I heard "Put aside your personal issues and turn the tide." If a billion people lit candles and stood outside at night, the light would be visible from outer space. This is a small example of our collective power.

At the beginning of November I experienced whirling in the Ashram. It felt glorious. As we spun, we created vortexes of colour. We were told to build the Temple of Solomon and were given complex geometric instructions. We were also told to change our thinking. We say it is going dark when in fact we are spinning away from the Sun and are entering the indigo area where we can see the infinity of space. During the day we are blinded by the Sun but we say this is when we are awake. What we call being asleep is when we are most awake! I wondered why it is always light in the Ashram. Maybe it is because it is beyond space-time. I glimpsed a dimension opalescent like a pearl and another one like a nebula.

A week later I heard "The hills are alive with the sound of music" and found myself in a lush green meadow, full of wild flowers, high up in the mountains. This meadow is one of Vivian's favourite places. I heard "Everything is alive and has its own song." We were told to enter the silence and hear the songs our Souls are seeking to sing. When we allow the Soul to sing its song, our lives become joyous and we feel fulfilled. The Soul's song causes the cells in our bodies to form beautiful harmonious patterns.

In the same meditation Willem heard Vivian reminding us that we are not alone in our Triangle. Our connection with the Ashram brings us within the Heart of Christ. Separation is an illusion. Willem felt a glow in his heart. Vivian told him not to feel guilty when in doubt or not well-aligned. She also missed a lot when on Earth. "When the gates open, the Eye also opens, and we can SEE."

On December 18th we were sitting with Vivian outside her

adobe house when she told us she would be moving on. She pointed across the water to the golden spires, domes and shimmering light of the Golden City. I remembered a recent dream in which she was going to be 'executed' and I was searching through her papers in an attempt to prevent it from happening. I had a similar dream about my mother after she died. It signifies the death of the personality. She said we could still tune in but it would be with Viva, her Soul, not Vivian.

I have wondered why Vivian recreated and stayed so long in her adobe house on Spirit Mountain. I think there are three reasons: she had missed it during the two years she was unable to move, and she may have been 'on hold' until she could move on to a higher plane. The third reason may have been to stay in touch with us.

In the same meditation I noticed a beautiful boat, shaped like a swan, sailing across the water to the Golden City. It was being watched by a multitude on both shores and was the passage of a great Soul. It was Eileen Caddy (co-founder of the Findhorn Community) who died last week. We watched and knew it would soon be Vivian's turn to sail to the Golden City. It was exactly six years since she had left her physical body.

(See Eileen Caddy in the Glossary of Terms.)

When an old person dies, their transition is much quicker than when a young person dies, mainly because they have had a long life and are ready to move on. When we die young, we still have strong bonds with people on the physical plane and want to remain connected to them. Therefore, it takes longer to detach from the personality.

At the end of 2006 we received this message:

"The clamour and conflicts of the mundane world do not exist in the Ashram. Tibetans and Chinese are one. Israelis and Palestinians unite. Muslims and Christians are brothers. There is no division or warring conflict in the Ashram. A keynote of

life in the higher realms is brotherly love.

"Try to reflect this in your daily life in the mundane world. Love the differences as well as the similarities, the dissonance as well as the harmonies. Love those who feel enmity towards you and those you dislike, for they are your best teachers! See the 'evil that men do' and love them nevertheless. For you are part of the same human family. Love all, serve all."

2007

In 2007 I continued copy-typing Roberto Assagioli's book *Transpersonal Development* into my laptop in order for it to be re-translated and reprinted. It was a healing process and an absolute joy. It was one of the books I had inherited from Vivian but it was now out of print.

Our Triangle started to change and we were not able to meditate in the old way. We were being asked to bring what we were learning into our daily lives. Although Viva felt more distant, she still spoke to us: "You know we will always be connected through the heart. You do not need my help or my intervention to make the connection with the inner Ashram and beyond."

Willem saw the image of an arrow shot from the arc of our fiery determination. After he blew out the candles at the end of the meditation he heard: "You may blow out the candles but our inner contact and vibration will prevail."

In January we were shown how our Triangle has a specific mission with regard to the Reappearance of the Mother. In March Frances saw a female Bodhisattva over-lighting, enclosing and embracing our Triangle. She heard, "Do not give energy to the thought-forms of your imagined faults and flaws. Energise the more empowering thought-forms." In the same meditation I saw a cascading waterfall but it was light cascading to Earth with rainbows in it. "It is always here for you to bathe in, but you do

everything to avoid bathing in it," I heard. "It flows from the source of your being."

At the beginning of April Frances received this message in our meditation: "On waking up draw light into your body and ignite the joy in your heart – Joy supernal and the joy of being alive! Before you go out wear your cloak of light and let the flame of joy burn in your heart. Thus do you bring Light into the world, and delight and joy to all the people you meet. Infect others with joy."

At the end of April I heard: "Life is not what it appears. The trials, tribulations and problems you face are about developing qualities. What qualities are you developing?" I suspected that mine are trust and focussed intention. "If you merely trust but do not focus, it is not enough. If you focus but do not trust, you may create something but it may not be right for you. Trust and focussed intention is a perfect combination."

In May I was shown how over many lifetimes we sculpt a unique being out of the raw materials we are given. I was shown the Earth as an example and how it takes aeons to change its form. We may feel we are not changing but we are. We come into each life with what we have already become and in each life we work on what we are destined to be. Growth is not measured by achievements but by how we deal with problems and setbacks. The most profound growth occurs through "overcoming" and seeing through the illusions.

On May 21st I found myself in a beautiful green meadow, full of bright red poppies, high in the mountains. We were there for a specific purpose. Viva appeared with a group of beings. She wore a white robe with a silver belt and looked radiant. We were told to recline in the grass and take in the colours. The sky was a beautiful shade of blue and I heard heavenly music. I felt joy and peace. Viva reminded me that we can always meet in this beautiful place. All it requires is an act of will and imagination.

At the end of May, when I recited The Affirmation of the Disciple at the beginning of our meditation, I became aware of a beautiful fragrance. I was told that fragrance is a direct manifestation of divinity. It can elevate us and it is our destiny to be fragrant. I realised that I can smell any fragrance I am able to imagine. The fragrance of roses filled my being.

We were told to make the Ashram our home. Everything else is fleeting, illusionary and impermanent. "Act as if you are living within the Ashram and act accordingly. Within the energy field of the Ashram we bathe in its atmosphere of joy and brotherhood."

Frances heard: "We know only joy. We live in joy. With the quality of joy we nourish our own and our brothers' hearts. Joy is a quality of the Soul. You can seek earthly happiness and yet not find joy. The happiness experienced by the personality is transient. You can be unhappy and yet be full of joy. Happiness is of the personality. Joy is of the Soul. Bliss is experienced by the Monad. Be blessed and live in joy!

"The harmony and peace of the Ashram is the result of an ordered rhythm. Everyone plays a part and the Law of Love prevails. Everything has its consequences and is what right action teaches us, but what is right action? It means living within the flow of the natural rhythms of nature regulated by Mother Earth and the cycles of the constellations as they move in stately rhythm in the heavens.

"Live in harmony with the Self, with nature and with the cosmic cycles, and you live in right action, as we in the Ashram live. Listen with the voice of intuition and develop the ability to discriminate. Living in harmony with yourself and the environment is the best service you can render to the One Life and the One Soul."

At the end of May Willem was shown how we are prisoners of thought. Our thoughts create ideas, structures and systems in order to control our lives and for us to feel safe. Our thoughts

are like partitions, which prevent us from advancing and flowing freely. The partitions create numerous barriers, enclosing subjects, like our ideas on Hierarchy and the Masters, but the Ashram is free of such ideas. Only when there are no preconceptions, nothing to hold onto, can we enter cosmic dimensions. We were told to look at our thoughts with compassion, without harshness or judgement, and once we have detected the partitions, we will be able to penetrate the veils with our inner eye. On the other side pure freedom of spirit awaits us.

At the beginning of July I was engulfed in a beautiful blue colour/light. It was almost a substance. We were in the Ashram invoking this blue 'substance' coming from Sirius and bathing the Earth to heal and elevate it. It was both an invocation and a distribution. In the same meditation Frances also perceived a blue light radiating from a chamber with a partially open door. She knew it was the door to a Masonic Lodge and saw three beings from Sirius dressed in white robes standing in front of the door and closing it. We are not ready but one day we will truly stand outside this door, knock, and ask for admission. We both saw Viva in this meditation.

In another meditation Viva appeared in the Ashram gardens when we were being taught how to inhale and exhale fragrance. I heard: "Each Soul has its own fragrance with subtle differences. The Masters have their own particular fragrance. It is possible to recognise each person or being by their own unique fragrance." I was overwhelmed and intoxicated by fragrance!

A week later Viva told us: "It is not the outer circumstances of life that are important but the inner process. Pay attention to the inner process and do not think that outer circumstances are making you happy or unhappy. Develop inner peace so that the events of your life do not affect you. This is the secret of life and enlightenment. The last two years of my life were more profound than you realise."

At the end of July I found myself in a round boat, like a cor-acle, on a beautiful lake. It was still and translucent, like a mirror, and was surrounded by high mountains. There was a circular temple on the shore, which I have seen before in other medita-tions. It looks as if it is made of alabaster with columns and steps leading up to it. Viva was standing on the steps with some beings. Frances, Willem and I each had our own little boat anchored in the lake, like the water lilies around us. I felt that we were being anchored in our hearts and that it was a pictorial representation of an inner process: a symbolic activation and/or opening of the heart chakra. Frances also experienced peace, calm water, high mountains and stillness in this meditation.

A week later we were being taught about Pure Being, which is beyond feeling, thought and imagery. Everything we perceive, feel and think is an illusion. Imagery is also an illusion. It is a 'scene' to help us understand abstract concepts. Even the world is a form of imagery, which we all perceive differently, but which provides the equipment for integration and growth. Pure Being is where we truly exist. I experience it rarely and mostly through the music of J.S. Bach. Immediately after Vivian died, I played Bach's Gold-berg Variations in order to experience the cool clear light and not to burden her with my grief as she made her transition.

On August 13th I experienced a gathering in the Inner Sanc-tuary at the centre of the Ashram with Lord Maitreya who was sitting on his golden lotus throne. We were in the outer circle and Viva was closer to the centre with her group. We were reaching up to Shamballa in a meditation ending with the words "Thy Will Be Done". It was as if the energy from Shamballa was being utilised to bring peace into the world. I felt a strong Soul connection with Viva and did not want to return to the room where Frances and I were meditating. She also experienced being in the Inner Sanctuary with Lord Maitreya, seated on his golden lotus throne, and members of the Ashram sitting within their

Ray groups. It appeared to be a continuous meditation to bring peace and equilibrium to those areas of unrest in the World. We were asked to meditate every day and see ourselves standing within the New Group of World Servers and the Hierarchy to radiate peace out into the world as a dedicated group.

(See Shamballa and the New Group of World Servers in the Glossary of Terms.)

On August 20th I saw the large building with the columns, triangular roof, and veranda overlooking the mountains. I recognised it as the Hall of Higher Learning and Service. Inside I saw Viva with Roberto Assagioli and John Cullen, Vivian's friend and mentor, who has also died. We had been invited into this class for more advanced students and were shown how to watch world events with loving detachment, and to radiate love and goodwill to the world in order to help and heal.

A week later I found myself in the coracle-like boat floating on the still lake with the water lilies. I was being shown a way to centre myself. I saw a thread going from my heart up into the Sun and another thread down into the Earth. I felt peaceful and centred. Frances also experienced deep peace in this meditation as if held in the arms of the Cosmic Mother.

At the beginning of September we were in the light and freshness of the Ashram with Viva. Energies were streaming in from Sirius and there was a constant transmission of energies from the Ashram to the Earth. We walked in the gardens and saw the Temple of Healing in the distance where the healing angels appear.

In another meditation I heard Viva say she would continue to keep the Triangle appointment with us. I heard "It's time to build another bridge – a bridge to the Far Distant Shore." We were told to climb the Mountain of Aspiration, which is high and steep. We climbed and reached a high place where we could see the Far Distant Shore - the Golden City – the Kingdom of Souls. Having made the ascent, we were faced with the descent where

we are always tested before we can proceed. Viva was very present in this meditation.

At the end of October we were again in the Hall of Higher Learning and Service. Assagioli was talking about the cultivation of joy, and many people were listening. "It lifts the spirit and is contagious," he said. "We all need to cultivate inner joy especially when life is difficult." Frances also experienced being inside this building with the open veranda and views of the surrounding snow-capped mountains. It is a place where meetings, meditations and rituals occur.

In November I went to Southern Spain and rented a house in an urbanisation called Alhambra with beautiful gardens and stunning views of the sea and the mountains. Transpersonal Development was ready to go to the printer and I needed a holiday. However, the house I rented was then sold and I had to find another rental. A stranger knocked on my door and offered me a house called Casa Angel in the same urbanisation. It belonged to a Swedish movie star and was full to the rafters with angel figurines. They were above the bed, in the kitchen, and even in the bathroom. I was totally surrounded by angels and I could not help but feel that I had been given this lovely house as a gift.

On November 12th I experienced being in the Ashram and being told why we build bridges. Everyone in the Ashram is involved in bridge-building because it helps us to grow in consciousness. A bridge does not just go up and over, it also goes down. For every upward movement, we have to make a corresponding downward movement in order to avoid inflation and grandiosity.

A week later Viva told us not to feel guilty if we miss an appointment. "Meditation is a state of being," she said. "Nourish each other with the Love of the Heart. This is most needed. Fan the Fire of the Heart."

At the end of November we all experienced being in the

Ashram. Frances received this message: "The Ashram and those who dwell therein are always busy. Yet a serene calm pervades all. Try in your daily life to cultivate serenity within all circumstances: serenity in action, thought, and repose. Observe what brings you out of that balanced state, trace its origin and cause. On dark grey days visualise golden light flooding the inside of your head. This will stimulate the light receptors in the brain and counteract so called SAD symptoms."

In the same meditation Willem saw that we were being invited to a meeting of the High Council with one of the Masters who told us to drop our inferiority complexes and accept who we are. We too often identify ourselves with our weaknesses and shortcomings as human beings instead of acknowledging the fact that we are being invested with Ashramic responsibility. This investiture enables us to "hold" a position in the "externalisation" process. While the Master was transferring his thoughts, Willem could feel the three of us being well-aligned and embodying the responsibility of our job. It is not a job as human society sees it but rather a deep knowing of essence – the Purpose that can be realised through the Divine Plan.

My meditation was full of joy – the joy of angels – soaring – ecstatic joy - with wings of fire!

(See Externalisation in the Glossary of Terms.)

On December 10ᵗʰ I experienced the love the Masters and Higher Beings have for us. It is profound and caused tears to roll down my cheeks. This love is totally unconditional, ever-present and patient. It pervaded my being and I felt it as a living vibrating substance in which I am suspended. All we have to do is let go and surrender to it.

In the same meditation Frances saw us with Viva on a lush green lawn under some flowering rhododendron bushes in the radiant light. We were watching a festive celebration, someone making intricate patterns with two long brightly coloured

streamers of a brocade-like material, whirling them up and around with skill.

Willem saw us walking the Path with clear focus. Becoming and Being the Path filled him with joy and responsibility. He saw that if we get rid of the programs and the mundane stuff whirling around and pervading us every day, silence and space can enter, and we can feel who we are instead of thinking of what we should be doing.

A week later I saw that we were in a procession and all the various Ashram members were wearing stunning robes. Usually they wear white robes with coloured sashes or belts, but these were salmon pink, turquoise, sapphire blue and colours I did not recognise. We were in a procession to attend a ceremony involving Lord Maitreya. In the same meditation Frances saw Maitreya in deep meditation being given power from a source deep in space. She heard "Nothing is what it appears. When you think you understand, then expand your consciousness. More forces are flowing into the Earth than ever before. Rest in the heart of Christ, love, and lift your consciousness to the Divine."

On Christmas Eve we were watching an outpouring of energy from the Sun, looking like the Northern Lights, but in exquisite shades of pink, yellow, blue and other colours I did not recognise. These lights were bathing the Earth.

On New Year's Eve we were concentrating on Gratitude; not just for food, shelter, warmth and friendship, but planetary gratitude in particular for Jupiter and the Moon, for without them life on Earth could not have evolved. Jupiter is Earth's guardian protecting it from being hit by asteroids. Without the Moon we would have no regulated climate. The Earth would oscillate between being frozen and fried. The Moon stabilises the Earth and prevents it from wobbling.

2008

On January 1st the proof copy of the newly reprinted Transpersonal Development arrived at Casa Angel. I was thrilled with the cover: the Coronet constellation on the front and a photo of Roberto Assagioli on the back. I danced joyfully around the house. It had taken three years to complete and had helped me to work through my grief. It was one of the books I inherited from Vivian and I had worked on it in three different places: California, Scotland and Spain.

In our meditation on January 7th Frances saw three beings dressed in white robes waiting for us in the Ashram. They were full of joy and were transmitting their purity of being to us in the clearest of white light. They want us to carry this sacredness within us in our daily lives. In my meditation I experienced being taught how to soar. We were full of joy as we were lifted up into the light. Willem experienced leaving our incarnated state and floating in an opalescent white light. There were no sounds or words – only the harmonious movement of soaring in the light. We were meditating in three different countries but had very similar experiences.

A week later we were walking across a bridge with huge arches spanning an abyss so deep, I could see nothing when I looked down. We crossed the bridge and entered the Golden City with its opalescent buildings, golden spires and crystal windows deflecting the golden solar light into dancing rainbows. It is a heavenly place full of peace and fragrance. Following a winding path to the top of a hill, upon which the Golden City appears to float, I felt we had a mission to fulfil.

Our meditations were now taking place within the Ashram with Viva who told us "In the dimension where I am, we are in a state of Being. This is difficult for you to imagine because you are conditioned by time and space. You often ask what the Mas-

ters, Initiates and Disciples are 'doing' but there is no such thing as 'doing' in the Ashram. There are rituals and gatherings but they are 'appearances'. Telepathy is their way of communicating and impulses are given. Life is subtle and harmonious. It can only be compared to music."

Viva was smiling and Willem received a glow in his heart when he registered the thoughts that she was transmitting. Through our contact with Viva, we are able to see the beauty and refinement of the Ashram: its radiant colours, glorious manifestations of the Nature Kingdom, and the exquisite sound of the angels. We were asked to bring the perfume of the Ashram back with us into the world.

On January 21st we were again with Viva in the Ashram. Frances heard: "Attune to your own finest, subtlest vibration and observe what you find there. Take the perfume of the Ashram back with you into the world. Be Blessed." Viva dissolved into a petal soft light, flowing and dancing with a subtle perfume, an interplay of constantly moving colours and light.

A week later Viva took us to where she is with Roberto Assagioli in the Golden City. He looks much younger and radiates joy. This meeting may have been arranged because I reprinted his book regardless of the many obstacles blocking my way. He was working on this book when he died and I had felt a subtle collaboration with him when I was typing it.

He was working with us on a process I can only call 'elevation' because we were 'elevating' other souls incarnated on Earth. This may be why Willem heard "Start gathering the flock." We were in a place bordering on bliss causing me to weep throughout the meditation. I was not sad. It was simply my body's reaction to the high vibration. I stayed in the meditation for an hour with tears streaming down my cheeks.

On February 5th Frances and I had very similar meditations although we were meditating in different countries. Frances

experienced being in the light of the Ashram with Viva. She was advised to dwell within the light of the Ashram. All we need to do is lift our consciousness to that level. We know how to do it. We just have to remember to align ourselves during the day, before we go to sleep at night, and when we wake up. Frances asked if Pan is there. "Yes, Pan is of the Angelic Kingdom and is an expression of the sentience of nature."

She asked if animals are there. "As this is the Kingdom of Souls, only an animal Group Soul can find expression at this level within the law governing the Nature Kingdom. Exceptions are those whose vibrational frequency is high enough, usually through their unconditional love for humans, which has allowed them to individualise to a degree which includes having developed the beginnings of mental activity."

I also experienced being in the Ashram with Viva. It was light and fragrant, and I wanted to stay there. I was told I could. I just have to remember to carry it within me. I was shown that we have a similar relationship with animals to the one the Masters have with us. We elevate the Animal Kingdom just as the Masters elevate the Human Kingdom. By bringing animals into our homes as pets, we help them to individualise. Animals belong to a Group Soul but can achieve an individual Soul life through being in loving relationships with humans. The Masters bring humans into the Ashram in order to elevate us into the Fifth Kingdom of Souls, of which Pan is a member. The Masters are in a similar relationship with the Lords who elevate them to a level we cannot even imagine. Pan is the Lord of the Nature Kingdom, which has reached a high level of perfection. We only have to look at nature to see that it brings through divinity in the form of beauty, colour and fragrance.

I remained in this meditative state for a week and observed my distractions, mostly of an emotional nature, and about the future. I was having to vacate Casa Angel at the beginning of

March, having experienced three months of absolute joy. In this meditative state I realised that I am always in the right place at the right time.

On February 25th in my meditation I found myself in front of a large building with big double doors. It looked like a temple. We had been invited to a ceremony taking place in the higher Ashram where Assagioli is. It was by Invitation Only and we were privileged to be there. In the centre was an arena with a wheel but it was composed of members of the Ashram. The one in the middle was turning slowly. Those forming the outer circle were whirling but they were greatly affected by the one turning slowly on the central hub of the wheel. We were being shown how the Soul spins slowly on the central hub, just as the Sun shines in the centre of our solar system, but its influence is great. Each of us, with our different lives, is whirling so quickly on the outer rim of the wheel, we do not notice when the Soul faces us and gives us its attention. This is a great moment in our evolution – a moment to be celebrated and cherished. Everything in the universe is dancing on this Wheel of Life.

On March 17th Willem heard "Heaviness increases, violence grows, materialism appears to hold humanity in its grip. Lightness of Being is the antidote." Willem could not have known that "Lightness of Being" was one of Vivian's favourite phrases.

In my meditation we were taught how to 'hold' the world. It is a bit like holding a safety net for someone who is jumping off a tall building. Everyone is needed to hold a piece of the safety net in order for the person to land safely. The world is in crisis and we are asked to hold a safety net. We are holding the tension and it is hard work.

A week later the safety net had grown and was spread around the planet. Many people are holding it but only those in physical bodies can do the work. It requires holding the tension on the physical plane.

On April 14th Willem saw us standing on a mountain with some Brothers who were backing and protecting us. We held one arm outstretched, our hands touching above a flame. We were swearing an oath for inner action, swearing that nothing can stop us. We are Warriors of the Spirit and, at the same time Magicians, knowing our strength and our ability to bring the death of false systems, treason, lies and corrupted forms. "Let Life prevail on Earth." The Brothers of Light protected our short ritual. Our hearts became one in the Greater Heart.

I also experienced a fiery meditation in which we took more responsibility. We were shown that, compared to the majority of people in the world, we have our heads above the clouds. We see what is invisible to others. We have direct experience of the spiritual world and are aware of our work in the Ashram. Now we are asked to take more responsibility, to teach by example, and to lead others whose heads are still in the clouds. We also have our feet on the ground, giving us more responsibility towards our human family.

At the end of April we were sailing in a boat to the Far Distant Shore where Viva and Roberto Assagioli were waiting for us. Viva is now studying within his Ashram, and because of our connection, we are invited to where the higher Ashrams are located. This is where our teachers study. We are being prepared to bring new Souls into the Ashram. The keyword in this meditation was "Preparation".

On May 19th Willem had a very close contact with Viva. He felt that he could almost touch her. She told him about her life in the Greater Life and asked him to "hold on" and not think about leaving the planet. We all have a specific task and our Triangle is a vehicle of light - it is our chariot of fire!

A week later I was walking through the quiet corridors of the Ashram and feeling the tranquillity of the place. Viva appeared and we went to a quiet place where we talked about our lives

and work. Viva is still teaching but now studies in Assagioli's Ashram in the Golden City. She also enjoys music and the extensive library.

At the beginning of June I saw hundreds of prayer flags billowing in the wind. I found myself in a beautiful place where prayers are gathered. Many beings were meditating in deep silence and with strong focus. I was shown how prayers are gathered. This is not the same as answering prayers but more a matter of being totally present for the people saying the prayers. This showed me that prayers are received by beings devoted to being present for those in desperate need of help and support. When we pray, someone hears us. It was a profound experience.

Two weeks later Willem saw Viva coming out of the inner sanctuary of the Ashram. She advised us to create cocoons of light and remain in them for as long as we are in our physical bodies. In this way we can remain in the Ashram within our hearts and minds. In the same meditation I saw that we were involved in a ritual, wearing ceremonial robes, and making a figure of eight in constant motion. Maybe we were spinning the cocoons!

A week later we were outside the Tibetan monastery high in the mountains. Master Morya was there and called it "the Ceiling of the World". He was showing us how to send blessings to the world through intricate hand gestures.

Master Morya appeared again in a meditation at the end of June in which he was talking about dedication. He invited us to be dedicated. I saw beings sending blessings to the world just as there are beings listening to prayers.

(See Morya in the Glossary of Terms)

At the beginning of July I saw that the spaces between the Sun and the planets are not devoid of life. Between the Earth and the Sun the Ashrams are stretched like pearls strung out on threads of light. I saw how the other planets are also schools of

learning. The sacred planets are guardians of the solar system. All of the planets looked like lotus flowers on a lake of translucent light. This is why it is always light in the Ashram.

A week later we were striving to contact our Souls through study and meditation in the Ashram and in our lives. Our Souls appeared to be in deep meditation waiting for us to contact them.

On July 21st Frances saw four shafts of radiant golden light moving upwards from four corners, forming a pyramid with a square base and meeting at the apex. With Viva, we form the four shafts of light. The apex of the pyramid opens like a flower and a shower of light flows out to the planet and into space. We heard "The higher you go, the further your light radiates." A great angel watches over our Triangle of blue light shot through with soft green and white.

At the end of July we were taken by Viva to a special meditation in her Ashram, which we would not be able to attend as individuals, but we have formed a strong group. The meditation was to enable us to contact our Souls, and it was profound. During this meditation I visited my dear old friend May who died recently. She was pleased to see me and showed me her legs, which are now the same length. One of her legs had been shortened in a disastrous hip replacement operation. I could visit her and still be in the meditation with Viva, Frances and Willem.

At the beginning of August we were sitting in a huge round auditorium, open to the sky, which was dark and thick with stars. We were listening to the music of the spheres.

A week later we were given a technique for meditation which each one of us received but experienced in a slightly different way. In my meditation we were standing on top of a mountain looking across a chasm to another mountain where Viva was waiting for us. To cross the chasm we had to walk across a thread as fine as spun silk. As we followed each other across the chasm, I realised that if I elevated my entire being, I could soar across

the chasm without touching the silk thread with my feet. In this state of 'perfect poise' there was no fear of falling into the chasm. I spent the entire meditation in this uplifted state and did not want to stop. Later Willem found a quote from Master Morya describing my experience:

> "They will ask thee how to traverse life. Answer: like crossing
> an abyss upon a taut string - Beautifully, carefully and fleetly."
> Leaves From Morya's Garden I

In Willem's meditation we were riding in a golden chariot with Viva hovering above us and encouraging us to increase our speed. He could feel the fiery energy running through his heart, sweeping like a wave. Later he found another quote by Master Morya:

> "The attraction to Our Heart can increase so greatly that it
> would be impossible to restrain it. This is called 'The Fiery
> Chariot'."
> Super Mundane 1.60

Frances was also lifted above her personality. She saw Viva with a star above her head connected to Sirius through the Sun.

A week later Frances felt a strain in her head when meditating. Viva showed her how to avoid strain. Frances saw an eye forming at the ajna centre with a lighter energy field around it. Images appeared in the lighted centre of the eye, which became a window through which she could see vivid and precise images. Viva asked her not to think but just to observe the images without trying to identify them.

At the end of August Willem saw us in our light bodies with thousands of Earth disciples advancing with a huge battering ram to break through the wall imprisoning humanity and the world. In my meditation I heard the word "Focus". We were being asked to focus on what we can contribute towards planetary change.

We are ALL being asked to focus on what we can do. One person alone cannot break down the wall imprisoning humanity, but many can. In the same meditation Frances saw us with a group of disciples and initiates standing between humanity and the Hierarchy. She felt the solidarity of the group, our place, and our work. She remembered the Maitreya Sangha Meditation:

> *"We stand with calmness, forever unperturbed, linking the heavens and the earth, the inner world of meaning and the outer world of form."*

In September I scattered the ashes of May, my 93-year-old friend, in the sea along with dried rose petals and fragrant flowers. Later that day in my meditation I saw the rose petals and the flowers being washed up on another shore for my friend's enjoyment. As flowers exist in the physical and ethereal realms, they can be sent and received.

In the middle of September in our Triangle meditation we were in a meadow full of poppies. There was a stream running through it and mountains in the distance. I realised that we were inside the cover of Vivian's book Being Here When I Need Me. She said she had brought it alive through 'imagery' and that everything is imagined into existence. Nothing exists that has not been imagined first. Then we were walking through the Ashram, which appears to be constructed of stone and marble. It feels solid, ancient and eternal but Viva told us it has been 'imagined' into existence. Then we were in the Golden City, which appears to be constructed of alabaster, mother of pearl and gold. From a distance it is not unlike the Kremlin in Russia. It is much more ethereal and appears to float on the Far Distant Shore. Finally, we were in a place composed of light, colour and fragrance. In this place there is no separation. There appears to be nobody there but we are not alone. It is an experience of total unity. I wondered if I was now inside the mind of the One who

imagines. Viva gave us a powerful experience of existence and how the physical world is only a denser manifestation of Divine imagination.

At the end of September I bought a house in Alhambra where I had been living since the previous November. In the first meditation in my new home I heard the word "Illumination".

In another meditation I saw curtains of light all over the planet. It was like the Northern Lights. I heard "A crisis unites people. It makes change inevitable." There was a financial crisis in the world but joy in the Ashram where there is an atmosphere of gladness, good humour and expansive joy. Frances heard "Do not take yourselves and life so seriously. Bring humour, joy and playfulness into your lives. Dance along skilfully with the irresistible forces of change, living as you do in the stream of abundance. Fear is not relevant."

A week later we met in the Ashram gardens where Frances saw a bird fluttering above us. It was a bluebird. It led us along a steep path through dense green shrubbery. Suddenly we were high up on a mountainside with a panoramic view of the valley below where we saw a river, woods, meadows, lakes and foothills rising up into the mountains. She sensed that we find the elusive bluebird of happiness through the daily practice of appreciation.

On October 27th I met Viva in a cave. It was dark and mysterious with soft lighting. Viva was enjoying the space and conveying a sense of the importance of dark places for meditation and reflection. After the meditation I called Frances, who was staying in my house in Spain while I was in Scotland, and she told me she had been down in the caves that day. I had taken Vivian into these caves in 1996 when she visited me in Spain. She loved them so much, she was reluctant to leave, and we were almost locked in. Somehow Viva knew that Frances was visiting the caves and in our meditation conveyed it to me by meeting me in a cave. I had no idea Frances was in the caves that day. In

the photographs she took inside the caves there are huge globes of light everywhere.

In a later meditation Frances linked into the caves where the energy is deeply sacred and like being inside the womb of the Great Mother. Viva was with us in this meditation. Willem then found this quote:

> *"We are now on the point of entering the cave wherein the new birth can take place. And therefore the stage of life's journey is nearly completed."*
> *From Bethlehem to Calvary* by Alice Bailey

In the pre-American elections in November Frances saw an image of Barack Obama's head and shoulders with the American eagle above his head. There was a meditation in the Ashram for the 'right outcome' and the Hierarchy was engaged in holding back the dark forces, so there would be no unlawful interference in the elections.

On November 17th Frances was asked to be more aware of the angels, who are all around us, and to consciously work with them. She saw an image of Mary dressed in white with a diadem of seven stars around her head.

In the same meditation Viva took me to an octagonal room with stained glass windows depicting angels. Light was streaming in through the stained glass windows and I sensed it was a healing room. I was not feeling well, so I let the colours enter and heal me.

At the end of November Frances saw a sheer rock face with a person laboriously climbing with much effort and hardship. Then she saw a mountain goat leaping lightly from one foothold to the next. There are two ways to approach the climb to the spiritual heights: we can see it as a heavy task or as a joyous one. She heard: "Deal with life's karmic lessons with optimism and lightness of heart, knowing the obstacles are there to be cleared.

Attitude is the key. Learn to become lighter."

At the end of 2008 Viva proclaimed: "Love the skin you are in" accompanied with fireworks and party streamers. "You are embodied on the physical plane and must love the bodies you are in."

2009

At the beginning of 2009 we were told, "You are in the world but not of it. You have reached the point where you are aware of the spiritual realms. Not many people have reached this point. It is important to embody what you know, so that others will want to follow. Most people live beneath the clouds but you can see above them to where the Sun is always shining."

In our meditation on January 12th I said the Affirmation of the Disciple, which I love. The final verse caught my attention:

"And standing thus, revolve, and tread this way the
ways of men, and know the ways of God.
And thus I stand."

I saw a spinning wheel with the Soul standing on the central hub. From this central position, it can view any of its many lives, which it sustains, but this particular life is catching its attention. We have become aware of each other. This is a pivotal life for all of us.

Afterwards I looked in A Treatise on White Magic and found this quote on pages 108-9:

1. *The Solar Angel begins the work of initiating the personality.*
2. *It withdraws its forces from soul enterprise in the spiritual kingdom, and centres its attention on the work to be done.*
3. *It enters into deep meditation.*
4. *Magnetic rapport with the instrument in the three worlds is instituted.*

5. The instrument, man, responds, and also enters into meditation.
6. The work proceeds in ordered stages and with cyclic activity.
7. The light of the soul is thrown downwards.
8. The light of the vital body and the physical form is synchronised with that of the head.
9. The centres swing into activity.
10. The light of the soul and the two other aspects of light are so intense that now all life in the three worlds is illumined.
11. Alignment is produced, the work of discipleship and of initiation becomes possible and proceeds according to the Law of Being.

A week later Viva was again very present. Frances heard that the need to 'visualise' a place after death has caused us to create the astral planes. On the highest of these the Ashram of the Christ is 'imprinted' in the malleable ethers of the etheric. When we raise our consciousness, it's this 'imprint' that we experience. After leaving the earth plane, we go to the astral plane onto which is reflected the Kingdom of Souls. We remain there until we are no longer attached to dwelling within form and can move into the greater reality of pure consciousness. This is where Viva is now.

In my meditation Viva was also very present and told me our connection is now on the Higher Mental plane. She encouraged me to write and begin a report on what happened to her after she died. It would take me another two years to compile this report.

At the end of January I saw Viva in a meadow full of bright red poppies. She said she had created it for us, adding that it is important for us to 'visualise' and how 'visualisation' is used in the higher realms. This is probably why Roberto Assagioli placed so much importance on it in Psychosynthesis. Viva said it is the Soul that creates the form when spirit and matter meet on the

physical plane. It is easier to create on the spiritual plane because it's instant. She loves to create beautiful images and caused some mountains to appear behind us. It reminded me of a quote from the Bhagavad Gita:

"I become manifest through the magical power of the soul."

At the beginning of February Willem found himself sitting with Viva within the cosmic vault. She said two things to him: "Marilyn's action with regard to the common endeavour of the past years is an excellent initiative. It will enable you to better understand certain aspects of the Ashramic way of working." She was referring to the Triangle Meditation Report I had started to compile. Secondly, Viva said we should focus our attention on the information on the subject of meditation, which Willem received and transmitted in the Triangle on June 14th 2004. She said it will help us to grow, to advance, and go beyond accepted thought-forms on meditation. This is what Vivian said to Willem in that meditation:

"Through your endeavour to create a relay for us, an Ashramic platform, please consider meditation in that perspective: through meditating you are open and in contact. The link is permanent, yes, while the short moment of contact enables us to transmit impulses. Now and then, if it needs to be, we help you to balance, to find equilibrium. I know of course how precarious the situation is for the three of you. Hold on and be lucid!"

When Willem made this contact with Viva, I experienced her presence the entire evening.

A week later Viva appeared and I asked her about her life. She told me she contemplates, studies, teaches and listens to music. Her intuition guides her. She talked about sound and music, which makes beautiful geometric patterns she can now see when

she listens to music. Vivian loved listening to music and often joked to her friends that she forced me to listen to Mozart, which I loved. She said more about sound but it was too complicated for me to comprehend. It is related to creation and the higher planes.

In the middle of February, Willem heard that when we are in our spiritual centre we have limitless possibilities around us. We are the point in the circle. We break through thought-forms and barriers (illusions) and reach spacious and timeless universes of creation.

In my meditation Viva talked about discrimination and gave me some feedback. I had stopped writing because a friend was staying with me. She said I need to put my work before the needs of others. Vivian always put her work first. She said she is studying music and sound because it unites and sustains creation. I was now feeling her presence on a daily basis.

A week later I asked Viva where the spiritual planes are located. She told me they stretch from the Earth to the Sun. After death we find ourselves on a plane similar to the Earth with houses and gardens. As we ascend, the light increases because we are nearer to the Sun and our solar angels who are with us every day in sunlight. Not many people realise that sunlight is a living substance. When we are reunited with our solar angels, a crisis occurs because we have to make a choice. We have to turn away from the Sun and take one of the paths out of the solar system. I wondered if this is "the taut string above the abyss" from Master Morya's quote. In Willem's meditation he heard "the taut string above the abyss." Maybe he was hearing the answer to my question!

At the beginning of March Willem was assaulted by doubts. Would he be able to hear, see or make contact? Would he be able to formulate what he experienced? Viva appeared and said, "You ARE in the Ashram right where you are sitting now, Willem. You are being lured by your physical senses, emotions and thoughts.

Reality is beyond form – and you know it." He started to breathe freely, realising that no effort is needed. He can just BE.

I started to meditate before our arranged time, feeling 'called' and I immediately became aware of a warm golden glow surrounding me. I was in what appeared to be a cathedral full of golden light. I looked up and saw that it had no roof. There was a shaft extending upwards for what appeared to be forever. The golden light was coming down through the shaft and filling the cathedral-like building. Then I saw Viva. She was in a choir and they were singing up through the shaft of light. It was an invocation: a 'calling forth' to Christ, which was beautiful and melodious.

A week later I was back in the Golden Cathedral where Viva is now studying the chakras in her music studies. She explained how the chakras can be played like musical instruments – like harps. Maybe this is why angels are portrayed playing harps!

The following week I was accusing myself of inventing what happens in my meditations. So in this meditation absolutely nothing happened. Viva gave a message to Willem for me to "Regain confidence".

A week later we were told to "integrate" and not to separate our meditations from our daily lives. We need to make our lives into a "walking meditation" and to know there is NO separation. We are always in the Ashram. We need to carry this knowledge with us wherever we are. It is a constant practice; not just when we sit down to meditate.

At the end of March Willem saw a City of Light in the distance. He came closer and was in a timeless dimension of permanent meditation. This is not like the meditation that we do. It is a state of alignment and permanent enlightened consciousness. He heard the word "Glory" – a bliss that he could almost touch.

At the end of March Willem tried to contact Viva but she did not appear. A few hours later she told him: "Do not linger on

images of the past or ask where I am now, and what I am doing. The person I was has left its outer robe. Our Soul contact is what really matters. It is deep and needs no comment. Our Soul contact is part of a vaster Reality. We are united in the One Work."

In the same meditation I found myself sitting alone in the Ashram gardens. I wanted Viva to appear but was told that we are to be in a state of permanent alignment and enlightened consciousness. We all felt that Viva was closer to us but not in a personal way. It was happening at a Soul level.

At the beginning of April in our meditation I was in a boat on a wide expanse of water. It looked like Kashmir. The water was like glass. It was very peaceful, and I had the insight that the physical world is a negative - like a photographic negative – of the spiritual world. The Universe, 96% of which is invisible to us in our physical bodies, supports the mere 4% that we are able to see!

A week later I had a meditation about water, which is a substance as magical as light. Water is a living substance. Without it there can be no life. Viva showed me the pools and fountains in the Ashram gardens. I remembered the pool in Maitreya's garden, with the lotus growing in it, and how the stem is rooted in the Earth. It occurred to me that water connects. After death we travel through cosmic liquid to the astral plane. Viva travelled across a wide expanse of water to the Far Distant Shore when she moved to the mental plane. The various planes are connected by water but it is not wet like the water we drink. There is liquid everywhere on the spiritual planes and maybe the water we have on Earth is a mere reflection of it. The pool in Maitreya's garden connects him to the world. He sits by the pool and keeps watch over his people. There is a great secret about water and fire. There can be no life without either of them. They are as opposite as night and day, but when they combine, an alchemical process occurs.

A week later Frances had a meditation about fearlessness. She

was lifted up to a higher level where Viva is. She felt an inflow of the energy of the Ashram of Christ. Reflecting on fearlessness on the mental and emotional levels, she realised that the best way to overcome fear is to draw in and become infused with the Love-Wisdom of the Christ. As we draw on that reservoir of Christ love, fear is no more and negativity evaporates. We can draw from this reservoir at all times.

In another meditation we were with Viva in a no-man's land between her reality and ours. Frances saw a radiant sun and was reminded of the initiates in the Ashram of Christ who see our radiance and not our personalities. The amount of light we radiate reveals how useful we are in service.

At the beginning of June Frances felt Viva's presence and heard "Take refuge in the Ashram. Thought can be powerful. Plant only good seed thoughts and the abundance of their flowering will be available to the collective."

In the middle of June I saw a beautiful ceremony involving music, bells, flowers and fragrance. Imagine my surprise when I attended the Summer Solstice ceremony at the Lodge of The Holy Grail the following Sunday and saw the same ceremony. It was one of the most beautiful and inspiring experiences of my life. I've seen similar ceremonies in the Ashram but to see it taking place on the physical plane was a huge privilege. Frances was taking part in it, as she is a member of the Lodge of the Holy Grail.

In a later meditation I heard "You do not see the whole picture. It is as if you are looking at the back of a tapestry. You see only the knots. Open your eyes and see the bigger picture from its true perspective."

At the end of June Viva appeared and reminded me of the boat imagery she had given me. I sat in my boat on the beautiful lake, dropped anchor, and soaked in the silence and the stillness. I aligned myself with the Sun and felt steady: anchored in the

waters of life and held steady by the Sun.

At the beginning of July Viva sat with me in my boat on the wide lake surrounded by meadows and mountains. She said she had created the scenery for me and that it is a place to meet and share with each other. I asked her where she lives now and she replied that she no longer needs to live anywhere. Her home is within. We need homes when we have physical bodies. After the car crash she had longed for her adobe house on Spirit Mountain. So she recreated it and lived in it until she no longer needed it. She said it was an emotional need, and if we die with a strong emotional need, we manifest it on the astral plane. This is why it's important to deal with our emotions when we are in a physical body because they are much stronger after death. On the physical plane we can distract ourselves with food or alcohol, but we cannot do this after the body has died. Our emotions create the climate and the scenery we find ourselves in after death. I wanted to stay with her and she indicated that I can be there with her as well as here!

In the same meditation Frances also experienced being in a boat with Viva. She had spent the day gardening and received this message: "Weeds and humans are only harmful if they are in the wrong place. Every plant, every being, has its season and its place. If planted in the right place, it benefits all of creation. Then it can grow and radiate, come into flower, and not take nourishment from others. Planted in the right place, it will feel a sense of peace and rightness. Then it becomes a blessing for its environment. Radiate the perfume of the Ashram in your daily living, so that all around may receive its uplifting fragrance. May you be blessed."

A week later we were again with Viva who urged us to notice the qualities of the Ashram and to carry those qualities into our daily lives. "The Ashram is a place of abiding joy, profound peace, deep calm and love eternal."

Frances experienced fresh energy, like water gushing from a spring. Her lungs expanded, her heart opened, breathing the purifying air of the Ashram. Swirling colours of radiant indigo to purple filled her head.

On my 64th birthday I had a meditation about detachment. One day we will have to leave everything behind, and we do not know when that day will be. Instead of waiting for that day, we need to start practising detachment now.

In the same meditation Frances felt the energy of gratitude and the following dropped into her mind: "Gratitude is an aspect of love. All beings in the Ashram remain in an open state of joyous gratitude for the divine blessings flowing in from still higher realms. Love is like a diamond with many facets, all of which are an expression of it. Gratitude is one facet. Joy, beauty, truth are other facets. Peace is the essence of its emanation, as is fire." We both felt Viva's presence.

A week later Frances had a meditation about the Deva evolution. It was filled with spaciousness, clarity, and a clear light. Soft pink and rose: the colours and quality of rose petals. She felt an expansion into a lightness of being and awareness on several levels at the same time. She saw the four of us journeying together as a group and heard: "As you raise your consciousness into lighter finer dimensions, from the fifth dimension onwards, your connection with the deva evolution becomes closer and more conscious. Those who dwell in the Ashram are from both evolutionary streams and thus Maitreya is 'the Master alike of angels and men'. Pay more conscious attention to the devas around you. The physical world is the result of their activity under the guidance of the Mother. This includes your own physical vehicle. Aspire to a level where there is no more separation." We all experienced Viva's presence in this meditation.

(See Devas in the the Glossary of Terms.)

At the beginning of August Frances heard Viva say, "The

connection is well established. We journey together a small group of four travellers." Frances asked, "Where do we meet?" Viva replied, "Try to release the need for an image of a place, rather attune to a plane. What is the plane in consciousness on which we meet? Think of a plane of pure consciousness, a place of mental clarity. You may perceive light and sense a particular quality, but it is not a place which you can see - only touch with other senses. This is the plane of pure consciousness where we can learn to communicate mind to mind. You are learning true telepathy."

In the same meditation Willem heard a call to stand in our power. He saw an image of 'She Who Leads' by the Russian artist Nicholas Roerich in which a woman is leading the way. He felt the power of womanhood, the restoration of the balance within and without.

A week later Willem again felt Viva's presence. He took the opportunity to thank her. She said "Thank you Willem, but there is no time for thanksgiving or congratulations. There are Sirius matters at hand. We all need to focus with accuracy and react promptly when needed." This pun on serious/Sirius is something Vivian often did although Willem could not have known this. He only met her once!

In the same meditation Frances heard: "Time is relative. On the Buddhic plane all becomes one, time as you know it is no more. Past, present and future are one. However, in all the realms there is a principle of timing. There is a 'right time', a window of opportunity for everything. Learn the skill of recognition, of knowing when the moment is there, and act on it. Then you will find that all things will flow with much more ease – even on the third dimensional plane."

On August 24th Willem saw a fountain of gold. A thick liquid ready to solidify came out of the skies and splashed into our midst. In my meditation we were being bathed in golden light.

It filled my being and invigorated me.

On September 7th all three of us received a similar message from Viva. In my meditation I saw Viva on the veranda of the building with the columns. She told us to detach from the personality and connect with the Soul. In Willem's meditation he saw Viva and heard her say that we need to detach ourselves from the past, from all the things that are so dear to us, which we cling to; from all the heady stuff, from all the clever knowledge. Everything we need for our journey is within. "Just go!" said Viva. We went joyfully and courageously.

Frances saw Viva and heard "The faculties of imagination and visualisation are powerful tools. By acting 'as if' something were true, it eventually becomes a reality. Ask yourself how different your life would be if the Soul, not the personality, was in control? All conflict would end because the personality will have aligned itself with the will of the Soul. Can you imagine the inner peace this would bring? You are truly of the kingdom of Souls, yet dwelling as you do in a three-dimensional world, it is difficult to maintain that high ground in the daily round. When the tyranny of the separated personality takes hold, try to act 'as if' the Soul were taking over, and before you know it, it will be so."

On September 14th Willem and I both experienced time as an illusion. It only exists because we live on a planet rotating on its axis and revolving around the Sun. It gives us the illusion of moving through time.

During this time I was packing up the house I had lived in for twenty three years.

In October Willem's mother died at the age of one hundred. Several images of his mother were sweeping through his mind when Viva said, "Break the image." It helped him to connect at a Soul level. Viva added, "Let our meditations be heart contacts. It helps to solidify the heart bridge between the worlds."

On October 19th Frances reviewed all of the places we have

visited in our meditations: the Halls of Learning, the large terrace outside the Greek temple-like building, the high snow-covered mountains beyond, the Ashram gardens and the valley beneath. All fell away as we came to a place where there is only energy and consciousness; a place beyond the known. All four of us were in a place of peace near a source of radiant golden light. Could we have moved beyond the Mental plane to the first of the Buddhic planes? This is now where Viva is. In the same meditation I found myself in a place beyond form or image. I asked Viva how we recognise each other after death and she said that it is through the essence, which is developed over many lifetimes, and through our heart connections with each other. This essence makes each Soul unique and easily recognised.

At the beginning of November I had an experience of unity in which there was no separation; not even from the flies that were everywhere because of unseasonably hot weather in Spain. It was beautiful to be free of the usual sense of separation. After this meditation I found a fly drowning in my glass of water and I decided to save its life after such a profound experience of unity. That night I dreamt I had an audience with the Dalai Lama who taught me how to communicate with a dog, which is god spelled backwards. The Dalai Lama was laughing all the way through the dream and I woke up feeling light-hearted.

A week later Willem experienced strong presence radiating from Frances and me in the Triangle. When he thinks of us on a Soul level he activates a positive, nourishing, and uplifting energy current. In the same meditation Frances and I felt Viva's strong presence, which is now always with us. Frances felt a sense of the Ashram of Christ from where we are sent out into the world and to which we shall return. We were asked to express our spiritual will – the will to good. In the previous dispensation it was to anchor Christ love. Now we are asked to engage the dynamic will.

"The Ashram of the Christ is your true home. In your daily activities in the world endeavour to act as if you are expressing the quality of life within the Ashram."

In a later meditation I saw how much more there is yet to know. It is as vast as the universe and would fill a billion libraries. I was in awe and felt Viva's excitement at embarking upon this voyage of discovery. One could never be bored or run out of things to learn.

At the end of November Willem saw Viva with Master Morya but when he tried to call to them, no sound came out. Viva asked telepathically: "Why do you want to call us, Willem? Why do you want to reach us? We are already in your heart. So close!" Willem's heart was bursting with joy.

In the middle of December I heard the word "elevate" and was shown how to expand my consciousness to include other realities and dimensions. I felt my energy field expand. The further I extended my awareness, the more abstract it became. It was both ethereal and crystal clear. I can only compare it to Bach's music, which is so abstract there are no images when listening to it – just an ethereal clarity. Certain music elevates.

On December 21st I witnessed a celebration of the Christ Mass but not the way Christmas is celebrated. In the Ashram of the Christ it is a celebration of Christ consciousness entering the world, not just through the birth of Jesus, but through the heart of humanity. It is a beautiful powerful time. Viva was very present in this meditation. Frances felt us lifted into the energy field of the Ashram and a great outpouring of Light flowed from there through our unified hearts.

A week later Viva told me she is continuing with her musical studies and that everything is vibrating according to its own particular note. Even the atoms are vibrating, forming patterns of creation according to a particular notation, like a musical score. This is difficult to explain and understand but I remember seeing

patterns in sand formed by different sounds. Patterns can also be seen in water crystals when music is played. Beautiful music forms the most exquisite patterns just as discordant music forms chaotic patterns. Apparently, Hebrew is the only language that forms the pattern of its sound when vibrated.

In the same meditation Frances was trying to see the Ashram as it looks from the astral plane. Viva said, "You are still trying to see a physical vision of the Ashram. It is true that there is a visual counterpart imprinted on the higher astral plane but this too is an illusion. The true Ashram is non-physical and non-astral."

2010

At the beginning of 2010 Viva suggested that we practise discrimination and detach from the people who drain us and distract us from our work. She said we have "crossed a line" and are moving towards discipleship where the work of the Ashram is more important than the pursuits of the personality. I felt a big shift and a turning away from personal issues in 2010. There was a power within me I had not experienced before – like Shiva!

A week later Frances sensed Viva's presence and the energy field of the Ashram. She was reminded that on the higher planes devas and humans work closely together. "Try from where you are in your daily life to develop a closer connection and relationship with the devic kingdom. Cultivate the link, for as you raise your awareness that connection will become closer. When healing, writing or being engaged in artistic activity, ask for the aid of the devas, and you may find that the work you do is enhanced and inspired."

In my meditation Viva was also very present and gave me a glimpse into her life in the higher realms. Her home is now the Ashram and, as she does not need to sleep or eat, she studies, meditates and sings. All is done with great joy and delight. I felt

blissful in her presence. She still aspires to raise her consciousness, just as we do. Willem also felt a heart contact with Viva.

In a later meditation Frances experienced a falling away of
old systems and patterns. In our consciousness we are now part
of the New Earth, which has a totally different frequency. Our
task is to continue releasing old outmoded patterns and habits,
which prevent us from moving into the new, much lighter, fre-
quencies. The New Earth is light, joyful and full of energy. The
old is heavy and drags us down. We were advised to visualise
breathing in light, to take flower essences to help transform and
release the old, and to have fresh flowers in our homes. "Just be
in joy! Look at everything you have learned up to now, and with
new eyes, discard or transcend what seems too limited and dogmatic. We are all in free fall – enjoy the ride!" Frances felt
buoyant, light, full of joy and dancing lightness of being.

In my meditation Viva appeared and took my hand. She led
me to a huge library larger than the Hermitage in St. Petersburg.
It is even more beautiful and contains everything that has ever
been written – even the books that have been destroyed. There
were corridors, staircases and more books than I have ever seen.
The Akashic Records are on the top floor but Viva said we would
need permission to go up there. She took me to a place where
the hand-written illuminated manuscripts are kept. They were
hand-written and illustrated by monks before the printing press
was invented. She showed me some, and with great delight, said
I had created them in another life. I have always felt that I was
involved with these beautiful hand-written illuminated manuscripts. I saw myself as a monk in a monastery where I worked
through the daylight hours carefully writing and illustrating. It
was exacting work. If I made a mistake, the manuscript was
ruined. I was content with my simple life and loved the work.
Even now nothing gives me more pleasure than writing and illustrating. This may have been why Viva showed me this past life.

She was delighted to have found the manuscripts.

A week later I was told I could no longer waste my time and energy. In my own life there was a purge. People who took my time and energy were dropping away. I was feeling totally alone. There appeared to be nothing to hang onto. My old way of being in the world no longer worked. I felt like Arjuna!

At the beginning of February we were told to hold the Earth steady as it goes through a major transformation. We could see this in the earthquake in Haiti. Although it is considered a major disaster, it is pushing us towards the 'critical mass' that will change the world forever. It is another 'mass movement of the heart' in which many are sacrificing their lives.

In the same meditation Frances was given this message: "The road to heaven is through the heart. The mind can be the 'slayer of the unreal', examine where motivation is coming from; is it the warmth and tolerance of the heart or the analytical mind? The heart knows, the mind thinks it knows. Rest in spaciousness."

A week later Viva told me that all of our lives leave an impression on the aura, which is how we recognised each other when we met in Pasadena. This explains how people are attracted or repelled depending upon past-life experience. She said she is not Vivian any more and does not need a name where she is now, but we can continue to call her Viva.

In my meditation a week later Viva was leading us across a high bridge. It was like a Roman aqueduct with huge arches. It was so high we could not see the ground beneath it. I had vertigo and did not want to go across. "Do not fear the heights," said Viva. We followed her across the bridge in single-file. It reminded me of a Roerich painting.

At the beginning of March I saw Viva singing in a choir in the great soaring cathedral-like building. It has enormous arched windows through which light is streaming in. We were part of a congregation listening to this heavenly choir, which sounded like

angels singing. Viva looked so radiant and joyous. They were all wearing white robes with different coloured sashes. It was a glorious sight and sound. We had been invited to hear the singing, which was part of a ceremony.

In the same meditation Frances saw the goddess Quan Yin with her robes billowing out towards the light. Then a stream of deliciously scented golden yellow flower petals moved around her and our Triangle. It was uplifting and purifying. Frances realised that we could use this visualisation to purify our homes and raise the vibration in order to dispel negativity and heaviness. Quan Yin emanated an energy field of great refinement, purity, delicacy and spaciousness. The delicate scent remained. I suspect that we were attending the same ceremony but brought back different parts of it.

In the middle of March I experienced everything as being alive: the furniture and the buildings as well as the trees and the flowers. We are all alive, a part of the Earth, and at various stages of evolution. It was a profound experience in which I knew I am not alone. It was an experience of Unity.

In the same meditation Frances heard "You may see yourselves as small specks but you are part of a much larger movement and all are needed. More and more are rallying to the 'Call', multitudes are being mobilised now to help build the New Earth. Do not give a backward glance to the old or the sufferings of those who are tied to it. Remain firmly focussed in the New and root yourselves there. Be with us, builders of a new and radiant Earth! Ally yourselves with all the groups – and there are many – who are building a new and radiant future. You will recognise your brothers and sisters when you encounter them from all races, cultures and points of the planet. You will recognise them by their willingness to work for the greater whole. Together you are a huge unstoppable force. Each of you has chosen to die to the old and live for the new. This has given you renewed life

force. Use it well!"

In a later meditation Viva led us to a place of white gold light and told us not to try and interpret with our minds. It was difficult to switch off the mind.

At the end of March Frances was aware of a multitude of light-workers standing in serried ranks within the fiery energy pouring through the Sun via Shamballa. We were sitting cross-legged with Viva in a triangular formation around a fiery vortex. We each had a flame above our heads. Then we were enveloped, each in our own column of fire, which kept expanding and growing into a vortex of fire in the centre of our Triangle until all was fire!

At the beginning of April Viva was present and said she is now without form. She is pure consciousness. Frances saw only golden light within her ajna centre but it had depth to it, like a veil, which could lift at any time and reveal what is beyond. She could almost see beyond it. She received assurance that this is the Christ light, He is here and we are serving Him. In the same meditation Willem had an impression of gentleness, soft colours, pure sounds – silence touched by a subtle wing in the realm of angels. He heard that we deserve to be gentle with ourselves. Our subtle bodies need to be nurtured with love!

A week later Willem experienced an overdose of fire in his heart and had difficulty breathing. He heard "Radiate it!" and was bombarded with the fire of Spirit. In the same meditation I was shown that being in heaven is not the same as having heaven within. Being in heaven is beautiful and profound but having heaven within is true Nirvana when heaven is not a projection but a living reality. The Masters have achieved Nirvana. I wondered if Viva has, as I felt this information was coming from her. I can only liken it to having the Sun inside us, so that even on a cloudy day, the Sun still shines!

I sat down to meditate a week later feeling physically ill.

Immediately I experienced absolute bliss. It consumed me and I was told it is always available. It is the backdrop to our lives but we rarely take advantage of it. I promised to experience more bliss despite being bent double with back pain intensified by coughing.

At the end of April I experienced the relationship the trees have with the Earth and the Sun. It is profound and I realised that life is much sweeter when we are in relationship with our environment. This intimacy with one's surroundings can spread to include everything from the birds in the trees to the bricks in the wall. It can be extended to embrace everyone and everything.

In the same meditation Frances was aware of Viva and a spiralling energy in her heart centre almost too intense to bear. It spiralled back into peace and serenity. Whenever our energies are scattered, we must stop and spiral back to the centre.

At the beginning of May I experienced bliss and realised that it is Viva's bliss. She is now in bliss and wants us to know that it is where we all belong. Bliss is a place!

In June I found myself in a beautiful temple with columns and golden light. There was great peace, presence and a sense of purpose. "Emblazon!" I heard. "Emblazon the world. Do not hide your light. Carry the golden banners through the streets." We were being asked to bring something into the world that it desperately needs. "Banish the gloom! Blow the trumpets and beat the drum," I heard. "Sound the Note!"

In the same meditation Frances was in a high place observing the turmoil, change and upheaval in the world. We were standing in a circle, a small group within a greater group, within a still greater group. We were reminded not to allow ourselves to get sucked in by the many things happening. We were advised to "stay in your centre, form a 'ring-pass-not' around you. Remember you are disciples. Concentrate on your priority of service. Use your time well."

In my meditation in mid-June I saw golden trumpets with red and purple banners attached to them. The trumpets were being blown. It was a wake up call to humanity. Are we ready? I heard: "Yes, come forth O mighty One!" In the same meditation Willem was led to the Great Invocation from the 1940's:

"Let the Lords of Liberation issue forth.
Let them bring succour to the sons of men.
Let the Rider from the Secret Place come forth
And coming, save.
Come forth, O Mighty One!"

It's interesting that we both heard "Come forth O Mighty One!"

In a later meditation Willem heard "Let ardour be written on your banner!"

On June 21st I heard the word "Contact" and saw two triangles: one pointing up and one pointing down, their points touching. I also saw the painting of God reaching out to Adam. I was reminded that we are fortunate to have made "contact".

At the beginning of July I meditated on "I am a point of sacrificial fire focused within the fiery will of God" from the Affirmation of the Disciple. It was a powerful experience. I experienced a shaft of light coming from a single point within the mind of God, from whom we all emanate. Some are closer to this point of singularity. Others are further away. Most are unaware of where they really are. To sacrifice my personal will to the Will of God is to regain this Unity and to see separation as the ultimate illusion.

A week later I found myself in the Ashram where there is always peace and harmony. I saw it as my true home and soaked up the healing energy and high vibration. It rejuvenated me! This meditation helped me to return to my busy life and see it as a temporary experience, which is helping me to grow and develop.

At the end of July I found myself inside a red membrane. The

colour red was shining into this new and mysterious space. There were others and I sensed a golden light shining around us. In the same meditation Frances found herself on a plane she had never experienced before. It was a very high fine energy combining light, love and power, but above all great peace. She realised that when one lives in a purified energy field everything becomes transparent. Pure consciousness leads to unified consciousness. This is how the Masters communicate. They simply know each other's thoughts when tuning in. When there is no more personality, there is no separate self.

At the beginning of August in my meditation I found myself in a large impressive chamber with a golden throne in the centre. We were waiting for Maitreya to appear. When he did, he walked around the golden throne but did not sit on it. Instead he said, "Do not elevate me." Viva was also there.

In the middle of August Willem meditated on "I am a source of strength enabling them to stand" from the Affirmation of the Disciple. He felt how we, as a Triangle, are holding – or trying to hold - this strength in the same way that the light beings on the inner planes are a source of strength for us here on the frontline. In my meditation we were asked to be like a chalice in order to contain the energies. We are to distribute these finer energies out there in the world. The light beings on the inner planes need emissaries out in the world to hold and distribute. This work cannot be under-estimated.

A week later Willem experienced a lot of activity in the Ashram. Viva took us to one side and led us through an open gallery. She could not tell us what was going on but the effervescence in the ashram could be compared to the preparation for D-day in the headquarters of the allied troops in England. Frances also experienced being in the energy field of the Ashram with Viva nearby. She heard "Only when the personality kneels on the mountain top in humility and surrender does the disciple

become useful. Such a one can be trusted not to let the personality get in the way. Humility is unselfish, it gives of itself without thought of gain."

At the end of August Frances saw us standing outside a huge and very solid door waiting to be admitted. We were asked to honestly examine our own hearts to ascertain what is required to pass to the next level and to see if we are ready to be admitted. She heard "You are transmitting agents for divine forces. This Triangle is a receiving and transmitting unit as well as being nourished by the One Life. It is at its purest in the Ashram of the One Who is the heart of this planet."

At the beginning of September I saw a walled citadel in the Gobi desert protected by a high wall and huge double gates. Many people were entering the citadel including the three of us. Then the gates were closed and locked. Willem had a similar meditation in which he sensed that an ultimatum has been heard by those who have ears to hear. They have made the choice and are entering the City of Light.

On September 20th Willem saw us in a vessel of light cruising at high speed. At regular intervals we returned to the Mother Ship. We were being sent out to fish – like the disciples of Jesus – listening to calls – intuitively serving. It is busy work and we do not rest as before. We have been preparing for this job. In my meditation I also saw a vessel of opalescent light. It was an energy field of dazzling beauty. I sent some of its healing energy to a close friend I was visiting in a hospice at the time.

Frances experienced being in a place of deep peace. Viva was there and we were watching scenes through huge windows out into the world of terrible human suffering and destruction. In one place there was drought with starving multitudes. In other places floods, storms, tsunamis and earthquakes – the convulsions of the planet in the throes of change and rebirth. We were non-attached spectators, watching with immense compassion,

from a place of peace and serenity. We were shown that we are no longer a part of this reality, but that we are builders of the New Earth. To cope with living in the world at such a difficult time of increasing upheaval, we were advised to live "as if" we are in the Ashram. This will also help to raise those around us.

A week later Willem saw a golden shield to protect against all possible attacks which we were given on condition that we "hold this golden shield link within the Ashram of our hearts". Frances heard:"Expect the impossible. Things are happening which defy explanation. Reality as you have been taught to believe it, and think you know, is breaking down. Keep an open mind and rely on higher intuition to guide you." She saw an image of the shape-shifting Cheshire cat from Alice in Wonderland and heard "Beware of the false light. It is easier to be bamboozled as you journey into new realities, new dimensions. Look at 'old ideas' and concepts with new eyes, expand your horizons but venture not into the astral realms."

On October 4th in my meditation I saw huge red dragon doors through which we entered into an enormous space full of light with hundreds of monks meditating and chanting. I saw an immense golden Buddha as tall as a house and I had a feeling of immanence, which I had also felt in last week's meditation.

In the same meditation Frances heard "The pace of change is speeding up. All disciples are asked to gather their forces. Ask yourself, what is asked of me at this time? Then focus the will to hearken to the Soul's call. All work carried out on behalf of the Hierarchy is energised and blessed. Do the best you can in the place where you are."

A week later I saw an ethereal, abstract landscape composed of soft blues and pinks. Looking at this abstract landscape, I was aware of my friend's growing awareness after dying a week ago. She had started to develop as an abstract artist before she became terminally ill. I heard "Balance compassion with detachment. Be

in the world but not of it. You may be asked to leave without notice or a second glance."

On November 1st Frances saw images of Tibetan monks dancing in coloured costumes wearing fearsome masks with much clashing of cymbals and blowing of Tibetan horns. All the dancers represented some facet of the human condition. A huge golden sun disc appeared in front of the dancers and Viva said, "Step back and see: all the many facets of the personality are but shadow puppets dancing in the Sun."

A week later I experienced going up in a hot air balloon with Viva. As the landscape became smaller and more distant beneath us, I realised how much we magnify the trivia in our lives and are deluded by appearance. As we moved into space and saw the planet in all its glory as a single unit, I felt exalted. I was physically interrupted at this point and descended back to earth with a bump.

In the same meditation Frances heard "Cultivate My garden. Like a gardener preparing the soil for new seeds, prepare the Earth for My seeds. Nourish and encourage small beginnings so that they may be enabled to grow and flourish into large wisdoms. Let the flowers of My beauty open within you and let the fragrance and colour radiate out to all."

At the end of November I had a beautiful meditation in which I was able to ascend above the Maya and illusion surrounding me. I experienced a profound connection with higher beings and I saw how easily we distract ourselves from why we are here. I saw the need to ground this awareness. In the same meditation Willem experienced cosmic consciousness and asked if it was an exercise in detachment from the Maya and illusion surrounding and blinding us. He was told to develop the right perspective and remember who we really are. The Triangle boosts us.

In our meditation at the beginning of December I heard "Be in the world. The world needs you more than ever. Do not flee

from it or lock yourself away in a safe refuge. Be in the world." It was a forceful message at a time when I was being very reclusive!

In the same meditation Frances felt waves of joy and being uplifted. She heard: "New energy is now pouring into the world. Make way for the new! Release the old and be open to new energies, ideas and structures coming in. There is infinite hope for the world but all who are so motivated must play their part. Keep above the turmoil and remain uplifted as you are now."

A week later Frances was late for the meditation and sensed that Viva and I were already linked at the Ashramic level. There was much activity in the Ashram and she heard, "Wake up! Mobilise your forces. All are needed." Frances asked how we could help within our present circumstances. She heard, "Do not let personality concerns deflect you from the Purpose. Keep awareness high, listen and obey that inner prompting. Listen within!"

In the same meditation I experienced being in an arena where millions of souls were assembled. There were discarnate souls like Viva and incarnated souls like us. We, the incarnated souls, were each given an amber disc the size of an apple. They were bright and reflective. We were shown that if we all held them up together, we would be seen from outer space! We are to gather our forces and join together in unity to make a difference in the world. I thought of the Internet uniting people in order to bring about change, like the petitions I am always signing on line. The amber discs are similar. When placed together they light up the sky. The following morning I watched the Sun rise up out of the sea, like an amber disc, the speed of its ascent showing me the speed at which the Earth is spinning. The amber discs carry the power of the Sun and we are the custodians trusted to use this power wisely.

On December 20th Frances experienced a very powerful Christ energy flowing softly in waves of deep peace and stillness.

She felt as if she was sunbathing in the Christ light and wanted to turn her face up to receive its warmth. There was a sense of a massive wave of new energy flowing into the planet, bringing change relentlessly on its wings, dragging us along with it. There are a multitude of light workers standing by ready for the work of implementing this new energy for the new dispensation. All is very well but we are called to step up our commitment and our work. There is a sense of urgency as the forces of change sweep in relentlessly.

I spent the meditation with Viva who was very present and told me she is always with us in our Triangle. I feel privileged to have this ongoing connection with her and that any separation I may experience is an illusion. When Willem, Vivian and I began the Triangle in 1997, we did not know what an important link we were making with each other and the Ashram. Viva conveyed to us that it was planned.

2011

On January 3rd Viva told us she is now studying the Music of the Spheres. I later found this quote from Pythagoras:

"Let us set our hearts on the sublime symphonies of the Universe. Though our mortal ears be deaf to the Music of the Spheres, yet will it be heard in the extended ears of our souls."

On the night of January 10th I dreamt that Viva was telling me about precious stones. I later read in a book about guardian angels: "our precious stones are the angels' sense organs."

In our meditation we were told to bridge the gap between humanity and the spiritual world. Willem saw Viva and I weaving a path of light that bridges the worlds. The gap is closing.

Two weeks later we were in the Hall of Learning and Higher Service with Roberto Assagioli. We were looking at our readiness

to become disciples. We were questioned and our answers revealed how ready we are. Since our first meeting in 2007, this is what we are being prepared for. A hint of what this involves is in the Affirmation of the Disciple:

I am a point of light within a greater Light.
I am a strand of loving energy within the stream of
Love divine.
I am a point of sacrificial Fire, focussed within the fiery
Will of God,
　　　　And thus I stand.
I am a way by which men may achieve.
I am a source of strength enabling them to stand.
I am a beam of light, shining upon their way.
　　　　And thus I stand.
And standing thus, revolve
And tread this way the ways of men,
And know the ways of God.
　　　　And thus I stand.

At the end of January we attended a ceremony to celebrate the opening of the Bridge we have been building to the Far Distant Shore. We saw Viva and Maitreya on the other side of the bridge, which is long and straight.

A month later I asked Viva about Vivian whose presence I still feel in the Triangle. Viva replied that the Soul is individualised by its various incarnations otherwise all Souls would be the same. I realised that Vivian was 'Soul-infused' and to know such a person is a blessing. It has enabled us to remain in touch.

At the beginning of March Viva told me about her studies of the chakras and how they can be played like musical instruments. This indicates that she has chakras and is learning how to make music with them. Each chakra has its own note with which beautiful music can be played, like the Music of the Spheres.

At the end of March we were in the Cave of the Heart and were told to close the door to strife and turbulence.

On April 11th Viva transmitted to us that our task is to make the spiritual world "tangible and visible". We are now in the "School of Drastic Discipline".

A week later we were instantly with Viva who reminded us how easy it is to be with her now that we have built the bridge. She told us to "live in the moment between memory and imagination."

In May Viva showed us what it's like to BE music. She has found her Soul song which is ecstatic. This was a lovely meditation.

In June we were asked to "hold steady in the midst of chaos and turmoil". It is like standing on the deck of a ship in a storm. Willem heard: "Trusting God, stand steady in the eye of the storm. Be at peace in the midst of chaos."

On July 18th we were again in the alabaster temple with Viva and Morya. We were invited to step into a blue flame in which we were "purified and prepared".

It was during this time that I 'sensed' Viva was going to reincarnate. She had become increasingly abstracted. Distracted is the wrong word to use here but she obviously had a purpose which absorbed her.

Viva conveyed to me that she was going to incarnate in Switzerland. As I was the only one to receive this information, I wondered if I was imagining it. However, both Frances and Willem experienced Viva withdrawing.

Our meditations changed during this period. They became blissful and without images. I was aware of a radiant golden structure without windows. It reminded me of the Golden Sikh Temple in Amritsar, known as Harmandir Sahib, the Abode of God.

I later read in "The Causal Body" by Arthur E. Powell:

In the causal body the man needs no "windows" - which were formed by his own thoughts in the lower heavens - for this, the causal plane, is his true home, and all his walls have fallen away.

We now know that Viva was reincarnating and it was a process which held her attention. She was no longer available as she had been before. This reveals that the Soul is actively involved in the process of incarnation.

In the next couple of years Viva showed me the baby, and then the toddler, she embodied, who had a very close bond with her mother. In every meditation I saw this little girl and I wondered why Viva wanted me to repeatedly see her. Then I recognised her in a photograph on Facebook and wrote to her proud grandmother who confirmed that she was living in Switzerland.

Viva wanted me to meet her but I could not see how it would be possible, as I could not go to Switzerland. Imagine my surprise when her grandmother told me she was coming for a visit with her family. I met her just before her third birthday. She stood beside me with a toy telephone held to her ear, which was interesting considering how long we had been "communicating" with each other.

When her English grandmother sent me a copy of her birth-chart I was amazed by the similarities with Vivian's birth-chart. This degree of synastry cannot be a coincidence. She does have a very close relationship with her mother, as Viva had shown me.

Later Philip Lindsay, an esoteric astrologer, worked on the charts and was of the opinion that Vivian was meant to die at the time of the crash in September 1998. The transits and progressions at the time of the car crash indicated a sudden accident and a culmination of her work. It's very revealing that they have the same karmic lessons, with the South and North Nodes in the same signs and houses, and both have Mars in Cancer, Sun

conjunct Venus and Mercury. If Vivian had died in September, with the Sun in Virgo, she would have reincarnated in Virgo.

What convinces me is the alignment of Vivian's Part of Fortune at 29 degrees Leo with the Sun at 29 degrees Leo, and Vivian's Sun at 29 degrees Aquarius with the Part of Fortune at 29 degrees Aquarius. The Part of Fortune symbolizes good karma. When it's at the bottom of the chart, as it is in Vivian's chart, it indicates the sowing of good karma. When at the top of the chart it indicates the reaping of good karma. The good karma Vivian created in her life will be reaped in this new life, which makes perfect sense, and is a good example of how karma is carried forward from life to life.

If Vivian was meant to die in the car-crash, then the two years in which she could not move were like being in the Bardo. On reflection, I suspect that the whole point of our meeting was to go through this experience together and stay in touch between her death and rebirth. This would explain the repetitive dream I had in 1985, when I first moved into her home, about being in a house belonging to a man who cut up bodies, which is where I was staying when Vivian died in 2000. This house belonged to a pathologist.

We are still in contact with Viva but can only meet her where she is which involves elevating our consciousness.

If you want to break through the vault of the Universe, you may do so. Make yourself to grow to a greatness beyond measure; by a bound free yourself from the body. Raise yourself above all time; become eternity.
Hermes Trismegistus

Glossary of terms

The ASHRAM is the centre where the Masters (enlightened souls) gather aspirants and disciples for spiritual instruction and world service. The Ashram of Christ is presided over by the Christ, also known in the East as Maitreya, and is sub-divided into seven sub-ashrams, each presided over by a Master and imbued with the quality of one of the Seven Rays.

The ASTRAL BODY is another name for the emotional body. It is impressed with every passing desire and emotional reaction unless it is trained to register impressions from the intuition via the Soul. The aim is for the astral body to be still and as clear as a mirror in order to reflect the Soul.

The ASTRAL PLANE is the plane of illusion where most people in the world are busy working on astral matter with their desires. The ultimate aim is to be freed from the Astral plane with its illusions. The Astral plane appears to be real after the death of the physical body and reflects our desires back to us.

(Source: *The Astral Body* by A. E. Powell)

The AURA is an ovoid which envelopes us and is a reflection of our emotions, thoughts and spiritual aspirations or lack of them. The colours will depend upon our stage of development and attainment. Highly evolved beings have a golden aura.

The aura is like a set of Russian dolls, with the smallest doll symbolising the physical body, which is contained by the astral body, which is contained by the mental body, which is contained by the intuitional body. Each body is replaced by a higher body, as we progress, until there is no more containment. The final stage is cosmic consciousness.

The BURNING GROUND is the burning through of the etheric

web which surrounds and separates us from the various non-physical planes. We enter the Burning Ground through self-induced effort in order to progress, and it is often painful.

"Two factors tend to bring this about: the slow moving forward of the innate conscience into greater control, and the steady development of the 'fiery aspiration' to which Patanjali (The Light of the Soul, Book II, Sutra I, page 119) makes reference. These two factors, when brought into living activity, bring the disciple into the centre of the burning ground ... The burning ground is found upon the threshold of every new advance until the third initiation has been taken."

(*The Rays and the Initiations* – DK through Alice Bailey)

Humanity is going through the burning ground now and it's easy to see what is being burned up: selfishness and greed.

The CHAKRAS. When undeveloped they appear as small circles about two inches in diameter, but when awakened they are seen as blazing whirlpools, much increased in size, and resembling miniature suns. The seven major chakras are located parallel to the spinal column and are like spinning wheels. Chakra means wheel in Sanskrit. The first chakra is between the base of the spine and the pubic bone, and is called the Base Chakra. It is the seat of kundalini which, when aroused, awakens the other centres. The second chakra is situated behind and just below the navel and is called the Sacral. The third chakra sits in the V formed by the rib-cage and is called the Solar Plexus. The fourth chakra is in the middle of the chest and is called the Heart Chakra. The fifth chakra is located at the throat. The sixth chakra, called the Ajna centre or the third eye, is located between the brows. The seventh chakra, the Crown, faces upwards on top of the head. The chakras have a specific function, which is to absorb and distribute prana from the Sun and energy from the earth. When the centres are fully developed there is continuity of consciousness.

The Crown Chakra, when fully awakened, is the most resplendent, and is shown as a golden halo in paintings of saints. In Indian teachings it is called the Thousand Petalled Lotus although the actual number of radiations is 960. In addition it possesses a subsidiary whirlpool in its central portion, which has twelve petals. This is called the "Heart within the Head". When fully active, it is full of chromatic effects, and vibrates rapidly. The central portion gleams white, flushed with gold at its heart. A person with a fully opened crown chakra is enlightened and has direct access to the higher spiritual planes. The Masters have completed this process and are, therefore, radiant.

(Source: *The Chakras* by C.W. Leadbeater)

The DARK BROTHERHOOD functions on the astral and physical planes. The emphasis of their activity is upon the material aspect of manifestation and their aims are purely selfish. They want to subdue and control all living forms in all kingdoms, and sow the seeds of hatred and separation. The Dark Brotherhood is ruled on the physical plane by a group of six occidental leaders and six oriental leaders from the Black Lodge.

(Source: *Letters on Occult Meditation* – DK through Alice Bailey)

Dietrich Eckart was one of the seven founding members of the Nazi Party, a dedicated Satanist, and the central figure in a circle of occultists called the Thule Gesellschaft. Eckart was looking for a pupil who could be inspired to conquer the world and lead the Aryan race to glory. He found this pupil in Hitler, and Hitler considered Eckart to be the most important influence in his life. The inner core of the Thule group were all Satanists, who practised Black Magic, and were concerned with raising their consciousness through rituals. Because of Hitler's inability to hide his occult activities from Rudolf Steiner, an initiated Christian adept, he declared him to be the greatest enemy of the Nazi party, and attempted unsuccessfully to have him murdered

at Munich Railway station in 1922. Heinrich Himmler set up a school of occultism in Berlin and members of the SS and the Gestapo were ordered to attend. This became the Nazi Occult Bureau in which members of the SS took oaths of allegiance to Satanic powers. The Nazis demonstrated the demonic power of the Black Lodge, and evil entered the world during the Second World War when millions of innocent people died.

(Source: *The Spear of Destiny* by Trevor Ravenscroft)

DEVAS, also known as angels, grow and develop through feeling, and not through the power of conscious thought. The devas seek to "feel" just as man seeks to "know". They are active builders who work on the etheric levels. Nature Spirits work under the direction of the devas. The bird kingdom is specifically allied to the deva evolution, which is why devas are often depicted with wings. It is part of our evolutionary process to make contact with the devas to co-operate and co-create with them. Contact was made by Dorothy Maclean when the need to grow vegetables in sandy soil caused her to seek their advice through meditation. She wrote:

"Yes, I talk with angels, great Beings whose lives infuse and create all of Nature. In another time and culture I might have been cloistered in a convent or temple, or, less pleasantly, burnt at the stake as a witch ... Being a practical, down-to-earth person, I had never set out to learn to talk with angels, nor had I ever imagined that contact would be possible or useful."

(*To Hear The Angels Sing* by Dorothy Maclean)

Concrete proof of devas developed in the Findhorn garden, which became the basis for the development of the Findhorn Community in Scotland.

DJWAL KHUL describes himself as a Tibetan disciple living on the borders of Tibet where he presides over a large group of Tibetan lamas when his other duties permit. He describes his

work as spreading the knowledge of the Ageless Wisdom which he achieved with the collaboration of Alice Bailey, an English woman, who devoted forty years of her life to writing the books he dictated to her telepathically.

EILEEN CADDY was one of the founders of the Findhorn Community in north east Scotland. She received guidance in meditation which she called "the still small voice". Her guidance prompted her to "build a new world" and she wrote several books including *God Spoke To Me, Footprints On The Path, The Dawn of Change, The Living Word, Opening Doors Within* and her autobiography *Flight into Freedom*. Her books have been translated into many different languages. In 2001 she was named one of the most spiritually influential people in Britain on Channel 4's The God List for services to spiritual inquiry. She was awarded an MBE by the Queen in 2004.

www.findhorn.org

The ETHERIC BODY is an exact replica of the physical body. Its function is to store up rays of sunlight from the Sun and transmit them, via the spleen, to all parts of the physical body. When the physical furnace burns brightly, and prana is assimilated, the body functions well. The etheric body is the archetype upon which the physical form is built and is a web or network of fine interlacing channels. During physical life the etheric web forms a barrier between the physical and higher planes, which can only be transcended when consciousness has been developed through meditation. Then we become conscious of other subtler planes. It is through the etheric body that all energies flow, whether from the Soul or the Sun. One of the principle objects at the present time is the stimulation, purification and co-ordination of the etheric body which can then receive impressions through the awakened centres/chakras. Clairvoyance occurs when the Ajna centre has been awakened. Better etheric control is established

through an adequate amount of sunshine, a good diet, and the avoidance of fatigue and worry. The physical body is held together by the energies which compose the etheric body.

In appearance the Etheric body is a pale violet-grey or blue-grey. It is faintly luminous, coarse or fine in texture according to the fineness or coarseness of the physical body. It has two functions: to absorb prana or vitality from the Sun and distribute it to the physical body. Secondly, it acts as a bridge between the dense physical body and the astral body, transmitting the consciousness of physical sense contacts, and also transmitting consciousness from the astral and higher spiritual planes down into the physical brain. The Etheric double develops within itself certain centres by means of which we are able to see the etheric world and its phenomena. It is the connection between the brain and the higher consciousness. The etheric body leaves the physical body at night when we sleep, and finally at death.

(Source: *The Etheric Body* by Arthur E. Powell)

EXTERNALISATION began in the 1960s and is an important period of time when what was hidden, and only accessible to a few, will be revealed to the world. We see it in the popularity of meditation and yoga, and at Findhorn, predicted as "The Great Mystery School in the North" by DK in the Alice Bailey books. We see it in the current exploration of life after death, near death experiences, reincarnation and psychic research.

The externalisation of the trans-Himalayan Lodge, the White Brotherhood, their many disciples and aspirants, will begin to dissipate the "great heresy of separateness". The mantra of this great historical period is "We are One."

(Source: *The Externalisation of the Hierarchy* - DK through Alice Bailey)

GLAMOUR is the condition of being deluded and distracted from our true nature and purpose here in the world. This is a

world problem, which clouds perception, and is because the majority of people function emotionally/astrally. The aspirant has to learn to stand free from glamour and develop Intuition.

(Source: *Glamour: A World Problem* - DK through Alice Bailey)

HIERARCHY refers to the group of spiritual beings on the higher planes who oversee the evolutionary process. The Hierarchy is composed of Chohans, Masters, Adepts and Initiates working through their disciples in the world. The Planetary Hierarchy consists of Sanat Kumara, the Three Buddhas of Activity, and the Masters of the three departments of Will, Love-Wisdom and Creative Intelligence. These are overseen by the World Teacher, Christ, also known as Lord Maitreya.

INDIGO CHILDREN are believed to possess special supernatural traits and abilities. They tend to be creative, intuitive and empathetic, but can also be perceived as strong-willed and strange. They are often innately spiritual from early childhood and have a strong sense of purpose. They are intelligent and intuitive but because they resist authority, they do not function well in traditional schools. They are considered to be the next stage in human evolution and are here to create a New World.

INITIATION originates from the Latin word initiare, to begin. It is the entrance into a spiritual life and is embarked upon when we start working on building character and cultivating the qualities we lack. As a result we undergo an awakening and conscious expansion. At this stage we are called Aspirants.

The First Initiation involves taking the first step into the spiritual kingdom, having passed out of the purely human kingdom. It is the birth of the Christ within the Heart. What has previously been understood as love is superseded by love of humanity. The result is a loving dedication to serve, no longer allowing personal desires to take precedence, and not being ruled by the demands

of the body beyond natural sustenance. It is taking control of the physical vehicle and no longer being ruled by its appetites.

The Second Initiation, called the Baptism, occurs when the emotions have been understood and controlled. Emotions are tempered with clear discrimination. This is more difficult than the First Initiation and may take more than one lifetime to complete. The aspirant is now called a Chela.

The Third Initiation is called the Transfiguration and occurs when the distortions and illusions of the mind have been mastered. The mind becomes an instrument to be used by the Soul in order to express its wisdom in the world. The personality has been mastered and the entire lower self completely surrenders to the Soul. We are now accepted as Disciples.

The Fourth Initiation is called the Crucifixion. Enlightenment follows this difficult initiation. Karma has been worked through and perfection achieved. To the integrated Soul-infused personality the Causal body has been revealed, and now has to be released. The candidate must now transcend all limitations in order to reach the Monad, the Immortal Spirit, which had been obscured by the Soul. The sacrifice of what has been achieved over several life-times is extremely painful and caused Jesus to cry out on the cross: "Father, why hast thou forsaken me?"

(Source: *Initiation: Human and Solar* - DK through Alice Bailey)

INTUITION
"We are told by physicians and scientists that thousands of cells in the human brain are still dormant and, consequently, that the average human being uses only a small part of his equipment. The area of the brain which is found around the pineal gland is connected with the intuition, and it is these cells which must be roused into activity before there can be any real intuitive perception which, when aroused, will manifest soul control, spiritual illumination, true psychological understanding of one's fellowmen, and a development of the true esoteric sense, which is

the objective before you at this time."

(Quote: *Glamour: A World Problem* - Djwhal Kuhl through Alice Bailey)

The INTUITIONAL PLANE is also known as the Causal Plane and the Temple of the Soul. At the moment of individualisation, which is when we contact the Soul, its light becomes a flame. This causes the causal body to expand from being a colourless ovoid to containing all the colours of the rainbow within itself. It glows with an inner radiance and gradually, through many lives of suffering and endeavour, the flame pierces through the periphery. The content of the causal body is the accumulation, by a slow and gradual process, of the good in each life. The work of the personality is to beautify, build and expand the causal body which is sometimes referred to as building the Temple of Solomon. At a later stage upon the Path of Initiation, when the initiate has developed continuity of consciousness, the fusion is complete and the Soul is fully embodied. Continuity of consciousness occurs when we are conscious of the Soul and its activity on the Causal/Intuitional plane, which involves developing our intuition.

MAGIC is divided into white and black magic. Black magic is practised and actively encouraged by the Black Lodge and is the selfish pursuit of personal power and the enslavement of others. White Magic benefits others, is unselfish and evolutionary. The White Magician works through group centres and vital points of energy. The Black Magician works directly with substance and the forces of involution.

MAITREYA is that great Being whom the Christians call the Christ. He is known in the Orient as Lord Maitreya, the Bodhisattva, who relinquished His place in paradise to help

humanity. He is also the One looked for by devout Muslims under the name of the Iman Madhi. He is the great Lord of Love and Compassion, just as his predecessor, the Buddha, was the Lord of Wisdom. He is the World Teacher, the Master of the Masters, and the Instructor of Angels. Daily He pours out His blessings to the world and to those who seek to grow and aspire. The three departmental heads are focussed around the Christ and it is He who initiates at the First and Second Initiations.

The MANTRAM OF UNIFICATION was originally given by Djwhal Kuhl in September 1939 to members of his group of disciples to use with "heartfelt intent" in their meditation practice. The purpose was that, through a conscious and regular use of the Mantram, the disciples would begin to embody and express this sense of unity.

The sons of men are one and I am one with them
I seek to love, not hate
I seek to serve and not exact due service
I seek to heal, not hurt.

Let pain bring due reward of light and love.
Let the soul control the outer form, and life and all events,
And bring to light the love that underlies the happenings of the time.

Let vision come and insight,
Let the future stand revealed.
Let inner union demonstrate and outer cleavages be gone
Let love prevail
Let all men love.

(Source: *Discipleship in the New Age II* - DK through Alice Bailey)

MEDITATION

"Meditation when rightly carried forward is hard mental work for it means orienting the mind to the soul... It means that when you have learned to focus your mind on the soul you must hold it steady... and when you have learned to do that you must learn to listen in your mind to what the soul is telling you... Then you must learn to take what the soul has told you and form it into words and phrases and throw it down into your waiting brain. That is meditation, and it is by following that process that you will become a world server for you will then be the force of what you have accomplished. You will automatically find yourself overshadowed by that Great One whose mission it is to lift humanity out of darkness into light, from the unreal to the real."

(Lecture by Alice A. Bailey in 1936)

The MENTAL BODY is the vehicle through which the Soul/Higher Self manifests as concrete intellect in which are developed the powers of the mind, including memory and imagination. In later stages of our evolution, it serves as a separate and distinct vehicle of consciousness in which we can live and function apart from the physical and astral bodies. The mental body deals with Rupa (thought forms) and the causal body with Arupa (formless thoughts).

Theosophists call the mental plane Devachan. Christians call it Heaven. Devachan is an intermediate state between incarnations which is entered after separation from the physical and the astral bodies. The recognition of the Eternal Now is gradually developed from one life to the next and during the process of rebirth.

Concentration fashions the mind into an instrument which can be used to pierce the veil and achieve union. Concentration shapes the organ of perception. Meditation is its exercise. Anyone who is able to pay attention, without letting the mind wander, is ready for meditation. The mental body is the vehicle through which the Soul manifests.

The MENTAL PLANE is called Devachan or Heaven because it is experienced as blissful and joyous. This is because it is fuller and wider than the astral plane. The entire being is filled with light and harmony. Through the golden haze appear the faces we loved on earth. Nobody can adequately describe the bliss of the heavenly realms. There is no separation due to space or time, and there is a far closer communion between souls.

On the astral plane a familiar body is inhabited. The mental vehicle has to be developed. The time spent on the mental plane depends upon the materials brought from the earth-life. These include mental and moral faculties, and pure thoughts generated on earth. Although Devachan is to a certain extent illusory, it is experienced as having a far greater reality than life on earth. This is the realm often experienced and described by people who have near death experiences.

(Source: *The Mental Body* by Arthur E. Powell)

MASTER MORYA is a master of the ancient wisdom and one of the Mahatmas who inspired the founding of the Theosophical Society. His correspondence with A.P. Sinnett was published in *The Mahatma Letters*. He was also channelled through Madam Blavatsky and Helena Roerich. His previous lives were recorded by Annie Besant and C. W. Leadbeater, and includes Abraham, Melchior, one of the Wise Men who brought gifts to Jesus, King Arthur of Camelot, Thomas Becket and Thomas Moore. He ascended in 1898 and is the Chohan of the First Ray Ashram. He is now located in Dejeerling. Ascension occurs when the atoms of the physical body are transmuted so that physical death does not need to occur. The majority of Masters, who have taken the Fifth Initiation, either preserve their bodies or build a mayavirupa out of physical substance. It usually appears in the original form in which they took the Fifth initiation.

The MONAD is the threefold spirit on the Atmic plane. It is the unified triad of Atma, Buddhi and Manas or Spiritual Will, Intuition and Higher Mind. This is the immortal part of us which reincarnates in the lower kingdoms and gradually progresses to the final goal of individualised Spirit.

The MOTHER OF THE WORLD is the Feminine Principle in Creation, the Mother aspect of Deity, and the One who embodies our planet. She has many names: Isis, Ishtar, Sophia and the Holy Spirit. She is the Matriarch and Initiator of the Planetary Hierarchy and the spiritual mother of us all.

(Source: *Mother of the World* - Master Morya through Helena Roerich)

The NEW GROUP OF WORLD SERVERS are being gathered from every nation; not by the pull of ambition but through selfless service. The group now contains people from all races, of all types and tendencies. What they have in common is the need to be conscious servers. It has a specific mission to "externalise" on the physical plane the plan for humanity. Members must be willing to work behind the scenes and be sensitively aware of humanity without the need for recognition. It has no headquarters, no publicity and no creed. It is a band of dedicated workers and servers, obedient to their own souls, and to group need. All true servers belong to this group whether their line of service is cultural, political, financial, philosophical or psychological. They form part of an inner group of workers for the welfare of humanity. They believe in an inner world government and an emerging evolutionary plan. They are steadily cultivating an international spirit of goodwill and are convinced that an inevitable change for the better is on its way.

The mission of the New Group of World Servers is to receive and transmit illumination from the Kingdom of Souls, to receive

inspiration from the Hierarchy, and to go forth and inspire; to hold the vision of the Plan and to act as an intermediate group between the Hierarchy and humanity, receiving light and power. Then using both of these, under the inspiration of love, to build a New World. They are ushering in the New Age of Aquarius and are present at the birth pangs of a new civilisation and a new world outlook.

(Source: *Ponder on This* - DK through Alice Bailey)

NICHOLAS ROERICH was an artist and mystic who, with his wife Helena Roerich, travelled through China, Mongolia, Asia and the Gobi desert. When the Soviet cosmonaut Yuri Gagarin was asked to describe what the planet looked like from space, he said it reminded him of a Roerich painting. Roerich wrote thirty books and created over seven thousand paintings and theatre designs. Nicholas and Helena were Theosophists. They searched for the sacred site of Shamballa and for signs of the return of Christ. In the 1920s they co-founded what became the Agni Yoga Society (Agni = fire. Yoga = union with God). Helena Roerich was inspired by Master Morya who wrote several books through her.

In 1929 Nicholas Roerich was nominated for the Nobel Peace Prize for his work in creating the Roerich Peace Pact, signed by President Franklin Roosevelt and twenty three other world leaders, to protect the art treasures of the world. Roerich was a friend and advisor to heads of state, scientists, artists, writers, poets, and his work won the praise of Albert Einstein, Tolstoy, George Bernard Shaw, Tagore and others.

Nicholas and Helena Roerich were spiritual pioneers, ahead of their time, promoting equality for women and brotherhood among races and nations.

(Source: *Nicholas & Helena Roerich* by Ruth A. Drayer)

PLANETARY LOGOS. Our Planetary Logos dwells on the highest or divine plane of the cosmic physical plane. The Lord of the World, Sanat Kumara, represents Him on the level of the etheric physical plane of the Earth.

PSYCHOSYNTHESIS blends psychology, spirituality and philosophy. In practice it combines various psychotherapeutic tools and guided imagery to encourage the practice of presence, an aspect of the Soul. Its originator, Roberto Assagioli, an Italian psychiatrist born in 1888, drew inspiration from Jung, Freud and also Raja and Karma Yoga. He developed techniques for working with the unconscious and the Soul, which he referred to as the Transpersonal or Higher Self. He recognised that humans have an eternal aspect: a limitless source of love, will and creativity, which can be accessed and utilised in daily life. Assagioli developed the Psychosynthetic process which literally means the synthesis of the psyche.

SANAT KUMARA is the Lord of the World who is called "The Ancient of Days" in the Bible. From Shamballa, an etheric centre located in the region of the Gobi desert, he presides over the spiritual Hierarchy of ascended Masters in the Ashram of the Christ. He has chosen to watch over the evolution of humans and devas. He decides upon the advancements in the different departments and who shall fill the vacant posts. He meets in conference with the Masters and Chohans to authorise what shall be done to advance evolution. He is present at all the initiations and administers the oath at the Third, Fourth and Fifth initiations. Sanat Kumara and his three assistants have achieved the highest initiation and have offered themselves to the Planetary Logos as focal points. They are not in dense physical bodies but dwell in etheric bodies.

The SEVEN RAYS are streams of force from the Cosmos. They are divided into the First Ray of Will, the Second Ray of Love-

Wisdom, the Third Ray of Activity, the Fourth Ray of Harmony through Conflict, the Fifth Ray of Concrete Knowledge, the Sixth Ray of Devotion, and the Seventh Ray of Ceremonial Magic. A Ray determines the quality of the astral-emotional nature. It colours the mind and the physical body. It controls the distribution of energy and predisposes a person to certain strengths and weaknesses. It gives quality and tone to the personality and moulds the physical appearance. Certain attitudes are easy for one ray type but difficult for another.

(Source: *Ponder on This* - DK through Alice Bailey)

SHAMBALLA, where Sanat Kumara and his pupils reside, exists in the highest ethers of the physical plane and can only be seen when etheric vision has been developed. It is the headquarters for the mysteries where a group of Adepts and Chohans meet the needs of a rapidly awakening humanity. Lord Maitreya also resides there in the Residence of the Bodhisattva. He meets candidates for initiation in His garden.

(Source: *Ponder on This* - DK through Alice Bailey)

SIRIUS is the home of the mysteries and its effect is not felt until after the Third Initiation. The Great White Brotherhood is controlled from Sirius, the Ashrams are subjected to its cyclic flow, the higher initiations are taken under its stimulation, and it is where the Blue Lodge is located. Christ is the expression of a Sirian initiation. A large number of humans will become disciples in the Sirian Blue Lodge. To become a candidate in that Lodge, the initiate of the Third degree has to become a lowly aspirant "within the sunshine of the major sun."

(Source: *The Rays and the Initiations* - DK through Alice Bailey)

In his controversial book "The Sirius Mystery" Robert Temple postulates that beings from Sirius visited Earth many thousands of years ago and were partly, if not entirely, responsible for the

leap from a primitive state to the high standard of culture and civilisation achieved by the ancient Egyptians between 4500 and 3400 B.C. His hypothesis is based in part on the knowledge of the Sirius star system by the Dogon, African people living in Mali. The Dogon religion and its accompanying rites are built around the concept of the Sirian system which they are able to describe without the use of telescopes. They know about Sirius A and B, and describe Sirius C as the 'little sun' accompanied by a satellite planet they call the 'star of women'. The Dogon calculated the orbiting period of Sirius B around Sirius A as fifty years, the number fifty assuming a significant role in their sacred rites. Sirius A has always been associated with Isis, and Dogon information confirms the feminine nature of this beautiful blue white star. The Dogon are also aware of Jupiter's four moons and the rings of Saturn without ever having looked through a telescope.

(Source: *The Sirius Mystery* by Robert Temple)

The TRIANGLE MEDITATION work is a field of service in the "externalisation" of the Hierarchy. It requires commitment and consistency, and involves meditating once a week with two other people in the Triangle. This does not require the three people to meet physically but does require that they report back to each other regularly.

The network of Triangles being formed through the efforts of the Light Workers is closely related to the planetary etheric field described by Master DK:

"The inner web of light which is called the etheric body of the planet is essentially a web of triangles and when the evolutionary process is completed, it will have been organised. At present a pattern of squares is the major construction of the web but this is slowly changing as the Divine Plan works out. The etheric web of the sacred planets are largely triangles ...

"The effort on earth today (as seen by the planetary Logos) is to bring about a transformation of the web of the planet and thus slowly change the existing squares into triangles."
(Source: *Esoteric Astrology* - DK through Alice Bailey)

This Triangle work is built by esoterically trained meditators creating a link between each other, linking with the spiritual Hierarchy and the New Group of World Servers.

Meditation unifies, elevates and nourishes the field. By linking regularly with each other at the same time on the same day each week a spiritual unity is established. The core of the work takes place on a soul level. From the unity of hearts a pyramidal structure is created which enables electric fire to descend upon the safe transformation and distribution platform of the Triangle. This energy can then be used for service. Its intensity is so high that it can greatly speed up spiritual growth.

When a Triangle is started by three individuals, the formation has to be sealed and made with a shared commitment. This is called the Intonation of the Triangle. The following can be said:

I reveal my ardent power in the triangle formed by . . . . .
I reveal my energy of love-wisdom within the triangle
And I dedicate my Active Intelligence to the splendour
of the triangle.

Followed by three OMs.

How to proceed:
The same Activation of the Triangle can be used at the beginning of each triangle meditation. A heart connection is established between the three members of the triangle.

A level of consciousness is raised to the head centre beyond the personality into the clarity of the higher mental level.

Connection at the soul level at the apex of the triangle receives and sends out – like an antenna – and connects with the spiritual Hierarchy.

If the level of focus begins to drop, simply sound the OM internally and raise the consciousness back to the soul level.

Meditating once a week either together or apart is sufficient. The participants agree on a fixed time and day in which to link up. It is like making a regular appointment with each member of the triangle. Eventually the triangle connection is imprinted on the etheric level and is reactivated and ignited at each link up.

It is recommended that the participants strive to grasp the insights and/or experiences perceived, and try to formulate them either in writing or speaking.

When the reliability of the Triangle has been established the channel will gradually widen and it will be increasingly empowered.

(Compiled by Willem Reniers and Frances de Vries Robbé.)

WESAK is the annual festival of the Buddha, who is the embodiment of light and wisdom. It takes place in the Himalayas at the time of the full moon in May (Taurus). All the members of the Hierarchy attend the festival and wait for the brief appearance of the Buddha, who meets with Christ, and renews his touch and association with the work of our planet. It is a time of great spiritual power and is beneficial when meditators around the world tune in to receive the blessings and distribute them to the world in their field of service.